Assisted Reproductive Technologies

Assisted Reproductive Technologies

EDITED BY

Richard P. Marrs, MD

Director
The Institute for Fertility Research
Santa Monica, California

BOSTON

Blackwell Scientific Publications

Oxford • London
Edinburgh • Melbourne
Paris • Berlin
Vienna

Blackwell Scientific Publications

Editorial offices:

238 Main Street, Cambridge, Massachusetts 02142, USA

Osney Mead, Oxford OX2 0EL, England

25 John Street, London WC1N 2BL, England

23 Ainslie Place, Edinburgh EH3 6AJ, Scotland

54 University Street, Carlton, Victoria 3053, Australia

Arnette SA, 2 rue Casimir-Delavigne, 75006 Paris, France

Blackwell-Wissenschaft, Düsseldorfer Str. 38, D-10707
    Berlin, Germany

Blackwell MZV, Feldgasse 13, A-1238 Vienna, Austria

Distributors:

USA

Blackwell Scientific Publications

238 Main Street

Cambridge, Massachusetts 02142

(Telephone orders: 800-759-6102 or 617-876-7000)

CANADA

Times Mirror Professional Publishing

130 Flaska Drive

Markham, Ontario L6G 1B8

(Telephone orders: 800-268-4178 or 416-470-6739)

AUSTRALIA

Blackwell Scientific Publications (Australia) Pty Ltd

54 University Street

Carlton, Victoria 3053

(Telephone orders: 03-347-5552 or 03-347-0300)

OUTSIDE NORTH AMERICA AND AUSTRALIA

Blackwell Scientific Publications, Ltd.

c/o Marston Book Services, Ltd.

P.O. Box 87

Oxford OX2 0DT

England

(Telephone orders: 44-865-791155)

Typeset by Huron Valley Graphics, Inc.

Printed and bound by Braun-Brumfield, Inc.

© 1993 by Blackwell Scientific Publications

Printed in the United States of America

93 94 95 96 5 4 3 2 1

Library of Congress Cataloging in Publication Data

Assisted reproductive technologies/ edited by Richard P.
Marrs.

    p. cm.

    Includes bibliographical references and index.

    ISBN 0-86542-203-6

    1. Human reproductive technology. I. Marrs, Richard
P.

    [DNLM: 1. Reproduction Techniques. WQ 205
A84803 1993]

  RG133.5.A78 1993

  618.1′78—dc20

  DNLM/DLC

  for Library of Congress   93-1410

                          CIP

Contents

Contributors

Ricardo H. Asch, MD
Professor, Department of Obstetrics and Gynecology
Division of Reproductive Endocrinology and Infertility
Director, UCI Center for Reproductive Health
Assistant Dean, College of Medicine
University of California, Irvine
Orange, California

Jacques Cohen, PhD
Associate Professor of Embryology and Gynecology
    and Obstetrics
Scientific Director of Assisted Reproduction,
Gamete and Embryo Research Laboratory
The Center for Reproductive Medicine and Infertility
The New York Hospital/Cornell University Medical
    College
New York, New York

Alan DeCherney, MD
Luis E. Pasteur Professor,
Tufts University School of Medicine and
Chairman, Department of Obstetrics and Gynecology,
New England Medical Center
Boston, Massachusetts

John E. Grantmyre, MD, PhD
Halifax, Nova Scotia
Canada

Jamie Grifo, MD PhD
The Center for Reproductive Medicine and Infertility
The New York Hospital/Cornell Medical Center
New York, New York

Gary D. Hodgen, PhD
Professor and President
The Jones Institute for Reproductive Medicine
Department of Obstetrics and Gynecology
Eastern Virginia Medical School
Norfolk, Virginia

Anne E. Hood, MD
Outpatient Surgery Center
Los Angeles, California

John F. Kerin, MD PhD
Professor,
Department of Obstetrics and Gynecology
Flinders University Medical Centre,
Bedford Park, South Australia,
Australia

Gad Lavy, MD
Division of Reproductive Endocrinology
Department of Obstetrics and Gynecology
Yale University School of Medicine
New Haven, Connecticut

Larry I. Lipschultz, MD
Professor of Urology
Scott Department of Urology
Baylor College of Medicine
Houston, Texas

Henry E. Malter, PhD
The Center for Reproductive Medicine and Infertility
The New York Hospital/Cornell Medical Center
New York, New York

Richard P. Marrs, MD
Director
The Institute for Fertility Research
Santa Monica, California

David R. Meldrum, MD
Clinical Professor
ULCA School of Medicine
Director, Center for Advanced Reproductive Care at
    South Bay Hospital
Redondo Beach, California

Patrick Quinn, PhD
Tarzana Regional Medical Center
Tarzana, California

John A. Robertson, JD
Thomas Watt Gregory Professor
School of Law
University of Texas at Austin
Austin, Texas

Eric S. Surrey, MD
Director, Division of Reproductive Medicine
The Center for Reproductive Medicine
Cedars-Sinai Medical Center
Assistant Professor
Department of Obstetrics and Gynecology
UCLA School of Medicine
Los Angeles, California

Beth E. Talansky, PhD
The Center for Reproductive Medicine and Infertility
The New York Hospital/Cornell Medical Center
New York, New York

James P. Toner, MD, PhD
Assistant Professor
The Jones Institute for Reproductive Medicine
Department fo Obstetrics and Gynecology
Eastern Virginia Medical School
Norfolk, Virginia

Louis N. Weckstein, MD
Bay Area Fertility Medical Group
Co-Director, San Ramon Center for Reproductive
    Medicine
San Ramon, California

Preface

S I N C E the first success from in vitro fertilization and embryo transfer in 1978, a proliferation of associated technologies and a broadening of the indication for the use of these technologies has taken place. In the last calendar year, it is estimated that approximately 30,000 assisted reproductive technology procedures will have been performed in the United States. This is compared to 10 years ago when approximately 500–600 procedures were performed on an annual basis in this country. Not only have the number of procedures changed, but the types of procedures and the patient that we treat with these procedures have changed dramatically.

This compilation of writings from the leading authors in this field will bring you, the reader, up to date and focused on what the assisted reproductive technologies can, and should, do today. We have attempted to focus on not only the physiologic mechanisms and technological aspects of assisted reproductive technologies, but also have looked at the correlation of outcome to anesthetic protocols as well as the future of the various reproductive technologies. In addition, because these technologies have been utilized outside of the married couple, a focused discussion on third party involvement, such as donor oocytes and surrogate gestational carriers, is included in this book. Moreover, a discussion of the legal and ethical aspects of the advanced technologies is of utmost importance today, since the use of third party involvement and the long term cryopreservation of eggs, sperm and embryo is becoming a reality.

The authors who have provided the data are today the leaders in this field. The reader will enjoy the expertise of these individual authors and will certainly learn from the facts that are put forth. I hope that the reader finds this work beneficial, and I congratulate the authors in providing an excellent and factual account of today's assisted reproductive technologies.

Acknowledgments

I would like to acknowledge the tremendous effort put forth by Mr. Denny R. Cook in the preparation and organization of this book, as well as the authors who have contributed their time and expertise in preparing the chapters. Without the work of all of these individuals, this very important addition to our medical literature would not be available today.

Assisted Reproductive Technologies

1

Controlled Ovarian Hyperstimulation: Physiology, Techniques, and Controversy

Eric S. Surrey
John F. Kerin

Introduction

The successful application of controlled ovarian hyperstimulation (COH) techniques to naturally ovulatory women has resulted in an increase in the number of mature oocytes available for application to the assisted reproductive technologies, thus allowing for an increase in pregnancy rates (1). A dazzling variety of regimens and agents have been used to achieve this end (Table 1.1). An overview will be presented in this chapter. Unfortunately, comparison between even seemingly similar stimulation protocols is hampered by subtle differences among individual investigators, an overall lack of uniformity among laboratory techniques, and a paucity of prospective randomized designs.

Recovery of mature human oocytes from natural cycles was first described by Steptoe and Edwards in 1978 (2). The ability to time aspiration of a mature oocyte from a preovulatory graafian follicle capable of in vitro fertilization (IVF), cleavage, and successful implantation was based on careful monitoring of the duration of the preovulatory surge in luteinizing hormone (LH) by frequent radioimmunoassay of serum or urine samples. The administration of human chorionic gonadotropin (hCG) to induce a surrogate LH surge according to follicular size and serum estradiol (E_2) levels in such unstimulated cycles has enjoyed a slight resurgence of interest with some success as well (3). However, the majority of centers providing assisted reproductive technologies have shifted to the use of ovarian stimulation prior to oocyte aspiration, given the strong correlation between pregnancy rates and both number of oocytes aspirated and number of embryos transferred (1,4–6).

Table 1.1   Regimens for controlled ovarian hyperstimulation

Natural cycles ± human chorionic gonadotropin (hCG)
Human menopausal gonadotropins (hMG) + hCG
Follicle-stimulating hormone (FSH) + hCG
Clomiphene citrate (CC) ± hCG
CC + hMG + hCG
CC + FSH + hCG
FSH + hMG + hCG
Gonadotropin-releasing hormone (GnRH) agonists (GnRHa)
    + hMG + hCG
GnRHa + FSH + hCG
GnRHa + hMG + FSH + hCG

Controlled ovarian hyperstimulation in a uniovular species

The human female has an integrated cortical-hypotha-lamic-pituitary-ovarian feedback system that protects her from the potential hazards of superovulation and multiple pregnancy. Many of the problems concerning controlled hyperstimulation in the human relate to the in-herent programming for uniovulatory cycles in women under natural conditions. From an evolutionary point of view, any natural or familial tendency toward multiple ovulation in the human has been minimized by a higher incidence of early and late pregnancy losses through spontaneous abortion and perinatal morbidity and mor-tality due to premature birth and its related hazards (7). The natural blocking mechanisms to multiple dominant follicle growth in the human and other primate species, the process of follicle atresia, and the time frame of growth cycles of primordial follicles through to ovula-tion have been clearly documented (8,9).

The primary aim of controlled ovarian hyperstimu-lation (COH) is to maximize recovery of oocytes with full developmental capacity while minimizing asynchro-nous maturation of multiple follicles. The time is limited during which early follicular phase levels of follicle-stimulating hormone (FSH) can be sufficiently elevated to recruit a maximum number of follicles from the available pool but still allow for adequate synchro-nous maturation. After this point, rising E_2 levels suppress further increases in endogenous FSH release by exertion of negative feedback mechanisms at the level of the pituitary gland, thus resulting in atresia of secondary follicles (Fig. 1.1). The stimulatory agents used do not create a larger cohort of recruitable follicles than the

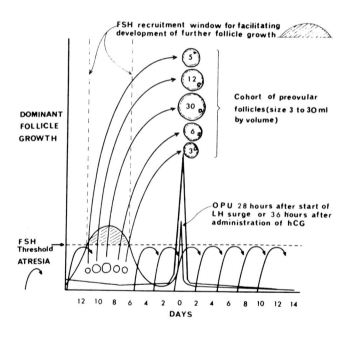

Fig. 1.1   Diagram of a proposed mechanism for the timing and limitation of synchronous follicle recruitment in the hu-man. OPU, oocyte aspiration.

Reproduced with permission from Kerin JF, Warnes GM, Quinn P, Kirby C, Godfrey B, Cox LW. Endocrinology of ovarian stimulation for in vitro fertilization. Aust N Z J Obstet Gynaecol 1984;24:121–124.

ovary has already preselected but, rather, provide a mechanism by which the selection process for atresia within the ovary is overridden. Although the optimal outcome would be to recruit and mature the entire cohort of preselected follicles in a given cycle, the result may be an unacceptable widening of the "FSH window" with an excessive degree of asynchrony (10). This may lead to a suboptimal endocrine environment with subsequent defects in luteal phase, fertilization, cleavage, and implantation. Whichever regimen is used, the stimulation should ideally be sufficient to promote the development of at least six to eight mature follicles capable of adequate fertilization at the time of oocyte aspiration.

Monitoring follicular development during controlled ovarian hyperstimulation

Major advances in our understanding of follicular development in both the natural and the supraovulatory cycle have allowed for more intensive monitoring and the ability to predict normal as well as suboptimal responses. More cumbersome and indirect traditional methods of monitoring such as measurement of cervical mucus scores or assay of urinary estrogens have been supplanted by more reliable approaches. The ability to measure directly and precisely incremental growth of the cohort of preovulatory follicles by serial ultrasound examinations in conjunction with rapid assessment of peripheral serum E_2 concentrations using radioimmunoassay techniques has been a major advance. Although follicular growth progresses in a generally linear fashion in the days immediately before ovulation, oocyte maturity appears to be attained over a wide range of mean follicular diameters varying from 14 to 30 mm in the natural or stimulated cycle (11–14). With the use of clomiphene citrate alone for COH, maturity occurs with mean diameters in the range of 18 to 20 mm (2,15);

with human menopausal gonadotropin (hMG), mature oocytes are obtained at a mean follicular diameter of 16 to 18 mm (9,16); in natural cycles, ovulation has been noted when follicular diameters of 18 to 27 mm were measured (12).

Serum estradiol (E_2) also correlates with follicular development. Peripheral E_2 levels on the order of 150 to 350 pg/ml can be attributed to each mature follicle larger than 18 mm (11,12,16,17). It is important to understand that serum values only indirectly reflect follicular E_2 production and are a product of the number, relative sizes, and maturational state of each of these follicles, as well as the metabolic clearance rate for each individual. Nevertheless, as a general rule, when at least two leading follicles are 16 to 20 mm in diameter in the presence of an adequate E_2 response, 10,000 IU of hCG can be administered with oocyte aspiration scheduled 34 to 36 hours later.

Various patterns of follicular phase E_2 levels have been described and categorized by the Norfolk group (18) (Fig. 1.2). Pregnancy rates per cycle were highest when E_2 levels progressively rose until after hCG administration (pattern A, 27% pregnancy rate) and when levels increased until the day of hCG administration but subsequently declined (pattern G, 16% pregnancy rate). Other patterns demonstrated progressively lower pregnancy rates with no pregnancy obtained when E_2 levels precipitously declined prior to hCG administration (patterns D and E). Thus, decline in E_2 levels during COH reflects suboptimal stimulation with a high likelihood of poor outcome.

There is good evidence that early follicular phase serum FSH levels greater than 20–25 mIU/ml obtained prior to COH are associated with poor cycle outcome as well (19). This may reflect increasing ovarian follicle insensitivity or "occult ovarian failure" as reproductive age increases. Schoolcraft and colleagues have suggested that early signs of premature luteinization as evidenced

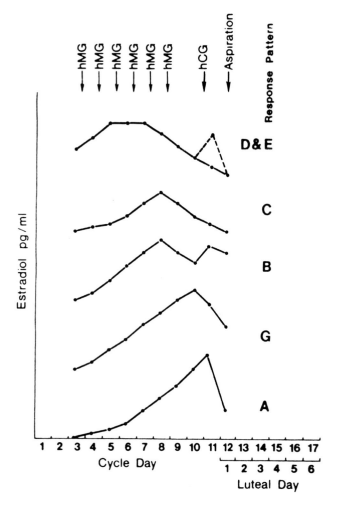

Fig. 1.2.   Representation of various peripheral serum E_2 patterns in conjunction with administration of hMG, hCG, and oocyte aspiration.

Modified and reproduced with permission from Jones H, Acosta A, Andrews M, et al. The importance of the follicular phase to success and failure in in vitro fertilization. Fertil Steril 1983;40:317–321.

by subtle rises in serum progesterone levels may also serve to predict unfavorable results (20).

Thus, taken in isolation, neither ultrasound measurements nor assays of individual hormones alone are sufficiently accurate to allow for prediction of follicular maturity and optimal timing of hCG administration and oocyte retrieval in the face of a stimulated group of asynchronous follicles. It behooves the clinician, therefore, to use a combination of parameters that are specific to each stimulation regimen including ultrasound assessment of follicular size and number, serum E_2, and perhaps progesterone levels to determine the adequacy of response. Despite the most scrupulous monitoring and careful timing of oocyte aspiration, there is evidence that some oocytes may still be immature and require individualized incubation times in vitro prior to insemination for optimal fertilization and embryo development to occur (21).

Controlled ovarian hyperstimulation with human menopausal gonadotropins

Purified urinary extracts of human menopausal gonadotropins (hMG) serve as potent stimulants of folliculogenesis. With great success hMG alone has been used to achieve maturation of multiple oocytes as an integral part of the assisted reproductive technologies after initial attempts by Steptoe and Edwards were abandoned due to excessive follicular asynchrony (2).

Pioneering work on the use of hMG alone within the confines of an in vitro fertilization–embryo transfer (IVF-ET) program was reported by Jones and associates in 1982 (22). The "low-dose" stimulation regimen used by the Norfolk group consisted of daily intramuscular (IM) administration, beginning on cycle day 3, of two ampules of hMG (Pergonal; Serono Laboratories, Randolph, Mass.), which contains 75 IU of both FSH and LH per ampule (23). Cycles were monitored by a combination of daily measurements of follicular size by ultrasound, end-organ estrogen response, and serum E_2 levels. Three overall categories of patient E_2 responses were described, low, intermediate, and high, and were correlated with alterations in peripheral biologic estrogen responses (karyopyknotic index and cervical mucus score), which were termed a "biologic shift." In "high" responders, hMG was discontinued when the serum E_2 level reached 300 pg/ml and a biologic shift occurred. In "low" responders, hMG was discontinued once the biologic shift had been present for 3 days even if serum E_2 values failed to reach 300 pg/ml. If the largest follicle had progressively developed and reached a mean diameter of 14 mm as judged by ultrasound, 10,000 IU of hCG was administered IM 50 hours after the last injection of hMG, and oocyte recovery was undertaken 36 hours later. Pregnancy rates per cycle varied among the three response groups, with the highest success (21%) achieved among the "high" responders. It is important to note that only 50% of the women whose embryos were transferred received more than one embryo.

In an effort to enhance pregnancy rates by increasing the number of oocytes obtained and thus embryos transferred per cycle, Laufer and associates used a relatively high dose of hMG in their stimulation regimen (24). Patients received three ampules (225 IU) of hMG daily beginning on cycle day 3 for 5 days. The dose was then increased in a stepwise, individualized fashion. Ultrasound measurements of mean follicular diameter were thought to be paramount over E_2 levels in the assessment of oocyte maturation. When at least two follicles with a mean diameter of more than 16 mm were visualized, hCG was administered, and oocyte aspiration was scheduled 36 hours later. Although at least two cleaved embryos were obtained in more than 80% of patients undergoing embryo transfer, the pregnancy rate per oocytes retrieved was comparable to that previously described with more conservative stimulation (22).

In a direct comparison between the low-dose and high-dose hMG regimens, Ben-Rafael and colleagues prospectively compared results from cycle initiation with two or three ampules of hMG (25). Although the mean number of mature oocytes recovered per cycle was identical for the two groups, pregnancy rates were higher in patients receiving two ampules daily (22.8% vs. 10.5%). This increase in pregnancy rate was primarily a function of those patients receiving low-dose hMG in whom the interval between hMG and hCG administration was extended to 48 hours. No pregnancies were obtained in either group when E_2 levels declined after hCG administration. It is important to note that in this protocol, hMG doses were not individualized to patient responses but were maintained constant throughout stimulation.

In a variation of the step-up high-dose regimen described by the Yale group, Meldrum et al. decreased the interval between the last hMG injection and hCG administration to 14 to 28 hours (26). In this protocol, E_2 production from mature follicles (14 mm or greater) was determined to contribute 150 pg/ml to peripheral levels, intermediate follicles (12–13 mm) to contribute 100 pg/ml, and lesser follicles to contribute 50 pg/ml. However, this approximation was not correlated with actual follicular fluid E_2 levels. An overall clinical pregnancy rate of 31% per oocyte aspiration was achieved, but strict adherence to protocol resulted in cancellation of 29% of cycles due to inadequate response, drop in E_2 levels, premature ovulation, or excessive stimulation.

A summary of these protocols is outlined in Table 1.2. One other variable that must be accounted for is the potential variation in bioactivity between lots of hMG, which may affect ultimate ovarian stimulation (27).

The use of hMG does not completely suppress endogenous gonadotropin secretion. Although Terrareti et al. suggested that cycling women treated with hMG did not demonstrate an endogenous surge of LH (28), others have disputed this observation. Glasier and coworkers noted that 86% of women receiving hMG alone mounted an LH surge (29). Vargyas et al. reported a 33% incidence of LH surge in a similar set of patients but noted a lower incidence when clomiphene was combined with hMG (30). Many investigators have recommended that the cycle be terminated in the event of an endogenous LH surge. No clinical pregnancies were reported by Lejeune and coworkers in such cycles (31). Others have suggested that not all such cycles need be abandoned. One set of investigators demonstrated that when the LH surge occurred less than 12 hours before hCG administration, neither oocyte number nor embryo cleavage rates were compromised (32). However, when the surge occurred more than 12 hours before hCG administration, embryo cleavage rates were significantly reduced, although oocyte recovery was unchanged. We have demonstrated that 45% of cycles undergoing a high-dose step-up hMG regimen managed by ultrasound and E_2

levels only were marked by an endogenous LH surge despite the absence of abnormal E_2 patterns or sonographic evidence of abnormal follicular development (33). No significant differences in fertilization, cleavage, or pregnancy rates were noted in comparison with patients without such surges. Thus, routine monitoring of serum LH levels may be unnecessary in the face of normal rises in E_2 and progressive follicular growth.

No consistent drug-related effects have been directly attributed to the use of hMG, and no increased incidence in congenital malformations compared to the population as a whole has been reported (34). Schwartz and Jewelewicz, in a retrospective review of the use of hMG for ovulation induction, described an increased rate of spontaneous abortions of 27.9% (35). However, in a large prospective study, Kurachi et al. reported a 19.4% incidence, which was not increased over that in the population as a whole (36). Most adverse reactions are due to the degree of ovarian responsiveness pro-

Table 1.2 Regimens of human menopausal and chorionic gonadotropins in controlled ovarian hyperstimulation

Reference no.	Initial hMG dose (IU)	Step-up	Monitoring	Timing of hCG	Cycles (n)	Cancelled failed retrievals (%)	Pregnancy rate per retrieval (%)
18,22	150	—	Ultrasound, E_2, biologic shift	50 h after hMG	175	17/	18.9
25	150	—	Ultrasound, E_2	24 or 48 h after hMG	57	NA	22.8
	225	—	Ultrasound, E_2	24 or 48 h after hMG	57	NA	10.5
24	225	Individualized (75–150 IU daily increase)	Ultrasound (E_2 secondary)	NA	63	12.7	17.3
26	225	Individualized (0–150 IU daily increase)	Ultrasound, E_2	14–28 h after hMG	119	29	31

NA, not available

duced. The primary complications are manifestations of the ovarian hyperstimulation syndrome. The incidence of severe manifestations of this disorder varies between 0.25% and 1.8% and, along with the issue of multiple pregnancy, will be discussed in detail below.

In summary, the use of hMG alone for controlled ovarian hyperstimulation prior to oocyte retrieval is an efficient means of obtaining multiple mature preovulatory oocytes when patients are meticulously monitored. Individualization of dosage regimens may enhance success rates, although cycle cancellation rates remain relatively high.

Controlled ovarian hyperstimulation: clomiphene citrate

After early failures with the use of menopausal gonadotropins (4), attention turned to clomiphene citrate (CC) as an agent to achieve controlled ovarian hyperstimulation. Clomiphene citrate is a nonsteroidal estrogen designed as a triphenylchloroethylene derivative (Fig. 1.3) and administered as a racemic mixture of *cis* and *trans* isomers. This agent interacts with estrogen receptors, displacing endogenous estrogen at the level of the hypothalamus and pituitary, thus resulting in an increase

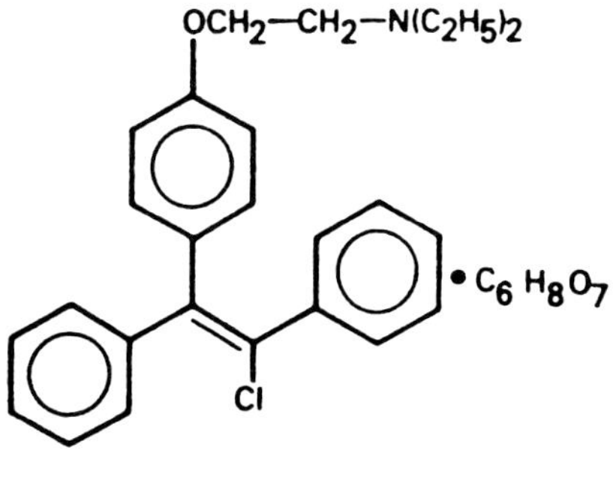

OCH$_2$—CH$_2$—N(C$_2$H$_5$)$_2$

• C$_6$ H$_8$ O$_7$

Cl

Fig. 1.3. Basic structure of clomiphene citrate, a nonsteroidal estrogen and triphenylchloroethylene derivative.

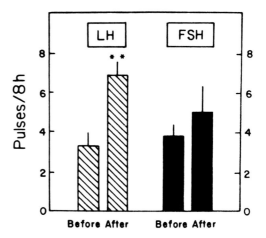

Fig. 1.4. Effect of administration of clomiphene citrate on gonadotropin pulses. $\star p < 0.05$.

Reproduced with permission from Kerin J, Liu J, Phillipou G, Yen S. Evidence for a hypothalamic site of action of clomiphene citrate in women. J Clin Endocrinol Metab 1985;61:265–268.

in endogenous gonadotropin secretion (37). Kerin et al. have suggested that a secondary increase in the pulse frequency of gonadotropin-releasing hormone (GnRH) may play a significant role (38) (Fig. 1.4). These pharmacologic actions may be primarily the result of an antiestrogenic action in which clomiphene antagonizes the negative feedback effect of estrogens (39).

Superovulation with clomiphene citrate with and without subsequent hCG administration in normally ovulatory women has been used successfully to achieve follicular synchrony resulting in aspiration of oocytes capable of fertilization in vitro and successful implantation (1,40–43). Employing a clomiphene dose of 150 mg daily from days 5 through 9 of the menstrual cycle and timing laparoscopic oocyte aspiration in 49 women either on the basis of hCG administration or by measurement of the endogenous LH surge, a 14%

pregnancy rate per aspiration was achieved in one series (44). A mean luteal phase length of 15.6 ± 0.3 days after hCG administration and 14.4 ± 0.3 days after monitoring the endogenous LH surge was obtained.

Other investigators have attempted to combine hMG with clomiphene to further enhance ovarian response (30,45–48). With slight variations, each protocol involves the use of these two agents in a sequential fashion with initiation of a fixed dose of hMG based either on completion of a course of clomiphene or in response to the primary E_2 rise initiated by clomiphene; hMG was administered either daily or every other day. Diamond and associates retrospectively compared protocols involving the use of hMG and clomiphene citrate alone and in combination (49). The combined therapy consisted of administration of 50 to 100 mg of clomiphene on cycle days 3 to 7 and 150 IU of hMG daily beginning on cycle day 6 or 7. Although oocyte yield and

fertilization rates were high in those receiving the combined regimens, pregnancy rates were not improved.

Nevertheless, the rate of cancelled cycles in patients undergoing stimulation with CC only or CC plus hMG remains fairly high (10). The majority of cycles are cancelled for abnormal or poor endocrine response including slow E_2 rises, poor follicular growth, E_2 decline, or premature LH rise (Table 1.3).

The antiestrogenic properties of clomiphene may have a deleterious effect on endometrial receptivity. Clomiphene may induce luteal phase defects (50). Sharma et al. have demonstrated a significant degree of endometrial asynchrony and advanced morphologic development in patients undergoing sequential CC and hMG superovulation protocols (51). This finding has also been demonstrated in the murine model (52). However, others have been unable to demonstrate any adverse effect on endometrial maturation during clomiphene cycles (53,54).

Those side effects specific to clomiphene include induction of vasomotor symptoms secondary to the inherent antiestrogenic properties of the agent and an extremely low incidence of self-limited visual symptoms including blurred vision and scotomata (37). Despite evidence that multiple birth defects may occur in the offspring of pregnant rats administered clomiphene (55), the incidence of spontaneous abortion, chromosome abnormalities, or congenital anomalies among live births in women taking clomiphene citrate appears to be no higher than among women in the general population (34,36,56).

Table 1.3 Reasons for cancellation of laparoscopy (1982–1984), University of Adelaide, Australia, IVF Program

Total cycles tracked	597	100%
Total cycles cancelled	146	24%
Total laparoscopies	451	76%
1. Suboptimal endocrine/follicle response	35/146	24%
2. Spontaneous fall in E_2	42/146	29%
3. Abnormal endocrine response	28/146	19%
4. Untimed LH rise	9/146	6%
5. Poor compliance/miscellaneous	9/146	6%
6. Undetected LH rise/luteinized	6/146	4%
7. Abnormal follicle growth on scan	7/146	5%
8. Early ovulation (< 10 days)	5/146	5%
9. Long follicular phase (> 19 days)	5/146	3%

Reprinted with permission from Kerin JF, Warnes GM. Monitoring of ovarian response to stimulation in in-vitro fertilization cycles. Clin Obstet Gynecol 1986;29:158–170.

Controlled ovarian hyperstimulation: human follicle-stimulating hormone

The relatively recent availability of purified human urinary follicle-stimulating hormone (57) has provided new approaches for COH prior to oocyte aspiration for

IVF-ET, gamete intrafallopian transfer (GIFT), or zygote intrafallopian transfer (ZIFT) procedures. Schenken and Hodgen demonstrated that administration of FSH to cycling monkeys could induce development of multiple mature follicles with relatively infrequent spontaneous endogenous LH surges (58). In addition, one could hypothesize that the elimination of exogenous LH present in hMG might decrease stimulation of local ovarian androgen production and thus enhance follicular synchrony and oocyte quality.

A series of clinical trials using FSH alone or in combination with hMG have been reported (59–64). As previously discussed, comparison among the findings of these investigators is extremely difficult due to differences in control groups, specific protocols, and laboratory techniques. In one of the only randomized prospective studies comparing hMG to FSH in equivalent doses for COH prior to IVF-ET, Lavy et al. found no difference in peak E_2 levels, days of drug administration, incidence of spontaneous LH surge, number of oocytes obtained, or fertilization or pregnancy rates between the two groups (61). This finding has been confirmed by others (63,64). Navot and Rosenwaks could show no difference in cycle outcome between initial doses of FSH ranging from 150 to 300 IU and hMG 150 IU, with the exception of a significantly lower cancellation rate in patients receiving FSH (63).

Others have combined FSH with hMG in various study designs. Sharma and coworkers compared six different regimens involving FSH in a randomized prospective study (59). All patients received 150 IU of FSH per day, but commencing at varying times during the treatment or preceding cycle either alone or in combination with 150 IU of hMG per day, or 100 mg of clomiphene per day. Pregnancy and fertilization rates were highest in those patients receiving FSH from days 1 to 4 and hMG from day 5 until hCG administration, although this did not reach statistical significance

compared with other regimens beginning during the immediate treatment cycle. There was no advantage to initiation of therapy during the antecedent cycle. Although Muasher et al. described a 27% pregnancy rate per cycle by combining FSH and hMG for 2 days followed by stimulation with hMG only, in an uncontrolled trial (62), others have failed to show any clear advantage of similar combined regimens in controlled series (60,64).

Controlled ovarian hyperstimulation: the role of gonadotropin-releasing hormone agonists

The incorporation of gonadotropin-releasing hormone agonists (GnRHa) into various combinations of exogenous gonadotropins may impart specific advantages in COH regimens for assisted reproductive technology procedures (65–70). A reduction in treatment cycle cancellation rates due to inhibition of the spontaneous preovulatory LH rise and subsequent premature luteinization may result (Table 1.4). Improved pregnancy rates per cycle initiated may also stem from a higher degree of synchronous follicular development and improved endocrine responses (65,71).

The classic experiments of Knobil demonstrated that pulsatile hypothalamic release of GnRH is crucial for physiologic release of pituitary gonadotropins (72). Continuous GnRH infusion into the portal circulation of monkeys with lesions at the level of the arcuate nucleus resulted in a biphasic gonadotropin secretory response: an initial agonistic release of LH and FSH followed by a progressive and sustained decline. This phenomenon is a result of a decreased number of available or unoccupied GnRH receptors at the level of the pituitary gonadotrope. Receptors become saturated, are internalized, and fail to be replenished in a timely manner, thus decreasing cellular response. This process is called "down-regulation."

GnRH agonists differ structurally from native GnRH by substitutions at amino acid positions 6 and 10. The result is an analogue of heightened potency due to increased resistance to degradation by endopeptidases. For example, with leuprolide acetate (Lupron; TAP Pharmaceuticals, North Chicago, Ill.), the combination of the substitution of glycine for leucine at the 6 position and glycine for ethylamide at the terminal 10 position yields a GnRHa with an order of potency 15 to 20 times that of native GnRH. Most of the data obtained in this country have been derived from work with this agent, although we presume that results obtained using other agonist preparations should be comparable. The structures of several other GnRHa employed internationally are displayed in Table 1.5.

The initial rationale behind the use of GnRHa in conjunction with COH lay in a desire to suppress the endogenous progressive FSH rise that begins during the late luteal phase (73). If successful, this suppression might allow for the exogenous administration of gonadotropins to lead to more synchronous growth of the cohort of potentially codominant follicles. Furthermore, suppression of the endogenous LH rise may prevent premature luteinization and ovulation, leading to a decreased incidence of cycle cancellation and improved oocyte quality (65). As a result of gonadotrope down-regulation, GnRHa administration causes a decline of ovarian E_2 and testosterone production to a castrate range as reflected by peripheral serum levels within 7 to 14 days in the majority of patients: a "medical oophorectomy" (68,71).

Four basic GnRHa-gonadotropin regimens have been employed and are classified according to when in the menstrual cycle GnRHa administration is commenced in relation to initiation of gonadotropin administration and whether the aforementioned agonistic effect ("flare-up") is utilized or suppressed (Fig. 1.5). The GnRHa-gonadotropin regimens are as follows: 1) luteal

Table 1.4 Outcome by stimulation protocol and procedures: 1989 S.A.R.T. Registry

			IVF		GIFT	
Stimulation protocol	Cycles	Cancelled cycles	ET	Clinical pregnancies[a]	Transfer cycles	Clinical pregnancies[b]
HMG alone	658	154 (24)	209	31 (15)	184	65 (35)
HMG, GnRHa	2876	287 (10)	1538	334 (22)	619	200 (32)
HMG, clomiphene	940	228 (24)	446	80 (18)	155	37 (24)
HMG, FSH	953	257 (27)	296	44 (15)	250	83 (33)
HMG, FSH, GnRHa	1663	255 (15)	778	159 (20)	310	114 (37)
Other combinations	667	267 (40)	198	41 (21)	176	45 (26)
Total	7757	1448 (19)	3465	689 (20)	1694	554 (32)

Values in parentheses are percentages. S.A.R.T., Society for Assisted Reproductive Technology; Et, embryo transfer.
[a]Clinical pregnancy rates are expressed as a percentage of ET cycles.
[b]Clinical pregnancy rates are expressed as a percentage of GIFT transfer cycles.

Modified and reprinted with permission from the American Fertility Society: Medical Research International, Society for Assisted Reproductive Technology, American Fertility Society. In vitro fertilization–embryo transfer (IVF-ET) in the United States: 1989 results from the IVF-ET registry. Fertil Steril 1991;55:14–23.

phase GnRHa administration for gonadotropin suppression followed by initiation of gonadotropins (hMG and/or FSH) about 10 days later when serum E_2 levels fall into the castrate or near castrate range (less than 30–35 pg/ml); 2) "long" follicular phase GnRHa administration for gonadotropin suppression followed by onset of exogenous gonadotropin therapy when E_2 levels fall into the castrate range and the ovaries are free of functional ovarian cysts; 3) a "short" follicular phase "flare-up" regimen in which GnRHa are administered for 2 to 3 days beginning in the early follicular phase followed by gonadotropins; and 4) a "concurrent" flare-up regimen in which GnRHa plus gonadotropin administration begins simultaneously in the early follicular phase. Regimens 3 and 4 take advantage of both the initial endogenous release of stored pituitary gonadotropin as a result of GnRHa and the direct stimulatory effect of exogenous gonadotropins.

The initial use of GnRHa was based on a desire to suppress endogenous gonadotropin release prior to initiation of COH. In general, GnRHa administration was initiated in the midluteal phase and continued for 7 to 14 days or until gonadotropin suppression, as reflected by suppression of serum E_2 to a level less than 35 pg/ml, was achieved. At this point, exogenous gonadotropin stimulation was begun. This regimen has proved to be highly successful in patients who previously had suboptimal stimulation cycles with hMG only (65,68,74). A prospective randomized trial comparing this luteal phase GnRHa-hMG regimen with sequential clomiphene-hMG protocols resulted in higher numbers of oocytes per aspiration and higher pregnancy rates per transfer when GnRHa was used (75). The duration of hMG therapy and overall dose of hMG required were greater in patients receiving GnRHa, however. These findings have been supported by others (76), although

Table 1.5 Structural modifications of GnRH agonist analogues compared to the native GnRH molecule

Agent	GnRH amino acid positions									
	1 Glu	2 His	3 Trp	4 Ser	5 Tyr	6 Gly	7 Leu	8 Arg	9 Pro	10 Gly-NH$_2$
Leuprolide (Abbott)						D-Leu				NHET
Buserelin (Hoechst)						D-Ser (tBu)				NHET
Nafarelin (Syntex)						D-Nal(2)				
Decapeptyl (DeeBiopharm)						D-Trp				
Lutrelin (Wyeth)						D-Trp	NMe Leu			NHET
Goserelin (ICI Ltd)						D-Ser (tBu)				AzaGly
Histerelin (Ortho)						D-His (Bzl)				NHET
GnRHa analogue (Salk Inst.)						D-Trp				NHET

NHET, ethylamide, elimination of 10th amino acid; AzaGly, azaglycinamide some investigators found no differences between the regimens (77). When luteal phase GnRHa plus sequential hMG was compared with hMG only, a lower incidence of cycle cancellation was reported, and some investigators demonstrated higher fertilization and pregnancy rates as well (67,68,78–81). Sathanandan et al. obtained improved results using this regimen primarily among patients who were described as "abnormal" responders to previous hMG plus CC stimulation. These abnormal responders were characterized by elevated follicular phase levels of progesterone or LH or both, as opposed to "poor" responders with previous suboptimal E_2 levels and oocyte development (70). In any of these studies there is no evidence of any relative advantage to the use of FSH as opposed to hMG after suppression has been achieved (82,83).

Initiation of leuprolide acetate, 1.0 mg subcutaneously daily during the midluteal phase, resulted in more prompt suppression of ovarian estrogen production compared with initiation during the follicular phase (84). This may be the result of a 30% incidence of agonistic stimulation of follicle growth with follicular phase initiation of GnRHa (73). Moreover, there appears to be no inherent advantage to the "long" follicular phase protocol, which most groups have abandoned in favor of luteal phase initiation of GnRHa or concurrent regimens as described below.

The short follicular phase "flare-up" method at-

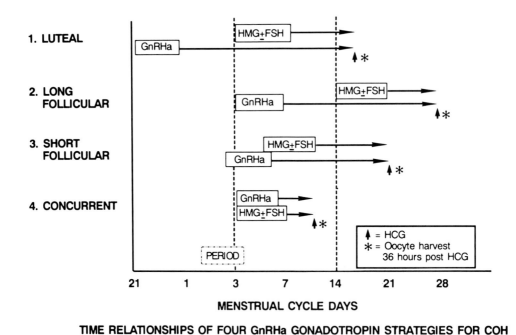

TIME RELATIONSHIPS OF FOUR GnRHa GONADOTROPIN STRATEGIES FOR COH

Fig. 1.5. Schematic representation of four basic GnRHa-gonadotropin regimens for controlled ovarian hyperstimulation in relation to the menstrual cycle. GnRHa, GnRH agonist; hMG, human menopausal gonadotropin; FSH, follicle-stimulating hormone.

tempts to take advantage of initial enhanced endogenous gonadotropin release induced by GnRH agonists followed by the administration of exogenous gonadotropins a few days later. A study comparing this method with the luteal phase administration of GnRHa followed by gonadotropin after down-regulation was undertaken by Garcia et al. (85). In this short follicular phase "flare-up" regimen, the GnRHa leuprolide acetate (0.75 mg/day for women < 75 kg and 1.0 mg/day for women > 75 kg) was begun on day 2 and continued until the day of hCG administration. Gonadotropins were commenced 3 days later on day 5, using a combination of FSH and hMG. FSH was discontinued when the E_2 rise was established (>600 pg/ml) and the leading follicle had reached 12 mm diameter. The hMG was continued until the day of hCG. In their luteal down-regulation regimen, GnRHa was commenced on day 3 to 5 of the luteal phase. The same method of FSH and hMG administration was started after menses when the baseline E_2 was less than 20 pg/ml. There was no difference in the number of follicles, mature oocytes, fertilization rates, or embryos transferred between the two regimens. However, the pregnancy rates for the short follicular phase "flare-up" and luteal down-regulation regimens were 41% and 28%, respectively, with abortion rates being 23% and 36%, respectively.

Despite these highly encouraging results, the efficacy of utilizing the initial agonistic effect of a gonadotropin-releasing hormone agonist during the follicular phase concurrently with the administration of a gonadotropin remains controversial (86,87). We have found that the outcome following a concurrent GnRHa and gonadotropin "flare-up" regimen is inferior to the luteal down-regulation regimen (73,88,89).

The primary intention of our investigation was to measure follicular and endocrine responses to the concurrent administration on day 3 of leuprolide acetate (Lupron, TAP Pharmaceuticals) and hMG (Pergonal,

Serono Laboratories) and compare them to those achieved following the more established pituitary desensitization regimen. A comparison of the numbers of oocytes harvested as well as fertilization and pregnancy rates was also undertaken.

In our investigation, women were matched for age (mean age 37 years) and infertility status and prospectively randomized into two groups for COH as follows. Members of group 1 (n = 20) were treated with Lupron, 1 mg per day by subcutaneous (sc) injection, commencing on day 21 of the menstrual cycle for at least 10 days or until E_2 levels were less than 30 pg/ml. The dose of Lupron was then reduced to 0.5 mg and continued until the administration of hCG. Pergonal, three ampules per day (225 IU), was initiated when suppression was achieved and was continued for 5 days. Doses were altered accordingly thereafter, depending upon the E_2 and follicle response. Members of group 2 (n = 19) were treated with Lupron, 0.5 mg sc daily from day 3 of the menstrual cycle until the day of hCG. Pergonal, three ampules per day, was commenced concurrently from day 3 for 5 days and altered accordingly, depending upon the E_2 and follicle response. Therefore, the only difference between group 1 and group 2 was the 10-day suppression with Lupron starting on day 21 of the previous cycle in group 1, prior to Pergonal stimulation (Fig. 1.5). Peripheral venous blood was obtained from all patients on the first day (hMG-1) and fifth day (hMG-5) of Pergonal administration and on the day of hCG administration. Mean levels of serum LH, FSH, E_2, progesterone (P_4), testosterone (T), and androstenedione (A) were measured by radioimmunoassay techniques.

The rise in E_2 was more rapid in the day 3 concurrent regimen (group 2) (Table 1.6). Although the levels were comparable at the time of hCG administration, it took another 2 to 3 days of Pergonal administration in group 1 to achieve such levels. The agonist effects of the day 3 concurrent regimen on LH and FSH

Table 1.6 Endocrine data for luteal phase (group 1) versus concurrent follicular phase (group 2) GnRHa–hMG regimens

Stimulation day:	hMG-1		hMG-5		hCG	
Group:	1	2	1	2	1	2
E_2 (pg/ml)	19±2.2	56±7.1[a]	247±40	510±117	1474±166	1811±240
P (ng/ml)	0.42±0.1	0.4±0.04	0.32±0.05	0.74±0.16[a]	0.64±16	0.78±0.12
LH (mIU/ml)	1.6±0.2	4.2±1[a]	1.3±0.2	4.3±0.6[a]	1.5±0.16	4.1±0.4[a]
FSH (mIU/ml)	4.6±0.9	8.7±1.3[a]	16±0.9	14.5±1.7	17.6±1.5	17.1±1.8
T (pg/ml)	179±11	183±12	219±15	327±24[a]	414±136	508±61
A (pg/ml)	811±53	871±55	1110±87	1460±87	1812±125	2138±125[a]

[a]$p < 0.05$ versus group 1

were evident. Elevation of LH persisted throughout the follicular phase following the concurrent administration of Lupron and Pergonal. This was reflected in an enhanced degree of androgen and progesterone production during the early days of stimulation that persisted until hCG administration. This phenomenon may have had a direct adverse bearing on oocyte quality.

Although the mean number of oocytes harvested and the fertilization rates achieved were comparable between the two regimens, the days of stimulation and overall dosage of hMG were significantly less with the concurrent day 3 regimen (group 2) (Table 1.7). However, pregnancy rates were higher with the luteal phase suppressive regimen (group 1). Several investigators have confirmed these findings (86–90), although this conclusion is not universal (91–93). One could hypothesize that enhanced androgen and progesterone levels during the follicular phase may have exerted a deleterious effect on endometrial receptivity or oocyte quality or both.

On the basis of these observations, we would recommend the day 21 midluteal suppression regimen before commencing gonadotropins for COH for IVF or GIFT procedures to 1) ovulating women, 2) women with preexisting functional ovarian cysts, or 3) women with preexisting endocrine disorders marked by estrogen and androgen excess such as polycystic ovary disease. We would reserve the day 3 concurrent GnRHa-gonadotropin regimen for women with hypogonadotropic hypothalamic-pituitary dysfunction who do not require ovarian suppression. The lack of hypothalamic GnRH stimulation in these women should prevent any agonistic release of endogenous gonadotropins due to depleted endogenous pituitary stores. This hypothesis, however, remains to be tested.

Table 1.7 Clinical data for luteal (group 1) versus concurrent follicular (group 2) phase initiation of GnRHa for COH with hMG

	Group 1	Group 2	p
Ampules of hMG	38 ± 5	26 ± 4	<0.01
Days of COH	8 ± 1	11 ± 1	<0.05
Oocytes recovered	8 ± 0.8	9 ± 0.8	NS
Fertilization rate	78%	83%	NS
Clinical pregnancy rate/ transfer	26%	13%	<0.005

NS, not significant

It is important to identify women with occult ovarian failure, since these patients do not benefit from GnRH agonist treatment and generally respond poorly to exogenous gonadotropin therapy (18,19,74,75). Women over the age of 35 are more likely to have occult ovarian dysfunction and can be identified by measuring their early follicular phase FSH levels. Response to GnRHa-gonadotropin regimens was analyzed in relation to women with elevated LH/FSH, normal LH/FSH, and elevated LH/FSH ratios. It was found that women with elevated LH/FSH ratios had poor responses to COH, indicating that the basis of their disorder was at the level of the ovary and not at the hypothalamus or pituitary (19,75). Such women may benefit from clomiphene citrate plus gonadotropins or from high-dose gonadotropins alone without GnRHa. If these strategies fail, then such women will benefit from the use of donor oocytes.

Although in our experience the luteal phase initiation of GnRHa appears to be more advantageous in terms of both cycle outcome and ease of cycle scheduling, two drawbacks remain. An increased incidence of ovarian cyst formation has been reported as a result of luteal phase initiation of the agonists (94,95). Despite a need for further prolongation of GnRHa administration until suppression is achieved, cyst formation has not been clearly shown to have an adverse effect on cycle outcome once resolution is documented. Second, care should be taken to exclude pregnancy in a woman who commences the day 21 luteal phase GnRHa regimen when there is tubal patency (96). Data from the pregnant baboon treated with GnRHa suggest that the incidence of spontaneous abortion may be heightened with GnRHa exposure in early pregnancy (97). However, there appears to be no evidence of teratogenicity of these agents in other primates (98) or in humans (96).

The predominant side effects of prolonged use of GnRHa are secondary to the hypoestrogenic effects induced by gonadotropin down-regulation. These include vasomotor symptoms, vaginal dryness, and evidence of reversible bone mineral density loss (99,100). The short period during which these drugs are used as adjuncts for COH should minimize such effects.

In summary, the use of GnRHa with gonadotropins significantly reduces the rate of cancelled cycles from approximately 20% to less than 5% due to a more predictable follicle response, inhibition of the endogenous LH surge, and better timing of hCG administration. GnRH agonists have led to a simplification of hormone administration, less midcycle monitoring, and an increased efficiency between cycles commenced, oocyte harvest, and pregnancy rate. From our experience in the use of Lupron with gonadotropins in more than 500 GIFT or IVF cycles, we now recommend its use in more than 90% of COH cycles in which gonadotropins are to be used. Furthermore, the incorporation of GnRHa with gonadotropins for COH is cost-effective and significantly reduces anxiety and uncertainty in both the patient and staff with respect to treatment cycle cancellation prior to oocyte harvest.

From our experience and that of others, it appears that one of the major benefits of GnRH agonists is the suppression of inappropriate endogenous gonadotropin interference with follicular maturation during COH. An effective way of accomplishing this is to administer GnRHa in the luteal phase to down-regulate the hypothalamic-pituitary-ovarian system before administering exogenous gonadotropin therapy. The concurrent "flare-up" regimen is associated with an unphysiologic elevation of follicular phase LH, progesterone, and androgen levels with an associated decline in pregnancy rates following IVF and GIFT. However, the slightly different technique described by Garcia et al. (85), using a short "flare-up" follicular phase regimen, appears most effective.

Controlled ovarian hyperstimulation: complications

Each of the agents used for effective COH is associated with an incidence of complications and side effects. Some of these are specific to the individual agent as described above, whereas others are unique to the assisted reproductive technologies as a whole.

Clinical pregnancy rates are enhanced by the presence of multiple oocytes (4) and transfer of multiple embryos (5,6). Unfortunately, the ability to obtain this goal through COH techniques is marked by an increased incidence of multiple pregnancy. Twenty-four percent of clinical pregnancies resulting from IVF-ET were multiple in the 1989 Society for Assisted Reproductive Technology (S.A.R.T.) Registry (6). The incidence of multiple pregnancy is generally correlated with the number of embryos transferred. The inherent complications of high-order multifetal gestation have been well described (101), and the decision to proceed with "selective reduction" of such pregnancies is not an easy one (102–104).

Ovarian hyperstimulation syndrome (OHSS) is a serious complication of COH, the pathogenesis of which has been reviewed in detail elsewhere (105,106). OHSS is manifested by symptomatic ovarian enlargement associated with luteinization of multiple follicles and stromal edema (107) (see Table 1.8). In progressively more severe forms, electrolyte imbalance, ascites, thromboemboli, pleural effusions, and hydrothorax may occur. The incidence of the most severe forms of OHSS is extremely rare with the use of clomiphene only (108), but is more common when gonadotropins are employed for induction of ovulation (109,110). Use of FSH has not consistently decreased this effect as was originally hoped (111). Some evidence was initially presented to suggest that the use of

GnRHa might decrease the incidence of ovarian hyperstimulation (112). Unfortunately, OHSS does occur despite down-regulation of pituitary gonadotropes and may be heightened in patients with polycystic ovary syndrome (113). The incidence of severe forms of this disorder may be somewhat lower when oocytes and luteinized follicular cells are aspirated during IVF, GIFT, or ZIFT procedures than when ovulation induc-

Table 1.8 Classification of ovarian hyperstimulation syndrome

Mild OHSS	
Grade 1	Chemical hyperstimulation
	Excessive ovarian estrogen and progesterone production
Grade 2	As above
	Ovarian enlargement up to 5 × 5 cm
	Abdominal fullness, swelling, pain
Moderate OHSS	
Grade 3	Increased abdominal pain and distention
	Ovarian enlargement up to 12 × 12 cm
Grade 4	As above
	Nausea, vomiting, and/or diarrhea
Severe OHSS	
Grade 5	Ovarian enlargement > 12 × 12 cm
	Ascites and/or hydrothorax
	Electrolyte imbalance
	Oliguria
	Hypovolemia
Grade 6	As above
	Severe hemoconcentration
	Coagulation abnormalities
	Thromboembolic phenomenon
	Pericardial effusion
	Anasarca
	Hypovolemic shock

Modified from Rabau E, Serr D, David A, Mashias S, Lunenfeld B. Human menopausal gonadotropin for anovulation and sterility. Am J Obstet Gynecol 1967;98:92–98.

tion alone is used, although this has not been clearly demonstrated.

The most ideal therapy is prevention. Correlation between OHSS and an ultrasound pattern of multiple intermediate-sized (9–15 mm) follicles during the immediate preovulatory period has been described (114,115). Haning et al. have shown that an increased risk of OHSS was associated with serum E_2 levels greater than 4000 pg/ml on the day of hCG administration (116). Whether or not such cutoff levels can be directly applied to cycles in which oocyte aspiration is anticipated has not been shown. We feel that a combination of maximum serum E_2 values, particularly associated with daily doubling, and the concomitant ultrasound pattern of multiple intermediate-sized follicles should be employed as predictive tools. Cycle cancellation by withholding hCG administration is the classic preventative measure. However, some investigators have recommended withholding gonadotropins while continuing down-regulation with GnRHa only, prior to reinstitution of gonadotropin stimulation, as a means of salvaging the treatment cycle (117). Others have suggested that hCG be administered, oocytes aspirated and fertilized, and resulting embryos cryopreserved while the patient is maintained on GnRHa in an effort to control the severity of OHSS (118). However, the safety of this approach has not been confirmed by other investigators or with sufficient patient numbers and, thus, cannot be endorsed by these authors.

Management of OHSS in its more severe forms requires hospitalization and demands meticulous attention to fluid and electrolyte balance to ensure adequate renal perfusion as well as prevention of thromboembolic phenomena. Paracentesis should be reserved for patients with severe respiratory compromise and used under skilled ultrasound guidance to avoid ovarian hemorrhage (119).

Conclusion

The application of various ovulation induction agents to the assisted reproductive technologies has provided a means of increasing the efficiency and success of any given treatment cycle. Careful monitoring of patient response is vital to achieve a high degree of safety and positive outcome. No single regimen is ideal for all patients. However, we feel that the adjunctive use of gonadotropin-releasing hormone agonists has enhanced our ability to obtain increased numbers of synchronous mature follicles while dramatically decreasing cycle cancellation rates. It is vital that the conflicting scientific reports in this rapidly evolving field are read with an extremely critical eye. We can only plead for increased numbers of well-designed and well-controlled multicenter randomized prospective trials to resolve the host of unresolved controversies within this discipline.

References

1. Trounson AO, Leeton JF, Wood C, Webb J, Wood J. Pregnancies in humans by fertilization in vitro and embryo transfer in the controlled ovulatory cycle. Science 1981; 212:681–682.

2. Steptoe PC, Edwards RG. Birth after the reimplantation of a human embryo. Lancet 1978;2:366.

3. Foulet H, Ranoux C, Dubuisson J-B, Rambaud D, Aubriot F-X, Poirot C. In vitro fertilization without ovarian stimulation: a simplified protocol applied in 80 cycles. Fertil Steril 1989;52:617–621.

4. Testart J, Belaisch-Allart J, Frydman R. Relationships between embryo transfer results and ovarian response and in vitro fertilization rate: analysis of 186 human pregnancies. Fertil Steril 1986;45:237–243.

5. Speirs A, Lopata A, Gronow M, Kellow G, Johnston W. Analysis of the benefits and risks of multiple embryo transfer. Fertil Steril 1983;39:468–471.

6. Medical Research International, Society for Assisted Reproductive Technology, American Fertility Society. In vitro fertilization–embryo transfer (IVF-ET) in the United States: 1989 results from the IVF-ET registry. Fertil Steril 1991;55:14–23.

7. Kerin JF, Warnes GM, Quinn PJ, et al. Incidence of multiple pregnancy after in vitro fertilization and embryo transfer. Lancet 1983;2:537–540.

8. Hodgen GD. The dominant ovarian follicle. Fertil Steril 1982;38:281–300.

9. Baker TG. A quantitative and cytological study of germ cells in human ovaries. Proc R Soc Br 1963;158:417–433.

10. Kerin JF, Warnes GM. Monitoring of ovarian response to stimulation in in-vitro fertilization cycles. Clin Obstet Gynecol 1986;29:158–170.

11. Kerin JF, Warnes GM, Quinn P, Kirby C, Godfrey B, Cox LW. Endocrinology of ovarian stimulation for in vitro fertilization. Aust N Z J Obstet Gynaecol 1984;24:121–124.

12. Kerin JF, Edmonds DK, Warnes GM, et al. Morphological and functional relations of graafian follicle growth to ovulation in women using ultrasonic, laparoscopic and biochemical measurements. Br J Obstet Gynaecol 1981;88: 81–90.

13. Buttery B, Trounson A, McMaster R, Wood C. Evaluation of diagnostic ultrasound as a parameter of follicular development in an in vitro fertilization program. Fertil Steril 1983;39:458–463.

14. De Crespigny L, O'Herlihy C, Hoult I, Robinson H. Ultrasound in an in vitro fertilization program. Fertil Steril 1981;35:25–28.

15. O'Herlihy C, Pepperell R, Robinson H. Ultrasound timing of human chorionic gonadotropin administration in clomiphene stimulated cycles. Obstet Gynecol 1982;59:40–45.

16. Hull M, Moghissi K, Magyar K, Hayes M, Zador I, Olson J. Correlation of serum estradiol levels and ultrasound monitoring to assess follicular maturation. Fertil Steril 1986; 46:42–45.

17. Marrs R, Vargyas J, March C. Correlation of ultrasonic and endocrinologic measurements in human menopausal gonadotropin therapy. Obstet Gynecol 1983;145:417–421.

18. Jones H, Acosta A, Andrews M, et al. The impor-

tance of the follicular phase to success and failure in in vitro fertilization. Fertil Steril 1983;40:317–321.

19. Scott R, Tower J, Muasher S, Oehninger S, Robinson S, Rosenwaks Z. Follicle-stimulating hormone levels on cycle day 3 are predictive of in vitro fertilization outcome. Fertil Steril 1989;51:651–654.

20. Schoolcraft W, Sinton E, Schlender T, Huynh D, Hamilton F, Meldrum DR. Lower pregnancy rate with premature luteinization during pituitary suppression with leuprolide acetate. Fertil Steril 1991;55:563–566.

21. Trounson A, Mohr L, Wood C, Leeton J. Effect of delayed insemination on in vitro fertilization, culture and transfer of human embryos. J Reprod Fertil 1982;64:285–294.

22. Jones H, Jones G, Andrews M, et al. The program for in vitro fertilization at Norfolk. Fertil Steril 1982;38:14–21.

23. Garcia J, Jones G, Acosta A, Wright G. Human menopausal gonadotropin/human chorionic gonadotropin follicular maturation for oocyte aspiration: phase II, 1981. Fertil Steril 1983; 39:174–179.

24. Laufer N, De Cherney A, Haseltine F, et al. The use of high-dose human menopausal gonadotropin in an in vitro fertilization program. Fertil Steril 1983;40:734–740.

25. Ben-Rafael Z, Benadiva C, Ausmanes M, et al. Dose of human menopausal gonadotropin influences the outcome of an in vitro fertilization program. Fertil Steril 1987;48:964–968.

26. Meldrum D, Chetkowski R, Steingold K, de Ziegler D, Cedars M, Hamilton M. Evolution of a highly successful in vitro fertilization–embryo transfer program. Fertil Steril 1987;48:86–93.

27. Stone B, Quinn K, Quinn P, Vargyas J, Marrs R. Response of patients to different lots of human menopausal gonadotropins during controlled ovarian hyperstimulation. Fertil Steril 1989;52:745–752.

28. Terrareti A, Garcia J, Acosta A, Jones G. Serum luteinizing hormone during ovulation induction with human menopausal gonadotropin for in vitro fertilization in normally menstruating women. Fertil Steril 1983;40:742–747.

29. Glasier A, Thatcher S, Wickings E, Hillier S, Baird D. Superovulation with exogenous gonadotropins does not inhibit the luteinizing hormone surge. Fertil Steril 1988;49:81–85.

30. Vargyas J, Morente C, Shangold G, Marrs R. The effect of different methods for ovarian stimulation for human in vitro fertilization and embryo replacement. Fertil Steril 1984;42:745–749.

31. Lejeune B, Degueldre M, Camus M, Vekemans M, Opsomer L, Leroy F. In vitro fertilization and embryo transfer as related to endogenous luteinizing hormone rise or human chorionic gonadotropin administration. Fertil Steril 1986; 45:377–383.

32. Punnonen R, Ashorn R, Vilja P, Heinone P, Kujansuu E, Tuohimaa P. Spontaneous luteinizing hormone surge and cleavage of in vitro fertilized embryos. Fertil Steril 1988;49:479–482.

33. Surrey E, Chisham P, Randle D, et al. Significance of serum luteinizing hormone levels during gonadotropin induced controlled ovarian hyperstimulation prior to oocyte retrieval [abstract 45]. Presented at the Annual Meeting of the Pacific Coast Fertility Society, 1989 Palm Springs, Ca.

34. Harlap S. Ovulation induction and congenital malformations. Lancet 1976;2:961.

35. Schwartz M, Jewelewicz R. The use of gonadotropins for induction of ovulation. Fertil Steril 1981;35:3–12.

36. Kurachi K, Aono T, Minagawa J, Miyake A. Congenital malformations after clomiphene-induced ovulation. Fertil Steril 1983;40:187–189.

37. Adashi E. Clomiphene citrate-initiated ovulation: a clinical update. Semin Reprod Endocrinol 1986;4:255–276.

38. Kerin J, Liu J, Phillipou G, Yen S. Evidence for a hypothalamic site of action of clomiphene citrate in women. J Clin Endocrinol Metab 1985;61:265–268.

39. Vaikutis J, Bermudez J, Cargille C, Lipsett M, Ross G. New evidence for an anti-estrogenic action of clomiphene citrate in women. J Clin Endocrinol 1971;32:503–508.

40. Lopata A, Brown J, Leeton J, McTalbot J, Wood C. In vitro fertilization of preovulatory oocytes and embryo transfer in infertile patients treated with clomiphene and human chorionic gonadotropin. Fertil Steril 1978;30:27–35.

41. Wood C, Trounson A, Leeton J, et al. A clinical assessment of nine pregnancies obtained by in vitro fertilization and embryo transfer. Fertil Steril 1981;36:502–508.

42. Hoult I, De Crespigny L, O'Herlihy C, et al. Ultrasound control of clomiphene/human chorionic gonadotropin stimulated cycles for oocyte recovery and in vitro fertilization. Fertil Steril 1981;35:502–508.

43. Lopata A, Martin M, Oliva K, Johnston I. Embryonic development and blastocyst implantation following in vitro fertilization and embryo transfer. Fertil Steril 1982; 38:682–687.

44. Kerin J, Warnes G, Quinn P, et al. The effect of Clomid induced superovulation on human follicular and luteal function for extracorporeal fertilization and embryo transfer. Clin Reprod Fertil 1983;2:129–142.

45. Rogers P, Molloy D, Healy D, et al. Cross-over trial of superovulation protocols from two major in vitro fertilization centers. Fertil Steril 1986;46:424–431.

46. Kerin J, Warnes G, Quinn P, et al. In vitro fertilization and embryo transfer program, Department of Obstetrics and Gynaecology, University of Adelaide at the Queen Elizabeth Hospital, Woodville, South Australia. J In Vitro Fert Embryo Transf 1984;1:63–71.

47. Quigley M, Schmidt C, Beauchamp P, Pace-Owens S, Berkowitz A, Wolf D. Enhanced follicular recruitment in an in vitro fertilization program: clomiphene alone versus a clomiphene/human menopausal gonadotropin combination. Fertil Steril 1984;42:745–749.

48. Diamond M, Wentz A, Herbert C, Pittaway D, Maxson W, Daniell J. One ovary or two: differences in ovulation induction, estradiol levels, and follicular development in a program for in vitro fertilization. Fertil Steril 1984;41:524–529.

49. Diamond M, Hill G, Webster B, et al. Comparison of human menopausal gonadotropin, clomiphene citrate, and combined human menopausal gonadotropin–clomiphene citrate stimulation protocols for in vitro fertilization. Fertil Steril 1986;46:1108–1112.

50. Cook C, Schroeder J, Yussman M, Sanfilippo J. Induction of luteal phase defect with clomiphene citrate. Am J Obstet Gynecol 1984;149:613–616.

51. Sharma V, Whitehead M, Mason B, et al. Influence of superovulation on endometrial and embryonic development. Fertil Steril 1990;53:822–829.

52. Nelson L, Hershlag A, Kurl R, Hall J, Stillman R.

Clomiphene citrate directly impairs endometrial receptivity in the mouse. Fertil Steril 1990;53:727–731.

53. Thatcher S, Donachie K, Glasier A, Hillier S, Baird D. The effects of clomiphene citrate on the histology of human endometrium in regularly cycling women undergoing in vitro fertilization. Fertil Steril 1988;49:296–301.

54. Punnonen R, Ashorn R, Heinonen P, et al. Endometrial maturation after sequential use of clomiphene citrate, human menopausal gonadotropin, and human chorionic gonadotropin in in vitro fertilization. J In Vitro Fert Embryo Transf 1988;5:112–113.

55. McCormack S, Clark JH. Clomid administration to pregnant rats causes abnormalities of the reproductive tract in offspring and mothers. Science 1979;204:629–631.

56. Adashi E, Rock J, Shapp L, et al. Gestational outcome of clomiphene related conceptions. Fertil Steril 1979;31:620–625.

57. Donini P, Puzzuoli D, D'Alessio I, et al. Purification and separation of FSH and LH from human postmenopausal gonadotropins. II. Preparation of biological apparently pure FSH by selective binding of the LH with an anti-hCG serum and subsequent chromatography. Acta Endocrinol 1966; 52:169–185.

58. Schenken R, Hodgen G. Follicle-stimulating hormone blocks estrogen positive feedback during the early follicular phase in monkeys. Fertil Steril 1986;45:556–560.

59. Sharma V, Riddle A, Mason B, Whitehead M, Collins W. Studies on folliculogenesis and in vitro fertilization outcome after the administration of follicle-stimulating hormone at different times during the menstrual cycle. Fertil Steril 1989;51:298–303.

60. Benadiva C, Ben-Rafael Z, Blasco L, Tureck R, Mastroianni L, Flickinger G. An increased initial follicle-stimulating hormone/luteinizing hormone ratio does not affect ovarian responses and the outcomes of in vitro fertilization. Fertil Steril 1988;50:777–781.

61. Lavy G, Pellicer A, Diamond M, De Cherney A. Ovarian stimulation for in vitro fertilization and embryo transfer, human menopausal gonadotropin versus pure human follicle stimulating hormone: a randomized prospective study. Fertil Steril 1988;50:74–78.

62. Muasher S, Garcia J, Rosenwaks Z. The combination of follicle-stimulating hormone and human menopausal gonadotropin for the induction of multiple follicular maturation for in vitro fertilization. Fertil Steril 1985;44:62–69.

63. Navot D, Rosenwaks Z. The use of follicle stimulating hormone for controlled ovarian hyperstimulation in in vitro fertilization. J In Vitro Fert Embryo Transf 1988;5:3–13.

64. Scoccia B, Blumenthal P, Wagner C, Prins G, Scommegna A, Marut E. Comparison of urinary human follicle-stimulating hormone and human menopausal gonadotropins for ovarian stimulation in an in vitro fertilization program. Fertil Steril 1987;48:446–449.

65. Serafini P, Stone B, Kerin J, Batzofin J, Quinn P, Marrs R. An alternate approach to controlled ovarian hyperstimulation in "poor responders": pretreatment with a gonadotropin-releasing hormone analog. Fertil Steril 1988; 49:90–95.

66. Meldrum D, Wisot A, Hamilton F, Gutlay A, Kempton W, Huynh D. Routine pituitary suppression with leuprolide before ovarian stimulation for oocyte retrieval. Fertil Steril 1989;51:455–459.

67. Chetkowski R, Kruse L, Nass T. Improved pregnancy outcome with the addition of leuprolide acetate to gonadotropins for in vitro fertilization. Fertil Steril 1989;52:250–255.

68. De Ziegler D, Cedars M, Randle D, Lu J, Judd H, Meldrum D. Suppression of the ovary using a gonadotropin releasing hormone agonist prior to stimulation for oocyte retrieval. Fertil Steril 1987;48:807–810.

69. Stone B, Serafini P, Quinn K, Quinn P, Kerin J, Marrs R. Gonadotropins and estradiol levels during ovarian stimulation in women treated with leuprolide acetate. Obstet Gynecol 1989;73:990–995.

70. Sathanandan M, Warnes G, Kirby C, Petricco O, Mathews C. Adjuvant leuprolide in normal, abnormal, and poor responders to controlled ovarian hyperstimulation for in vitro fertilization/gamete intrafallopian transfer. Fertil Steril 1989;51:998–1006.

71. Cedars M, Surrey E, Hamilton F, Lapolt P, Meldrum D. Leuprolide acetate lowers circulating bioactive luteinizing hormone and testosterone concentrations during ovarian stimulation for oocyte retrieval. Fertil Steril 1990;53:627–631.

72. Knobil E. The neuroendocrine control of the menstrual cycle. Recent Prog Horm Res 1980;36:53–88.

73. Kerin J. The advantages of a gonadotropin releasing hormone agonist (leuprolide acetate) in conjunction with gonadotropins for controlled ovarian hyperstimulation in IVF and GIFT cycles. Arch Gynecol Obstet 1989;246:S45–S52.

74. Droesch K, Muasher S, Brzyski R, et al. Value of suppression with a gonadotropin-releasing hormone agonist prior to gonadotropin stimulation for in vitro fertilization. Fertil Steril 1989;51:292–297.

75. Maclachlan V, Besanko M, O'Shea F, et al. A controlled study of luteinizing hormone-releasing hormone agonist (Buserelin) for the induction of folliculogenesis before in vitro fertilization. N Engl J Med 1989;320:1233–1237.

76. Segars J, Hill G, Bryan S, et al. The use of gonadotropin releasing hormone agonist (GnRHa) in good responders undergoing repeat in vitro fertilization/embryo transfer (IVF/ET). J In Vitro Fert Embryo Transf 1990;7:327–331.

77. Ferrier A, Rasweiler J, Bedford J, Prey K, Berkeley A. Evaluation of leuprolide acetate and gonadotropins versus clomiphene citrate and gonadotropins for in vitro fertilization or gamete intrafallopian transfer. Fertil Steril 1990;54:90–95.

78. Awadallah S, Friedman C, Chin N, Dodds W, Park J, Kim M. Follicular stimulation for in vitro fertilization using pituitary suppression and human menopausal gonadotropins. Fertil Steril 1987;48:811–815.

79. Dor J, Ben-Shlomo I, Lipitz S, et al. Ovarian stimulation with gonadotropin-releasing hormone (GnRH) analogue improves the in vitro fertilization (IVF) pregnancy rate with both transvaginal and laparoscopic oocyte recovery. J In Vitro Fert Embryo Transf 1990;7:351–354.

80. Lipitz S, Ben-Rafael Z, Dor J, et al. Suppression with gonadotropin releasing hormone (GnRH) analogues prior to stimulation with gonadotropins: comparison of three protocols. Gynecol Obstet Invest 1989;28:31–34.

81. Caspi E, Ron-El R, Golan A, et al. Results of in vitro fertilization and embryo transfer by combined long-acting gonadotropin releasing hormone analog D-Trp-6-luteinizing hormone-releasing hormone and gonadotropins. Fertil Steril 1989;51:95–99.

82. Edelstein M, Bryzyski R, Jones G, Simonetti S, Muasher S. Equivalancy of human menopausal gonadotropin and follicle-stimulating hormone stimulation after gonadotropin-releasing hormone agonist suppression. Fertil Steril 1990;53:103–106.

83. Bentiek B, Shaw R, Iffland C, Burford G, Bernard A. A randomized comparative study of purified follicle stimulating hormone and human menopausal gonadotropin after pituitary desensitization with Buserelin for superovulation and in vitro fertilization. Fertil Steril 1988;50:79–84.

84. Meldrum D, Wisot A, Hamilton F, Gutlay A, Huynh D, Kempton W. Timing of initiation and dose schedule of leuprolide influence the time course of ovarian suppression. Fertil Steril 1988;50:400–402.

85. Garcia J, Padilla S, Bayati J, Baramki T. Follicular phase gonadotropin-releasing hormone agonist and human gonadotropins: a better alternative for ovulation induction in in vitro fertilization. Fertil Steril 1990;53:302–305.

86. Bryzyski R, Muasher S, Droesch K, Simonetti S, Jones G, Rosenwaks Z. Follicular atresia associated with concurrent initiation of gonadotropin releasing hormone agonist and follicle stimulating hormone for oocyte recruitment. Fertil Steril 1988;50:917–921.

87. Katayama K, Roesler M, Gunnarson C, Stehlik E, Jagusch S. Short-term use of gonadotropin releasing hormone agonist (leuprolide) for in vitro fertilization. J In Vitro Fert Embryo Transf 1988;5:332–334.

88. San Roman GA, Surrey ES, Judd HL, Kerin JF. A prospective randomized comparison of luteal phase versus concurrent follicular phase initiation of gonadotropin releasing hormone agonist for in-vitro fertilization. Fertil Steril 1992;58:744–749.

89. San Roman G, Kerin J, Judd H, Surrey E. Differential steroid hormone and gonadotropin response of luteal phase (LP) versus follicular phase (FP) initiation of GnRH-agonist (GnRHa) for controlled ovarian hyperstimulation (COH) with human menopausal gonadotropins [abstract P-141]. Presented at the Annual Meeting of the American Fertility Society, 1990 Washington, DC.

90. Gindoff P, Hall J, Stillman R. Ovarian suppression with leuprolide acetate: comparison of luteal, follicular, and

flare-up administration in controlled ovarian hyperstimulation for oocyte retrieval. J In Vitro Fert Embryo Transf 1990;7:94–97.

91. Frydman R, Belaisch-Allart J, Parneix I, Forman R, Hazout A, Testart J. Comparison between flare up and down-regulation effects of luteinizing hormone-releasing hormone agonists in an in vitro fertilization program. Fertil Steril 1988;50:471–475.

92. Van de-Helder A, Holmerhorst F, Blankhart A, Brand R, Waegemaekers C, Naaktgeboren N. Comparison of ovarian stimulation regimes for in vitro fertilization with and without a gonadotropin-releasing hormone (GnRH) agonist: results of a randomized study. J In Vitro Fert Embryo Transf 1990;7:358–362.

93. Neveu S, Hedon B, Bringor J, et al. Ovarian stimulation by a combination of a gonadotropin releasing hormone agonist and gonadotropins for in vitro fertilization. Fertil Steril 1987;47:639–643.

94. Herman A, Ron-El R, Golan A, Nahum H, Soffer Y, Caspi E. Follicle cysts after menstrual versus midluteal administration of gonadotropin-releasing hormone analog in in vitro fertilization. Fertil Steril 1990;53:854–858.

95. Feldberg D, Ashkenazi J, Dicker D, Yeshaya A, Goldman G, Goldman J. Ovarian cyst formation: a complication of gonadotropin-releasing hormone agonist therapy. Fertil Steril 1989;51:42–45.

96. Serafini P, Batzofin J, Kerin J, Marrs R. Pregnancy: a risk to initiation of leuprolide acetate during the luteal phase before controlled ovarian hyperstimulation. Fertil Steril 1988;50:371–372.

97. Kang I, Kuehl T, Siler-Khodr T. Effect of treatment with gonadotropin-releasing hormone analogues on pregnancy outcome in the baboon. Fertil Steril 1989;52:846–853.

98. Sopelak V, Hodgen G. Infusion of gonadotropin-releasing hormone agonist during pregnancy: maternal and fetal response in primates. Am J Obstet Gynecol 1987;156:755–760.

99. Steingold K, Cedars M, Lu J, Randle D, Judd H, Meldrum D. Treatment of endometriosis with a long-acting gonadotropin-releasing hormone agonist. Obstet Gynecol 1987;69:403–411.

100. Johansen J, Riis B, Hassager C, Moen M, Jacobson J, Christiansen C. The effect of a gonadotropin-releasing hormone agonist analogue (Nafarelin) on bone metabolism. J Clin Endocrinol Metab 1988;67:701–706.

101. Lipitz S, Frenkel Y, Watts C, Ben-Rafael Z, Barkai G, Reichman B. High-order multifetal gestation-management and outcome. Obstet Gynecol 1990;76:215–218.

102. Berkowitz R, Lynch L, Chitkara U, Wilkins I, Mehalek K, Alvarez E. Selective reduction of multifetal pregnancies in the first trimester. N Engl J Med 1988;318:1043–1047.

103. Shalev J, Frenkel Y, Goldenberg M, et al. Subjective reduction in multiple gestations: pregnancy outcome after transvaginal and transabdominal procedures. Fertil Steril 1989;52:416–420.

104. Evans M, Fletcher J, Zador I, Newton B, Quigg M, Struyk C. Selective first trimester termination in octuplet and quadruplet pregnancies: clinical and ethical issues. Obstet Gynecol 1988;71:289–296.

105. Golan A, Ron-El R, Herman A, Soffer Y, Weinraub Z, Caspi E. Ovarian hyperstimulation syndrome: an update review. Obstet Gynecol Surv 1989;44:430–440.

106. Schenker J, Weinstein D. Ovarian hyperstimulation syndrome: a current survey. Fertil Steril 1978;30:255–268.

107. Rabau E, Serr D, David A, Mashias S, Lunenfeld B. Human menopausal gonadotropin for anovulation and sterility. Am J Obstet Gynecol 1967;98:92–98.

108. Polishuk W, Schenker J. Ovarian overstimulation syndrome. Fertil Steril 1969;20:443–450.

109. Crooke A, Butt W, Palmer R, et al. Clinical trial of human gonadotropins. J Obstet Gynaecol Br Commonw 1963;70:604–635.

110. Raj S, Berger M, Grimes E, Taymor M. The use of gonadotropins for the induction of ovulation in women with polycystic ovarian disease. Fertil Steril 1977;28:1280–1284.

111. Check J, Wu C, Crocial B, Adelson H. Severe ovarian hyperstimulation syndrome from treatment with urinary follicle-stimulating hormone: two cases. Fertil Steril 1985;43:317–321.

112. Fleming R, Haxton M, Hamilton M, et al. Successful treatment of infertile women with oligomenorrhea using a

combination of an LHRH agonist and exogenous gonado-tropins. Br J Obstet Gynaecol 1985;92:369–373.

113. Dodson W, Hughes C, Yancy S, Haney A. Clinical characteristics of ovulation induction with human menopausal gonadotropins with and without leuprolide acetate in polycystic ovary syndrome. Fertil Steril 1989;52:915–918.

114. Blankstein J, Shalev J, Saadon T, et al. Ovarian hyperstimulation syndrome: prediction by numbers and size of preovulatory ovarian follicles. Fertil Steril 1987;47:597–602.

115. Tal J, Paz B, Samberg I, Lazarov N, Sharf M. Ultrasonographic and clinical correlates of menotropin versus sequential clomiphene citrate: menotropin therapy for induction of ovulation. Fertil Steril 1988;44:342–349.

116. Haning R, Austin C, Carlson I, Kuzma D, Shapiro S, Zweibel W. Plasma estradiol is superior to ultrasound and urinary estriol glucuronide as a predictor of ovarian hyper-stimulation during induction of ovulation with menotropins. Fertil Steril 1983;40:31–36.

117. Forman R, Frydman R, Egan D, Ross C, Barlow D. Severe ovarian hyperstimulation syndrome using agonists of gonadotropin-releasing hormone for in vitro fertilization: a European series and a proposal for prevention. Fertil Steril 1990;53:502–509.

118. Amso N, Ahuja K, Morris N, Shaw R. The management of predicted ovarian hyperstimulation involving gonadotropin-releasing hormone analog with elective cryopreservation of all pre-embryos. Fertil Steril 1990;53:1087–1090.

119. Padilla S, Zamaria S, Baramki T, Garcia J. Abdominal paracentesis for the ovarian hyperstimulation syndrome with severe respiratory compromise. Fertil Steril 1990;53:365–367.

2

Male Factor

Larry I. Lipshultz
John Grantmyre

Introduction

Although media sensationalism repeatedly characterizes infertility as primarily "the woman's problem" and commonly associates this with the inevitability of a faltering biologic clock, in reality male factor infertility is equally common. In fact, statistics both in the United States and abroad have documented the fact that 30% to 50% of couples with primary infertility will be found to have significant male reproductive failure. In the last few years, we have witnessed increased understanding of the subtle abnormalities of gonadal and spermatozoal function that can contribute to seemingly unexplained male infertility. Newly emerging diagnostic tests may help define these previously obscure male factors. This chapter describes our approach to correcting and treating the infertile male, highlighting the areas that are innovative and potentially beneficial.

Although it has been recommended that clinical evaluation of an infertile couple be undertaken only after one year of unprotected intercourse, we believe that the initial screening for the man should occur whenever the patient comes to medical attention. While 85% of pregnancies will occur within one year of unprotected intercourse, the issue of fertility is fraught with strong emotional and cultural overtones, and the couple should be allowed the freedom to determine for themselves the urgency of their investigations (1). Nonetheless, the initial evaluation of the male partner must be rapid, noninvasive, and cost-effective. Several social factors have prompted earlier investigation of the male, and these may increase demand for fertility specialists in the future. One is the tendency in our society for later marriage; another is the increased role of women in the workplace. Both of these trends tend to delay the eventual age of childbearing. Although male fertility potential does not change appreciably with age, female fertility does decrease statistically over time. The result is that the current tendency to delay childbearing will increase the chance of infertility—the optimum age of fertility having passed. Reassessment of the previously held chauvinistic tendency to "blame" infertility on the female, and therefore to investigate her as the first and sometimes only patient, has now given way to earlier male investigation, especially since this is often easier from the patient's perspective. In addition to the factors already mentioned, a growing public awareness of improved treatments for infertility, bolstered by the modern trends of consumerism in medicine, have encouraged earlier assessment of the growing population of infertile couples.

Initial evaluation includes a detailed history and physical examination as well as semen and hormonal assessments. Because conception is a couple-dependent phenomenon, investigation of reproductive dysfunction should be undertaken concurrently in both partners. We encourage the presence of the couple during all discussions and discourage any sense of blame. Joint visits also help to improve general understanding of the information, which may be complex and formidable. Since infertility is a field with many recent technical advances, the presence of both husband and wife lessens or avoids the need for repeated explanation of the often complicated material.

History and physical examination

The history includes information about the duration of infertility, previous pregnancies with the current partner or previous partners, and documentation of any previous evaluation or treatment of infertility. If a female reproductive specialist has not been consulted previously, inquiries are made about the length and regularity of menstrual periods. A history of gynecologic or pelvic surgery, endometriosis, or pelvic inflammatory disease,

which could suggest the presence of a female factor, should prompt simultaneous female evaluation. The history obtained from the infertile male should cover not only the basic questions contained in any medical history but also those particular questions chosen to evaluate genitourinary function (Table 2.1).

A history of unilateral or bilateral undescended testes may be significant because, regardless of the patient's age at orchiopexy, semen quality is less than that found in normal men (2). Testicular torsion has also been associated with decreased fertility (3). A history of specific childhood diseases may also be relevant. Mumps do not appear to affect the prepubertal testis; after puberty, however, 30% of patients will have unilateral and 10% will have bilateral orchitis. Approximately half of the affected testes will become atrophic (4). Childhood surgery should be noted, especially infantile hernia repairs, since this procedure requires mobilization of the spermatic cord within the inguinal canal and iatrogenic damage to the vas deferens is possible. Surgery in the region of the bladder neck (particularly a Y-V plasty in association with ureteric reimplantation for reflux) can result in retrograde ejaculation (5). This surgery was popular in the early 1960s, and many of the men who underwent these procedures are now of reproductive age.

Past medical and surgical history may include a history of diabetes mellitus, multiple sclerosis, transverse myelitis, or retroperitoneal surgery. These conditions can affect the long sympathetic nerves that originate in the lower thoracic and upper lumbar spine and control emission and ejaculation (Fig. 2.1). Likewise a neuropathy, pelvic trauma, or surgery can cause impotence by damaging the delicate pelvic parasympathetic fibers and, thereby, indirectly affect fertility. A family history of cystic fibrosis is relevant since this condition can be associated with absence of the vas deferens and seminal vesicles. Immotile-cilia syndrome, which affects the cilia

Table 2.1 Infertility history

History of infertility	Pelvic injury
Duration	Pelvic, inguinal, or scrotal
Prior pregnancies	surgery
Present partner	Herniorrhaphy
Another partner	Y-V plasty, transurethral
Previous treatments	prostate resection
Evaluation and treatment of	**Infections**
wife	Viral, febrile
Sexual history	Mumps orchitis
Potency	Venereal
Lubricants	Tuberculosis; smallpox
Timing of intercourse	(rare)
Frequency of intercourse	**Gonadotoxins**
Frequency of masturbation	Chemicals (pesticides)
Childhood and	Drugs (chemotherapeutic,
development	cimetidine, sulfasalazine,
Undescended testicles,	nitrofurantoin, alcohol,
orchiopexy	marijuana, androgenic
Herniorrhaphy	steroids)
Y-V plasty of bladder	Thermal exposure
Testicular torsion	Radiation
Testicular trauma	Smoking
Onset of puberty	**Family history**
Medical history	Cystic fibrosis
Systemic illness (i.e., diabetes	Androgen receptor
mellitus, multiple sclerosis)	deficiency
Previous/current therapy	**Review of systems**
Surgical history	Respiratory infections
Orchiectomy (testis cancer,	Anosmia
torsion)	Galactorrhea
Retroperitoneal surgery	Impaired visual fields

Reproduced with permission from Sigman M, Lipshultz LI, Howards SS. Evaluation of the subfertile male. In: Lipshultz LI, Howards SS, eds. Infertility in the male, 2nd ed. Chicago: Mosby–Year Book, 1991; p 180.

of the respiratory tract as well as the sperm tail, leads to low or no sperm motility observed in conjunction with recurrent upper respiratory infections. Unexplained childhood deaths in the family or a history of precocious puberty can be associated with congenital adrenal hyperplasia, which is caused by a metabolic defect in androgen production and has been associated with infertility. Age at onset of puberty in relation to that of peers may be a clue to long-standing pituitary or hypothalamic causes of hypogonadism.

Previous testicular trauma and exposure to gonadotoxins must be documented. These include direct exposure to heat (as in regular use of a hot tub, but not the choice of underwear), environmental toxins (e.g., certain pesticides, specifically dibromochloropropane), and certain drugs, such as sulfasalazine, cimetidine, spironolactone, colchicine, marijuana, and anabolic steroids (6–11). In general, patients with drug-related infertility can expect excellent recovery of sperm function once these medications have been discontinued. This may not be the case with anabolic steroids; as they often are used in extremely high doses and in an unsupervised manner, permanent sterility can result (12). This is especially tragic when their use is prompted by social rather than medical concerns. Patients who have had therapeutic radiation treatment or chemotherapy usually will have a greater than 80% chance of infertility. There is evidence that many of these patients have had depressed semen parameters prior to their treatment (13). Recovery of sperm production may take as long as 4 to 5 years but can be anticipated in 50% of these patients (14). Cryopreservation of sperm prior to oncologic treatment is the only hope for those patients who fail to recover adequate sperm production; fortunately, this is being offered to an increasing number of these patients.

Febrile illness or infection occurring within 3 months of semen collection can alter the semen analysis. Spermatogenesis takes approximately 74 days from the initiation of type B spermatogonia to the appearance of mature spermatozoa and then an additional 11 to 15 days for passage through the ductal system before motile sperm are present in the ejaculate. Semen testing should be repeated in 3 to 6 months if significant illness has occurred in the period immediately prior to collection.

Sexual habits must be addressed during the initial evaluation, but this topic should be deferred until late in the interview after rapport has been established, which may improve the accuracy of information obtained. The most common problem is that the couple engages in intercourse either too frequently or too infrequently. Often the couple does not fully understand the signifi-

cance of the wife's menstrual cycle, specifically that the optimum time for intercourse is midcycle and that the optimum frequency of intercourse is every 48 hours. Sperm survive approximately 2 days in normal cervical mucus and cervical crypts; therefore, this coital frequency will promote the presence of viable sperm during the 12 to 24 hours during which the egg can be fertilized. Too-frequent ejaculation will lower the density of the sperm "bolus" that traverses the cervical mucus and, therefore, the number of sperm that can eventually fertilize the ovum. Spermatotoxic lubricants and periovulatory masturbation should be avoided. A history of impotence or premature ejaculation is often difficult to obtain when the couple first complains of infertility, but this has been estimated to affect approxi-

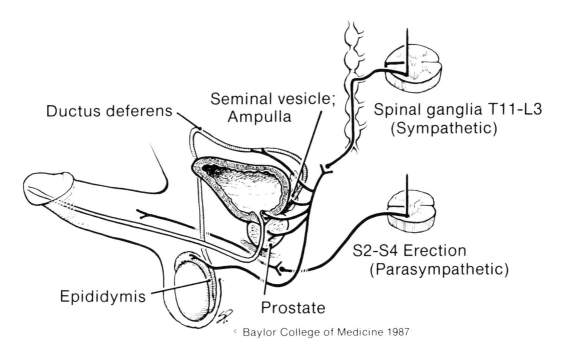

© Baylor College of Medicine 1987

Fig. 2.1 Diagram of nerve supply to bladder neck and erectile bodies. The long routed synthetic fibers (T11–L3) control ejaculation.

mately 5% of the infertile male population and should be addressed (15).

A past history of genitourinary infection, such as epididymitis, which can cause obstructive scarring or orchitis leading to atrophy of the germinal epithelium, is relevant. Symptoms of current infection such as prostatitis, urethritis, or cystitis are also significant since an increased number of leukocytes (more than $1.0 \times 10^6/cc$) has been shown to affect semen quality (16).

Finally, a thorough review of systems will rule out chronic disease conditions such as renal or hepatic failure. A history of headache, galactorrhea, or impaired visual fields, along with infertility, may indicate a prolactin-secreting pituitary tumor. Appropriate testing should be instituted (see below).

Physical examination of the infertile man should include a complete examination since any factor impairing one's overall health can theoretically affect sperm production and function. Inadequate virilization determined on the basis of genital size, hair distribution, or gynecomastia may suggest hormonal abnormalities and the need for further endocrine testing, including evaluation of testosterone and estrogen levels. Of course, emphasis of the examination should be on the genitalia. Penile curvature as well as malposition of the urethral meatus can result in improper placement of the semen in the vagina. Ventral penile curvature can be the result of chordee, usually in association with hypospadias. Dorsal curvature is more often seen in older men with Peyronie's disease. Hypospadias, with its abnormal position of the urethral meatus, can in its severe penile-scrotal form lead to semen deposition outside the vagina. Testicular size and consistency must be assessed because a decrease in testicular size is often associated with impaired spermatogenesis (17). This is not surprising since the germinal epithelium comprises 85% of the testicular volume. In the normospermic man, the testicles are firm to the touch, and the testicular length is

more than 4 cm. Evaluation of the peritesticular area is also critical and should include careful examination of the epididymis and vas deferens. An attempt to palpate a varicocele should be undertaken only after the patient has been standing for several minutes in a warm room. A Valsalva maneuver should be performed for documentation of smaller varicoceles. In our clinic those lesions that are equivocal on physical examination are routinely examined by high-resolution scrotal ultrasound. We consider dilatation of the panpiniform plexus to be significant on ultrasound if the diameter of the vessels exceeds 3 mm when the patient is standing and if there is evidence of increase in diameter of the vein with a Valsalva maneuver. Although many methods such as venography, Doppler ultrasound, radioisotope scanning, and thermography can demonstrate "subclinical" varicoceles, only those varicoceles diagnosed by clinical palpation have been repeatedly shown to influence fertility. For this reason, we use ultrasound (which is the most accessible and cost-effective method in our clinical setting) for *confirmation* of a varicocele only when we suspect one on clinical grounds—that is, physical examination. While varicoceles can be found in 15% to 20% of the normal population, this number approaches 40% in subfertile men (15). Varicoceles occur predominantly on the left side; however, we now identify bilateral varicoceles in up to 40% of those men affected. The examination is completed with a rectal examination to evaluate the prostate and seminal vesicles.

Laboratory evaluation

After the history and physical examination are completed, blood is drawn for hormone evaluation, and arrangements are made for a minimum of three semen specimens to be obtained at the couple's convenience. The semen should be analyzed within 2 hours of collection and after 48 hours of sexual abstinence. The bulk parameters that are routinely measured include the semen volume, the sperm density, the percentage of motile sperm, and finally, the forward progression, which is measured on a scale of 1 to 4. While computer-assisted semen analysis (CASA) is capable of analyzing large numbers of sperm, heterogeneity within the specimen is rarely a problem with manual analysis. Because debris and artifacts can be counted as immotile sperm by the computer, estimates of count and motility can be inaccurate, especially in patients with low sperm density. When a computer alone has been used, oligo-spermia has been diagnosed in azoospermic patients for the same reason (18). The standard hemocytometer is inexpensive and accurate in experienced hands. We have recently also employed the Micro-Cell 20-μm-depth semen analysis chamber (Fertility Technologies, Natick, Mass.), which has the benefit of using the same slide for both count and motility assessment. In addition to undergoing the routine examination, specimens are tested for the presence of antisperm antibodies by use of the direct latex agglutination method (immunobead) and for white blood cells by use of a specific monoclonal antibody stain. This stain is essential for differentiating white cells from immature sperm, which can have an identical gross histologic appearance. The essential parameters that are measured as well as their normal values are listed in Table 2.2.

Results from the three semen specimens together will indicate 1) normal bulk semen parameters, 2) azoo-spermia, or 3) abnormal bulk semen parameters. This classification has been helpful in categorizing subfertile male patients and, in conjunction with endocrine testing, in guiding our further evaluation and treatment.

The endocrine evaluation hinges on the intimate relationship between the hypothalamic-pituitary axis in sperm production by the gonad. The critical event, in terms of fertility evaluation, centers on the release of follicle-stimulating hormone (FSH) from the pituitary

under stimulation of gonadotropin-releasing hormone (GnRH) (see Fig. 2.2). Stimulation of the Sertoli cell by FSH increases germ cell production and local androgen binding. In the presence of normal spermatogenesis, inhibin is produced by the Sertoli cell and will feed back on the pituitary or hypothalamus and down-regulate FSH release. Patients who demonstrate even subtle elevation of FSH usually have impaired semen produc-tion. An elevation of FSH more than three times normal generally implies significant germ cell failure. In ad-dition to FSH evaluation, other serum hormones routinely assayed include testosterone, luteinizing hor-mone (LH), and prolactin, but it is rare to have a clinically significant abnormality of any of these other hormones in the presence of a totally normal FSH.

Normal semen analysis

Some infertile men will have normal bulk semen parameters. If pertinent historical factors such as poor coital timing are identified, these should be treated

---

Table 2.2   Semen analysis: minimal standards of adequacy

On at least two occasions

Ejaculate volume:	1.5–5.0 cc
Sperm density:	$>20 \times 10^6$/cc
Motility:	>60%
Forward progression:	> 2 (scale 1–4)
Morphology:	> 60% normal

And

No significant sperm agglutination
No significant pyospermia
No hyperviscosity

Reproduced with permission from Sigman M, Lipshultz LI, How-ards SS. Evaluation of the subfertile male. In: Lipshultz LI, Howards SS, eds. Infertility in the male, 2nd ed. Chicago: Mosby–Year Book, 1991; p 184.

appropriately. If no female abnormality has been found, more sophisticated sperm testing is recommended. The cross mucus test, which compares the activity of the husband's sperm and normal donor sperm after admixing with both the female partner's and a normal donor's cervical mucus, provides more information about sperm-mucus interaction than the standard postcoital test. If no abnormality is identified and sperm penetrate the mucus in a normal fashion,

adequate access to the ovum can be predicted. Subsequently, the sperm penetration assay (SPA) may provide valuable information regarding sperm capacitation. This test quantitates the capacity of human sperm to penetrate zona-free hamster eggs and has evolved as an important predictor of sperm function. We have modified and optimized the SPA so that more ova are penetrated and polyspermia is expected. The results are reported as the sperm capacitation index (SCI), which represents the number of penetrations per ovum (19). We believe that this is now a more reliable test of sperm function. Patients with a normal SCI have a significantly higher potential for eventual fertility than patients with an abnormal SCI. Another test of sperm function, the hemizona assay, is performed on *human* ova and may also evolve as a new, important test (20). The ova used have an intact zona pellucida and, therefore, assess a component of sperm function that is not seen in the SCI, that is, binding of sperm to specific sites on the ovum.

Azoospermia

It is essential to confirm a diagnosis of azoospermia by centrifuging the semen specimen to rule out severe oligospermia and also to check a postejaculate urinalysis to rule out retrograde ejaculation. As mentioned above, a marked elevation of the FSH (more than three times normal) implies extensive germ cell failure and suggests a poor prognosis. If the FSH is lower than normal, then testosterone, LH, and prolactin levels should be determined to establish a possible pituitary or hypothalamic cause of hypogonadism. Once azoospermia has been confirmed, repeating the scrotal examination to confirm the presence of both vas deferens is important because this lesion is found in up to 10% of azoospermic patients (21). Most commonly, with absence of the vas, the head of the epididymis is intact. Microscopic epididymal sperm aspiration (MESA) in conjunction with in vitro

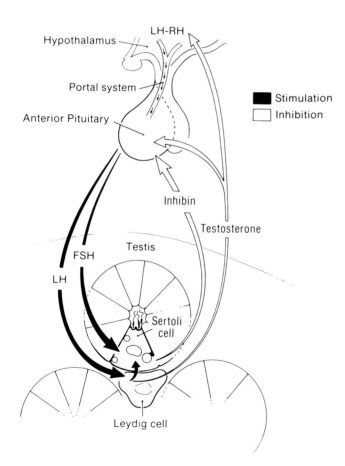

Fig. 2.2 Hypothalamic-pituitary-gonadal axis.

fertilization has been successful in achieving a pregnancy rate of up to 33% in some recent series (22,23). Those patients who have a normal hormone profile and a low semen volume undergo a transrectal ultrasound for further evaluation of possible obstruction of the ejaculatory ducts or seminal vesicles. In addition to aplasia of these structures, we have recently reported obstruction due to ejaculatory duct stenosis, stones, and impingement from prostatic cysts (Fig. 2.3) (24,25). In the past, seminal fructose has been used to assess low-volume ejaculate in an attempt to establish a seminal vesicle obstruction since it is a unique product of these glands. However, we have not found it to be a reliable marker especially when compared with transrectal ultrasound, which gives excellent anatomic detail of both the ejaculatory ducts and the seminal vesicles (26).

All azoospermic patients having normal or modest elevation of FSH and no evidence of ejaculatory duct or seminal vesicle abnormality are candidates for testicular biopsy and possibly for vasography. At the time of surgery a "touch preparation" of the biopsy is performed on a sterile slide prior to placing a specimen in Bouin's fixative. This "touch prep" is examined immediately after fixation and use of a routine hematoxylin and eosin stain for the presence of mature sperm. If mature sperm are observed, ductal obstruction is confirmed, and the epididymis and vas are meticulously examined. A vasogram can then be performed to delineate an

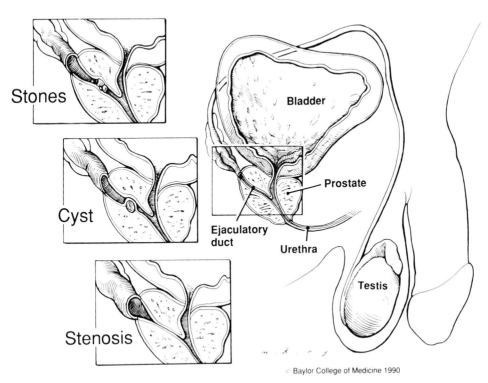

Stones

Cyst

Stenosis

Bladder

Prostate

Ejaculatory duct

Urethra

Testis

© Baylor College of Medicine 1990

Fig. 2.3   Obstructing lesions of the ejaculatory ducts.

upstream (abdominal) obstruction. Currently, vasography is used only if we are unable to irrigate the vas freely with methylene blue and recover it in the urine after a bladder catheterization. The absence of obstruction on the basis of easy irrigation obviates the need to subject the patient to radiography.

Obstruction near the testicular end of the vas or obstruction of the epididymis can be bypassed with either a microscopic vasovasotomy or vasoepididymostomy. Blockages at the level of the ejaculatory ducts can often be successfully treated with transurethral resection. If the "touch prep" fails to show sperm and the biopsy specimen shows a severe abnormality, such as germ cell aplasia (Sertoli only syndrome) or advanced peritubular fibrosis in association with maturation arrest, alternative means of pregnancy attainment should be considered, and the couple should be appropriately counseled.

Abnormal semen parameters

Nearly 55% of infertile patients will demonstrate a diffuse pattern of impaired bulk semen parameters (Table 2.3) (27). If the FSH is abnormally low, then the

Table 2.3 Distribution of semen abnormalities in 200 patients (%)

Azoospermia	8
Predominance of single abnormal parameter	37
Motility	26
Agglutination	2
Asthenospermia	24
Volume	2
Morphology	1
Oligospermia	8
All parameters normal	55

Reproduced with permission from Lipshultz LI. Subfertility. In: Kaufman JJ, ed. Current urologic therapy. Philadelphia: WB Saunders, 1980.

evaluation proceeds as in patients with azoospermia, to rule out a pituitary or hypothalamic cause. When the FSH is normal or elevated, a search for exposure to drugs, heat, stress or environmental toxins should be made, and these should be eliminated. The most common cause of diffusely impaired semen analysis is a varicocele (see below).

Isolated abnormal seminal parameters occur in 37% of all infertility patients. These include either high or low seminal volumes, hyperviscosity, impaired motility, and low sperm density. The most common isolated defects are aberrations in motility (26%), and the least common are aberrations in morphology (1%).

The initial step in evaluation of the semen is to measure the volume. When semen volume exceeds 5.5 ml, a split ejaculate or mechanical concentration followed by artificial insemination with the husband's semen can be considered. The benefit of a split ejaculate lies in the fact that the first few milliliters of semen contain sperm in the greatest density and of the highest quality. If the ejaculate volume is less than 1.0 ml, a collection error or retrograde ejaculation must be ruled out with a postejaculatory urinalysis. Normally, fewer than 10 to 15 sperm per high-power field will be present in a centrifuged urine specimen following ejaculation. Obstruction of the ejaculatory ducts and the seminal vesicles can also cause a low-volume ejaculate (Fig. 2.4). If this is noted in combination with severe oligoasthenospermia, a transrectal ultrasound should be performed to rule out the possibility of obstruction.

Human semen, after adequate liquefaction, is sufficiently fluid to be poured drop-by-drop. The inability to do so defines "increased viscosity." Increased seminal viscosity itself may not be pathologic; however, if it is observed in association with an abnormal postcoital test or cross mucus test, then treatment may be indicated. Precoital saline douches have been advocated to decrease cervical mucus viscosity and improve sperm-mucus penetration (28,29). In addition, aspirating and then ejecting the specimen through progressively smaller needles and syringes may be effective in initially breaking down the viscosity prior to insemination.

Asthenospermia, defined as a decrease in motility to less than 50% to 60%, can be due to many factors. Specimens must be examined when fresh (i.e., less than 2 hours from collection) and must be protected from extremes of temperature during transport. If antibodies are detected and found to be attached to more than 20% of the sperm on the basis of the direct immunobead agglutination assay, a brief course of corticosteroids can be useful. Several investigators have attempted sperm washing to remove the adherent antibodies, but this has not been successful (30). Failing a course of steroids, there is promise that in the future in vitro fertilization in combination with gamete micromanipulation may offer

a significant benefit to these patients (J. Stockton and L. I. Lipshultz, personal communication). This technology employs specially constructed micropipettes to cut or puncture the zona pellucida of the ovum. This allows intimate contact between the sperm and the oolemma and optimizes fertilization. If the sperm with attached antibodies are inherently normal sperm, then theoretically this should be an effective treatment as it obviates the motility problem.

In addition to antisperm antibodies, significant pyospermia may also affect sperm motility. Counts of more than 1.0 million white cells per cubic centimeter of seminal fluid are considered significant; the urethras of patients with such high counts are routinely cultured for *Mycoplasma* and *Chlamydia*. In addition, aerobic cultures of the semen are performed. Infection is an infrequent but easily treatable cause of decreased sperm motility. Once antisperm antibodies, infection, and hormonal causes have been ruled out, the remaining treatable cause of poor motility is partial obstruction of the ductal system. This can be at the level of the epididymis, vas deferens, or ejaculatory duct. Presumably, these obstructions may be partial and, hence, delay sperm passage and result in a large number of dead sperm in the ejaculate. Obstructive lesions of this nature usually produce a severe motility problem (less than 20% motile sperm) and generally require both a transrectal ultrasound to demonstrate more proximal obstructions and a scrotal exploration to demonstrate those in the epididymis or distal vas. Partial obstruction is a difficult diagnosis and should be treated only unilaterally because of the risk of causing total azoospermia if the operative procedure is not successful. When there is no demonstrable cause of asthenospermia, empiric sperm washing with or without a Percoll gradient in conjunction with in vitro fertilization or intrauterine inseminations may benefit a limited number of patients (31,32).

Polyzoospermia is defined as abnormally high

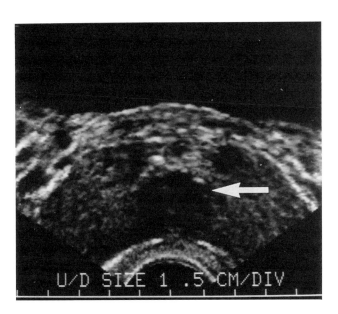

Fig. 2.4   Transrectal ultrasound of ejaculatory duct obstruction.

sperm density, greater than 250 million per cubic centimeter. It is not clear at this time that this is a "pathologic condition," but when associated with poor motility, it has been successfully treated with sperm dilution and intrauterine insemination (33).

Diminished sperm density or oligospermia that is idiopathic remains a perplexing problem. Once the various possible causes of testicular dysfunction and the presence of a varicocele have been ruled out, repeating semen analyses with longer abstinence may be worthwhile. Sperm count may improve in some oligospermic men; and if ovulation is accurately monitored, then insemination with the maximum number of sperm at precisely the time of ovulation may increase the chance of conception. In addition, as techniques of cryopreservation continue to improve, it may be feasible in the future to combine serial ejaculates to improve sperm density. It must be appreciated, however, that patients with abnormalities of sperm density and motility often have inherent sperm dysfunction, as has been demonstrated by comparing fertilization rates in vitro between normal men and those with oligospermia or oligoasthenospermia. Mechanical concentration by intrauterine insemination can benefit certain patients if the sperm motility is adequate or improves after processing (usually more than 5 million motile sperm), if the sperm tolerate the washing procedure, and if the SCI is normal. More often, decreased sperm density is part of a global picture of sperm dysfunction that also affects motility. The use of a silicone emulsion such as Percoll for sperm washing may improve the percentage of total motile sperm in specific cases. Failure of intrauterine insemination in idiopathic oligospermia (following three to six cycles of ovarian hyperstimulation) generally warrants a trial of in vitro fertilization. A course of empiric medical therapy (see below, nonspecific medical treatment) is often given prior to initiation of in vitro techniques, which have achieved limited success in these circumstances (34,35).

Surgical treatment

Varicocele

As mentioned above, a testicular varicocele is the most common surgically correctable cause of male infertility (see Table 2.4). It is also, fortunately, one of the most easily treated.

While varicoceles are found in approximately 20% of the normal male population, their incidence is at least doubled in infertility patients. Several theories have been proposed to explain the deleterious effects of these scrotal varicosities. These include reflux of adrenal metabolites down the left gonadal vein, venous sludging, and consequent hypoxia; however, overheating as a result of the venous "insulation" is generally the

Table 2.4 Distribution of final diagnostic categories found in male fertility clinic

Diagnosis	No.	%
Varicocele	159	37.4
Idiopathic	108	25.4
Testicular failure	40	9.4
Obstruction	26	6.1
Cryptorchidism	26	6.1
Volume	20	4.7
Agglutination	13	3.1
Sexual dysfunction	12	2.8
Viscosity	8	1.9
Ejaculatory failure	5	1.2
Endocrine	4	0.9
High density	2	0.5
Necrospermia	2	0.5
Total	425	100.0

Reproduced with permission from Greenberg SH, Lipshultz LI, Wein A. Experience with 425 subfertile male patients. J Urol 1978;119:507.

most accepted theory (36,37). While increased temperature appears to have a direct effect on spermatogenesis, experimental data have suggested that the varicocele may act as a cofactor leaving the testicle more susceptible to injury by gonadotoxins. Animal data have shown a gonadotoxic effect of both cyclophosphamide and nicotine that is increased in the presence of a varicocele. In clinical studies, patients exposed to certain pesticides had an increase in abnormal semen parameters if a varicocele was present (38,39).

It has long been accepted that the cooler temperature of the scrotal pouch is essential for optimum spermatogenesis. The normal scrotal temperature is 35°C, an average of approximately 2° cooler than body temperature. A varicocele has been demonstrated to decrease this temperature differential by approximately 0.8°C (40). This temperature aberration appears to result in abnormal spermatogenesis in the contralateral as well as the ipsilateral testis. Varicoceles typically produce a "stress pattern" in the semen analysis. The stress pattern is characterized by an increase in the number of immature sperm forms to more than 3% to 4% of the total. In addition to the increased number of immature forms, sperm motility is often affected by the varicocele; later in the pathogenic process, sperm production itself is often decreased.

The etiology of varicoceles is unknown but is probably related to the hydrostatic pressure developed by the valveless venous column in the panpiniform plexus when in the upright position. The venous column extends from the level of the renal vein on the left side to the gonad via the inguinal canal. On the right side the column is 8 to 10 cm shorter than on the left, since the right gonadal canal vein empties directly into the vena cava. The difference in length may account for the lower incidence of right-sided varicoceles.

Surgical repair is indicated for patients with decreased sperm density or motility after all other treatable causes of impaired testicular function have been ruled out. In addition, those patients with normal bulk parameters and a varicocele who have failed in vitro fertilization may benefit from a varicocele ligation (41,42). Varicoceles result from retrograde flow—that is, renotesticular or cavotesticular flow—and therefore can be decompressed by simple ligation of the affected veins. This can be performed by using a high scrotal, inguinal, or retroperitoneal approach. The scrotal approach is frequently more difficult, as a plethora of veins may exist at this level, and is mentioned only for historical purpose. The retroperitoneal approach may result in increased patient morbidity since this procedure requires mobilization of the peritoneum medially away from the gonadal vessels. Our preference is to use an inguinal approach (see Fig. 2.5). Optical loupes (3.5 ×) are used to ensure that during ligation of the two to

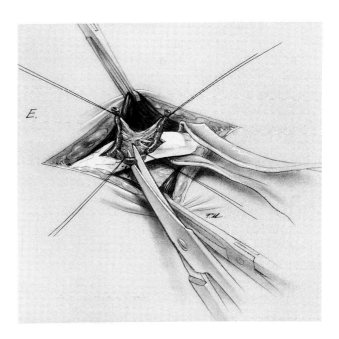

Fig. 2.5   Inguinal approach for ligation of varicoceles.

three branches normally seen at this level, there is no injury to the lymphatics, testicular artery, or the vas deferens. Magnification is essential in minimizing damage to the vascular or lymphatic supply that might lead to gonad atrophy or hydrocele, respectively.

Reports of postoperative improvement have varied widely between series. However, the larger series have demonstrated improvement in seminal parameters in 66% of patients with an overall fertility rate of 43%. This compares favorably with the 20% of "infertility patients" who will conceive spontaneously after similar follow-up (43).

Sterilization reversal

Obstructions to the normal passage of sperm can be congenital or acquired. Even though the former are being diagnosed with increased frequency, their numbers are dwarfed by the number of obstructions resulting from previous vasectomy. Vasectomies are performed in approximately 500,000 patients each year in the United States. The vasectomy procedure itself presents few complications and is usually performed with a local anesthetic as an outpatient procedure. For most couples it is seen as a more innocuous procedure than tubal ligation, and for this reason it has gained widespread popularity as a means of permanent contraception. The major indication for reversal of vasectomy is remarriage; however, a small number of couples have reconsidered their original decisions for reasons such as the death of a child. While there are no known systemic effects of vasectomy, biopsy studies have demonstrated that there are histologic effects in the testis of some men following vasectomy, and these may affect the "reversibility of the procedure" (44).

Vasectomy reversal can be performed by a variety of techniques; however, it seems that superior results are achieved with either a one-layer or a two-layer microsurgical reanastomosis (see Fig. 2.6). In experienced hands, these techniques result in patency rates in excess of 90%. The percentage of patients demonstrating sperm in the ejaculate and eventual pregnancy decreases with the duration of time between the original vasectomy and reversal. In a large multicenter study reviewing 1247 vasovasostomies, the patency and pregnancy rates for a vasectomy of less than 3 years' duration were 97% and 76%, respectively. For periods of 9 to 14 years' duration, the rates were 79% and 44%, and for longer than 15 years, 71% patency and 30% pregnancy. The median time to conception was 12.1 months from the time of reversal (45). The fall in pregnancy rates with the length of time from vasectomy is primarily the result of an epididymal "blowout" which is thought to be a result of back pressure distending and rupturing the delicate tubules of the epididymis. These "blowouts" heal as obstructing scars and block the epididymis, thus making a routine vasovasostomy ineffective. Clinical suspicion of epididymal obstruction based on the length of time from vasectomy and examination of the epididymis demonstrating gross engorgement is important. However,

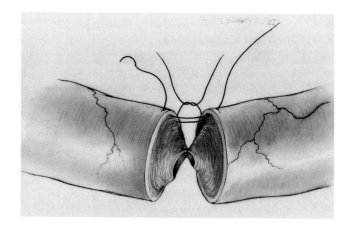

Fig. 2.6   Microscopic two-layer vasovasostomy.

only at the time of dividing the vas and aspirating the seminal fluid can one be certain that azoospermia exists and that an epididymovasostomy will be required (see Fig. 2.7). An epididymovasal microsurgical anastomosis is technically more difficult than a vasovasostomy. This difficulty and the incomplete functional maturation of sperm present in the epididymis result in decreased pregnancy rates of approximately 30% when

epididymal vasostomy is performed even by experienced microsurgeons (46,47).

Patients who fail to conceive after vasectomy reversal may have a technical failure, although this is believed to be less common than postsurgical stenosis of the vas lumen. These patients with stenosis may benefit from a surgical revision, although generally it should be postponed from 6 months to one year after the original surgery. This ensures that scar organization is complete and that any neovascularization of the surgical site has been established. Another cause of failure after vasovasostomy is development of germ cell dysfunction as a result of vasectomy, as has been suggested by biopsy studies (44). Antisperm antibodies are found in more than 50% of patients after vasovasostomy and, if sperm motility is low, should be quantitated by the direct immunobead technique. Recent studies have suggested that IgG antisperm antibodies may have less detrimental effect than IgA antibodies on eventual pregnancy. Meinertz et al. have shown that after vasovasostomy the presence of antisperm antibodies of pure IgG, IgG and IgA combined, and IgA alone have associated pregnancy rates of 85.7%, 42.9%, and 21.7%, respectively (48). A certain population of men known to be fertile prior to vasectomy will have developed a progressive testicular injury from an associated varicocele during the years since their original surgery. These patients may benefit from a concurrent varicocele ligation.

Alloplastic spermatocele

While vasovasostomy and vasoepididymovasostomy can be effective in circumventing some short obstructions of the vas or epididymis, these procedures are primarily indicated after vasectomy. Those patients with congenital absence of the vas deferens or long or more proximal obstructions are not candidates for such surgery. It is estimated that 10% to 15% of infertile

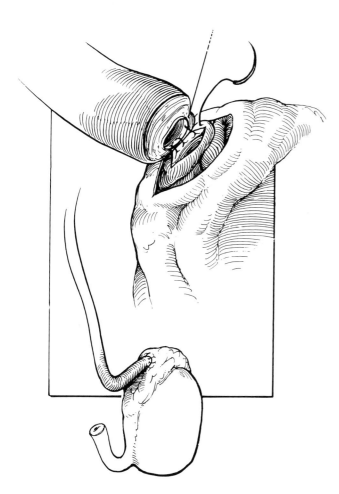

Fig. 2.7   Microscopic epididymovasostomy.

men with azoospermia have some form of obstruction of the efferent ducts and that congenital absence accounts for many of these. Because most with obstructive azoospermia have normal testicular function, much effort has been directed toward extracting sperm as they traverse the epididymis by creating a spermatocele.

The first attempts at creating an artificial spermatocele from which to aspirate sperm involved techniques using saphenous vein grafts (49). Although occasional pregnancies did result, other investigators could not reproduce this work. Artificial spermatoceles using tunica vaginalis have also been used effectively for sperm retrieval (50). Newer work has used alloplastic materials employing woven polypropylene and polytetrafluoroethylene vascular graft material (51,52). The most recent extensive review of world literature regarding a variety of alloplastic spermatoceles records seven pregnancies, four resulting in term infants, connected with the use of 130 spermatoceles (53). While the majority of implants did produce sperm initially, the motility was generally very poor, and the device was occluded within a few months after insertion. Work with spermatoceles continues and may have important implications for use of these devices in conjunction with in vitro fertilization because of the low number of motile sperm recovered. One pregnancy has been reported using this approach 3 months after implantation of an alloplastic spermatocele (54). In the meantime various investigators have used microscopic epididymal sperm aspiration (MESA) as a means of collecting sperm from an incised epididymal tubule to be used in concert with in vitro techniques of fertilization. Several pregnancies have been reported (22,23). At present, this approach is the most reasonable option for patients with congenital absence of the vas deferens or ductal obstruction that cannot be surgically corrected.

Electro/vibratory stimulation of ejaculation

While not a surgical procedure, this technology, which was pioneered in animal husbandry, has been an effective means of treating ejaculatory failure. The majority of patients treated have had spinal cord injuries; however, other patients with surgical damage to sympathetic fibers, neuropathy, or even psychogenic ejaculatory failure have been treated successfully.

Electrical stimulation delivered by a rectal probe is effective in obtaining sperm in either an antegrade or a retrograde fashion in more than 80% of patients (Fig. 2.8). Vibratory stimulation of the glans penis is less effective but warrants a trial prior to electrical stimulation because of its safety and ease of use. Although these methods are effective in inducing ejaculation and obtaining sperm, pregnancy rates have remained low, perhaps because so many of the patients have spinal cord injury and inherently poor semen quality. Many factors may be involved; among them are recurrent urinary tract infections, gonadal overheating associated with time

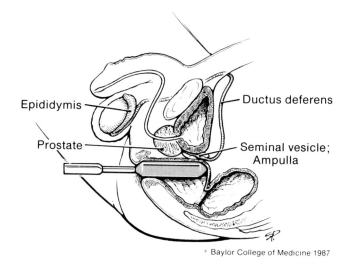

Epididymis

Prostate

Ductus deferens

Seminal vesicle;
Ampulla

© Baylor College of Medicine 1987

Fig. 2.8   Schematic of electroejaculation probe in position.

spent in the sitting position in the wheelchair, and the loss of thermoregulation from denervation, as well as previous surgery in the region of the ejaculatory ducts such as sphincterotomy (55). To date, more than 50 pregnancies have resulted from artificially induced ejaculation.

Specific medical treatment

Several conditions that result in male infertility can be effectively treated with medical therapy. Those that have been recognized to benefit from specific medical treatment include severe hypothyroidism, isolated testosterone deficiency, hypogonadotrophic hypogonadism (Kallmann's syndrome), congenital adrenal hyperplasia, hyperprolactinemia, asthenospermia in association with antisperm antibodies, retrograde ejaculation, and genital tract infection or colonization.

Hypothyroidism can cause infertility. It is generally accepted that only the more severe forms of this condition will affect fertility potential. Since these cases should be clinically evident, general screening for hypothyroidism is not warranted. Thyroxin replacement has been shown to restore fertility in many of these patients with documented thyroid deficiency (56).

Hypogonadism can result from an isolated testosterone deficiency, from an insufficiency of both testosterone and gonadotropins (Kallmann's syndrome), or more rarely from an isolated gonadotropin deficiency (i.e., LH or FSH). If low testosterone alone exists, intramuscular testosterone enanthate (200 mg biweekly) will restore testosterone levels and improve libido. However, the potential for improving spermatogenesis is poor because Leydig cell failure is rarely seen without significant dysfunction of germ cells. Oral androgens are erratically absorbed and should not be used for replacement therapy (57). If the cause of hypogonadism is pituitary or hypothalamic dysfunction, combinations of human chorionic gonadotropin (hCG), which has LH-like activity and human menopausal gonadotropin (hMG), which mimics FSH, at doses of 1500 IU three times weekly and 75 IU three times weekly, respectively, have been effective in initiating spermatogenesis in 30% to 50% of these men (58,59). Another, more complex treatment employs gonadotropin-releasing hormone itself (Facteryl). This approach has also produced sperm in more than 60% of patients with gonadotropin deficiency (60,61).

Bromocriptine, a dopaminergic antagonist, has been used effectively to lower prolactin levels in oligospermatic men with hyperprolactinemia. This has resulted in improved sperm counts and pregnancy in previously infertile couples. Prior to medical treatment, however, these patients must be screened for medications producing hyperprolactinemia (phenothiazines, dopaminergic gastrointestinal motility agents, e.g., Motilium) and have a magnetic resonance imaging scan of the sella tursica to rule out a prolactin secreting tumor that may require neurosurgical treatment.

The presence of antisperm antibodies in the seminal plasma can significantly affect sperm motility. This problem is especially apparent in the vasovasostomy patients, more than half of whom will have significant antisperm antibodies. Presumably, these antibodies are the result of long-term vasal obstruction or perisurgical spillage of sperm outside the blood-testis barrier and the epithelialized genitourinary tract and exposure to the host immune system. Testicular trauma, torsion, tumor, genital tract infection, and ductal obstruction have all been associated with the presence of significant antisperm antibodies (62). Antisperm antibodies are also seen in approximately 10% of the infertile population as a whole (63). Previous studies have demonstrated that this is a significant increase over the normally fertile population. Many approaches, such as temporary suppression of spermatogenesis and sperm washing, have been attempted and found to be ineffective. At present, steroids in high dose appear to be the most effective treatment, leading to pregnancy rates of 15% to 44% (62,64,65). However, not all investigators have shown improvement in pregnancy rates of subjects after steroid treatment for antisperm antibodies, and any benefit must be weighed against the possibility of disastrous complications such as aseptic necrosis of the hip, a possible result of high-dose steroid treatment (66). Both in vitro fertilization and intrauterine insemination have been used to bypass the cervical mucus and decrease the distance traveled by the sperm, but pregnancy rates have been approximately 15% (67). New techniques of micromanipulation of sperm in conjunction with in vitro fertilization may be a promising means of future treatment in patients with antisperm antibodies, since they circumvent the problem of ineffective sperm-egg fusion (associated with inadequate motility) that appears to be the primary abnormality preventing conception in these men.

Retrograde ejaculation is a result of failure of closure of the bladder neck at the time of ejaculation and is under the influence of α-sympathomimetic innervation. Problems with retrograde ejaculation are most often seen after surgery (such as retroperitoneal lymph node dissection) that affects these sympathetic fibers but can result from a neuropathy (e.g., diabetes), surgery in the region of the bladder neck (e.g., Y-V plasty), or spinal cord injuries (68–71). Alpha agonists such as phenylephrine and pseudoephedrine have been used successfully to achieve adequate sperm retrieval in 30% to 40% of these patients (72). Sudafed is the most common agent used in a usual dose of 60 mg four times daily; this medication should be continued for 2 weeks before assessing its effect. Those patients most likely to respond appear to be diabetic patients and those who have had retroperitoneal lymph node dissection. Many of these patients may have an associated failure of emission (passage of semen from the ejaculatory duct to the posterior urethra), and these patients may benefit from electroejaculation in combination with drug therapy. In addition, a variety of drugs used to treat psychosis, depression, and hypertension can also disturb ejaculation; these should be eliminated if possible (see Table 2.5).

Several studies have suggested a deleterious effect of urinary tract infection on sperm function. *Escherichia coli* has been shown to impair semen quality by causing clumping and agglutination. Studies that have demonstrated this effect, however, use a bacterial concentration of 10^8 to 10^{13} colonies per milliliter and may not be relevant to the much lower counts that are seen in the clinical setting (73,74). Bacterial prostatitis has been associated with changes in semen plasma quality. These changes include an increased pH with lowered concen-

Table 2.5 Commonly used medications associated with disturbances of the ejaculatory process

Antipsychotics
Chlorpromazine
Perphenazine
Thioridazine
Trifluoperazine hydrochloride

Antidepressants
Amitriptyline
Imipramine hydrochloride
Phenelzine sulfate

Antihypertensives
Guanethidine sulfate
Phenoxybenzamine hydrochloride
Prazosin hydrochloride
Thiazides

Reproduced with permission from Murphy JB, Lipshultz LI. Abnormalities of ejaculation. Urol Clin North Am 1987;14:583.

trations of zinc, citric acid, and fructose (75). Poor quality semen has been reported in conjunction with lowered seminal zinc concentrations. However, this may not be a cause-and-effect relationship since other studies in men with chronic prostatitis and low zinc levels have shown no abnormalities in semen quality (76,77). In general, gram-negative bacterial infections of the urinary tract in men are symptomatic and therefore are treated. As a result, considerable work has focused on those infections that are asymptomatic.

Both *Chlamydia trachomatis* and *Ureaplasma urealyticum* (or *T-mycoplasma*) are unique organisms in that they are bacteria but do not possess a cell wall. The incidence of both these infections is directly related to the number of one's previous sexual partners (78). Both *Chlamydia* and *Mycoplasma* can cause a mild to moderate urethritis, but between 10% and 25% of infected men are asymptomatic. Screening for asymptomatic *Chlamydia* or *Mycoplasma* infections in infertile men has not been rewarding. Reports relating the effect of colonization and fertility are contradictory (79,80). However, in a large study involving 268 infertile patients, Fowlkes and coworkers were able to show that those with positive *Mycoplasma* cultures had poorer semen counts and impaired motility as well as lower ejaculate volumes than those who were culture-negative (81). Swenson et al. demonstrated improved motility after successful doxycycline treatment in a culture-positive group compared to those with persistent infection with *Mycoplasma* (82). Some investigators have suggested empiric treatment instead of difficult and costly cultures. We limit urethral culturing to those with elevated white blood cells in the semen (more than 1.0×10^6). In addition, all patients who are entering an in vitro fertilization program have routine *Chlamydia, Mycoplasma,* and semen cultures performed, since contamination of the oocytes will ruin the procedure.

Nonspecific medical treatment of idiopathic oligospermia

It should be remembered that patients with idiopathic infertility constitute approximately 25% of the infertile male population (6). These patients often feel themselves to be in a desperate and vulnerable situation. Virtually all of the specific treatments mentioned above as well as a myriad of other drugs have been used with little scientific justification to "treat" these men. Corticosteroids, zinc, bromocriptine, and vitamins E and C are ineffective, and their use is irrational (83,84). Treatments that we will discuss are indicated only when there is no reversible cause of suboptimal semen quality and after a full evaluation of the female partner has been completed.

Antiestrogens

Several antiestrogens, especially clomiphene citrate and tamoxifen, have been used to treat idiopathic oligospermia. Their use is based on the dependence of spermatogenesis on stimulation of the Sertoli cell by FSH in concert with high intratesticular levels of testosterone. These tissue testosterone levels are 20 times higher than peripheral serum levels, and a deficiency at the site of spermatogenesis may not be recognized on the basis of the peripheral testosterone levels (85). In addition, the biologic activity of FSH may not always be accurately measured using traditional radioimmunoassay (86). For this reason, it is theorized that increasing the intratesticular testosterone levels or the serum FSH may benefit sperm production.

Normal regulation of FSH and LH is largely controlled by negative feedback of circulating androgens. This regulation occurs at the level of the pituitary and hypothalamus, and evidence suggests that the androgen effect occurs after aromatization to estrogens (87). Antiestrogens can block this feedback and decrease the inhibitory effects of androgens. This action will increase the release of both FSH and LH. It is postulated that this can lead to increased spermatogenesis caused by the stimulatory effect of FSH on the Sertoli cell and also to the effect of LH increasing intratesticular testosterone levels.

Clomiphene citrate is an estrogen analogue that acts as a competitive inhibitor of estrogen at the pituitary-hypothalamic level. Initial animal studies demonstrated a gonadotropin-inhibiting effect, and, as expected, early human use for male infertility was disappointing. Doses and patient selection have varied widely in clinical studies, making interpretation of data difficult. Doses of 25 to 50 mg a day of clomiphene citrate are effective in increasing FSH, LH, and testosterone levels, and monthly assessment of these hormone levels is essential for proper dose regulation. Failure of elevation of FSH will require an increased clomiphene dose, whereas an elevation of serum testosterone consistently above the normal range will override the effect of clomiphene at the pituitary-hypothalamic level and as a result decrease the sperm production. Patients most likely to respond to clomiphene are those with no prior elevation of FSH in association with their oligospermia (88).

Numerous studies of clomiphene treatment with conflicting results have been reported; however, many have demonstrated an improvement in semen parameters or fertility. Studies by Wang et al. and by Paulson using doses of 25 mg of clomiphene citrate per day achieved pregnancy rates of 36% and 35%, respectively, with the latter study showing seminal improvement in 70% (89,90). However, using the same dose, Sokol et al. achieved a pregnancy rate of only 9%, which was lower than that for the placebo treatment group (91). Clomiphene is an estrogen analogue and does possess some intrinsic estrogenic properties. Side effects are very uncommon but can include visual problems, hypertension, and fluid retention.

Overall, the use of clomiphene appears to benefit only a small subset of men with idiopathic oligospermia. One of the major drawbacks to a "trial" of clomiphene is its cost, especially since the usual dose is taken daily for a 6-month period. Despite reservations concerning efficacy, clomiphene remains the primary drug used to treat idiopathic oligospermia. Its use should be limited to those patients with normal FSH, as suggested by Wang et al. (89).

Tamoxifen, also an antiestrogen, but with lower estrogenic activity than clomiphene citrate, has also been used to treat oligospermia. The usual dose is 10 to 20 mg per day. While sporadic reports have shown improved sperm density, no controlled studies have shown an improvement in pregnancy rates (92,93).

Gonadotropins and gonadotropin-releasing hormone

As mentioned, the treatment of hypogonadotropic hypogonadism with gonadotropins has been very effective in treating infertility. The benefit of these same drugs, however, in treating patients with an apparently normal pituitary-gonadal axis is not established. Those preparations that mimic gonadotropins include human chorionic gonadotropin, which stimulates Leydig cell secretion of both testosterone and estradiol and lowers FSH by an inhibitory feedback mechanism. Human menopausal gonadotropin has both LH- and FSH-like activity. These drugs have been used in combination and individually in the treatment of oligospermia. The use of hCG and hMG alone has generally been disappointing, with the most optimistic studies quoting pregnancy rates of 30% (94). The majority of studies, however, demonstrate overall pregnancy rates of less than 17% (95–97). Likewise, combination therapy using both hCG and hMG has not shown benefit over placebo (98). The difficulty in the frequent parenteral administration adds further pessimism to the disappointing clinical results.

Gonadotropin-releasing hormone (GnRH, or LH-RH), which can augment or inhibit gonadotropin release depending on the dose and frequency, has gained popularity in the treatment of prostate cancer, endometriosis, and ovarian stimulation. A single controlled study using this modality for treatment of idiopathic oligospermia by Badenoch et al. did not demonstrate any benefit of treatment (99), and the most optimistic study had a pregnancy rate of only 24% (100). These drugs are extremely expensive and await further controlled clinical trials before being recommended for clinical use.

Androgens

As mentioned above, androgens have an inhibitory feedback on gonadotropin release and would be expected to worsen spermatogenesis in eugonadotropic men. This has been confirmed when the abuse of anabolic (and androgenic) steroids by athletes has resulted in oligospermia or azoospermia (12). Therefore, the therapeutic use of androgens to treat infertility has included only low-dose treatment. Mesterolone in doses of 25 mg per day has not resulted in more pregnancies than placebo treatment (101). Oral androgens are notorious for variable absorption and can have significant hepatic toxicity. To date, no convincing data support the use of androgens in the treatment of idiopathic oligospermia, and in light of adverse effects, these compounds are not recommended.

Other treatments

Several new and promising treatments have evolved along lines independent of hormonal treatment. These therapies attempt to affect metabolic function of the spermatozoa. The kinin family of polypeptides have a wide range of function in the body as mediators of inflammation and coagulation. Kinins also appear to have a role in sperm motility (102,103). Kinins are formed by kallikrein, an enzyme that can be orally administered. The only published double-blind study, by Schill, suggests an improvement in semen parameters and a pregnancy rate of 38% compared to 16% in the placebo group (104). Other uncontrolled studies have been less promising (105,106). However, this drug is well tolerated and may prove to be clinically useful. Another group of peptides, the prostaglandins, are well known for their ubiquitous nature, and elevated levels have been shown in vitro to have inhibitory effects on sperm motility (107). It has been theorized, therefore, that drugs that lower prostaglandin semen concentration, such as a nonsteroidal antiinflammatory group of cyclooxygenase inhibitors, may improve sperm function. Using indomethacin, 150 mg per day, Barkay et al. demonstrated a lowering of semen prostaglandin levels. Using a lower dose of 75 mg per day in a controlled study, they reported a pregnancy rate of 35% compared to 8% for a matched placebo control group (108). Because of the low toxicity of this drug in a population of predominantly healthy young men, a trial of indomethacin is frequently offered to patients with unexplained motility disorders.

Conclusion

The investigation of infertile men is largely an exercise of exclusion. Approximately 75% of those investigated will have an identifiable cause of male infertility while in the other 25% it remains idiopathic. In evaluation of such patients, it is essential that the physician be astute and thorough. The omission of any strategic step of investigation may cause the oversight of potentially effective treatment. The initial evaluation has been streamlined and can be completed at a reasonable cost within 10 days of the initial office visit.

When treatment is recommended, the patient must be clearly informed of risks as well as possible benefits. The medical or surgical treatments that may be recommended are entirely elective; therefore, any potential complications or failures must be understood. Each couple will establish the emotional and financial cost that they are willing to bear. The physician must then attempt to balance this with the realistic chances of attaining pregnancy for each treatment offered. A close relationship between reproductive urologists and gynecologists is essential in optimizing the decision making and in maximizing care of the patient.

References

1. Tietze C, Guttmacher AF, Rubin S. Time required for conception in 1727 planned pregnancies. Fertil Steril 1950;1:338.

2. Lipshultz LI, Caminos-Torres R, Greenspan CS, et al. Testicular function after orchiopexy for unilateral undescended testes. N Engl J Med 1976;295:15.

3. Bartsch G, Frank S, Marberger H, et al. Testicular torsion: late results with special regard to fertility and endocrine function. J Urol 1980;114:375.

4. Werner CA. Mumps orchitis and testicular atrophy. Ann Intern Med 1950;32:1066.

5. Oshsner MG, Burns E, Henry HH. Incidence of retrograde ejaculation following bladder neck revision as a child. J Urol 1970;104:596.

6. Lipshultz LI, Ross CE, Whorton D, et al. Dibromo-chloropropane and its effect of testicular function in man. J Urol 1980;124:464.

7. Levi AJ, Fisher AN, Hughes L, et al. Male infertility due to sulphasalazine. Lancet 1979;2:276.

8. Van Thiel DH, Gavalet JS, Smith WI, et al. Hypothalamic-pituitary-gonadal dysfunction in men using cimetidine. N Engl J Med 1979;300:1012.

9. Neuman F. Effects of drugs and chemicals on spermatogenesis. Arch Toxicol 1984;7(Suppl):109.

10. Ehrenfeld M, Levy M, Margllioth EJ, et al. The effects of long-term colchicine therapy on male infertility in patients with familial Mediterranean fever. Andrologia 1986;18:420.

11. Kolodny RC, Masters WH, Kolodny RM, et al. Repression of plasma testosterone levels after chronic intensive marijuana use. N Engl J Med 1974;290:872.

12. Jarrow JP, Lipshultz LI. Anabolic steroid induced hypogonadotropic gonadism. Am J Sports Med 1990;18(4):429–431.

13. Braken RB, Smith KD. Is semen cryopreservation helpful in testicular cancer? Urology 1980;15:587.

14. Sherins RJ, Brightwell D, Sternthal PM. Longitudinal analysis of semen of fertile and infertile man. In: Troen P, Nanakin H, eds. New concepts of the testis in normal and infertile men. New York: Raven Press, 1977:437.

15. Greenburg SH, Lipshultz LI, Wein AJ. Experience with 425 subfertile male patients. J Urol 1978;119:507.

16. World Health Organization. WHO Laboratory manual for the examination of human semen and semen–cervical mucus interaction, 2nd ed. Cambridge: The Press Syndicate of the University of Cambridge, 1987:27.

17. Lipshultz LI, Corriere JN. Progressive testicular atrophy in the varicocele patient. J Urol 1977;117:175.

18. Vantman D, Koukoulis G, Dennison L, et al. Computer assisted semen analysis: evaluation of method and assessment of the influence of sperm concentration on linear velocity determination. Fertil Steril 1988;49:510.

19. Smith RG, Johnson A, Lamb DJ, et al. Functional tests of spermatozoa. Sperm assay. Urol Clin North Am 1987;14:451.

20. Burkman LJ, Coddington CC, Fraken DR, et al. The hemizona assay (HZA): development of a diagnostic test for the binding of human spermatozoa to the human hemizona pellucida to predict fertilization potential. Fertil Steril 1988;49:688.

21. Charny CW, Gillenwater J. Congenital absence of the vas deferens. J Urol 1965;93:399.

22. Oates RD, Oshowitz SP, Krane RJ. Epididymal sperm aspiration (E.S.A.) in conjunction with gamete intra-fallopian transfer (G.I.F.T.) to achieve pregnancy [abstract]. Presented at the American Urological Association Annual Meeting, New Orleans, La. May 1990.

23. Silber SJ, Ord T, Balmeceda J, Patriozio P, et al. Congenital absence of the vas deferens. N Engl J Med 1990;323(26):1788–1792.

24. Marks JK, Shinohara K, Lipshultz LI. Correlation of transrectal ultrasound findings and ejaculatory duct obstruction. Presented at the 44th Annual Meeting of the American Fertility Society, Atlanta, Ga., October 1988.

25. Hellerstein DK, Meacham RB, Lipshultz LI. Transrectal ultrasound and partial ejaculatory duct obstruction in male infertility [abstract]. Presented at the American Urological Association Annual Meeting, Toronto, Canada, 1991.

26. Shinohara K, Lipshultz LI, Scardino PT. Transrectal ultrasonography of the seminal vesicle in the azoospermic patient [abstract 13]. Presented at the South Central Section Meeting of the American Urological Association, Guadalajara, Mexico, November 1985.

27. Lipshultz LI, Kaufman JJ. Subfertility. In: Lipshultz LI, Kaufman JJ, eds. Current urologic therapy. Philadelphia: WB Saunders, 1980:399.

28. Amelar AD, Dubin L. Special problems in management. In: Amelar RD, Dubin L, Walsh P, eds. Male infertility. Philadelphia: WB Saunders, 1977:191.

29. Bunge RG, Sherman JK. Liquefaction of human semen by alpha-amylase. Fertil Steril 1954;5:520.

30. Edeghe AJ-H. Effect of washing on sperm surface autoantibodies. Br J Urol 1987;60:360.

31. Confino E, Friberg J, Dudkiewicz A, et al. Intrauterine inseminations with washed human spermatozoa. Fertil Steril 1986;46:55–60.

32. Clarke GN, Lopata A, McBain JC, et al. Effect of sperm antibodies in males on human in vitro fertilization (IVF). Am J Reprod Immunol Microbiol 1985;8:62–66.

33. Quigley MM. Polyzoospermia with poor motility. In: Garcia CR, Mastroianni L Jr, Amelar RD, et al. eds. Current therapy and infertility 1984–1985. Philadelphia: BC Decker, 1984:179.

34. Matson PL, Turner SR, Yovich JM, et al. Oligospermic infertility treated with in vitro fertilization. Aust N Z J Obstet Gynaecol 1986;24:84.

35. Hirsh I, Gibbons WE, Lipshultz LI, et al. In vitro fertilization in couples with male factor infertility. Fertil Steril 1986;49:659.

36. You CH. Blood gas analysis of varicocele, spermatic vein and peripheral vein. Chinese J Surg 1989;January 27(1):37–38.

37. Goldstein M, Eid JF. Elevation of intratesticular and scrotal skin surface temperature in men with varicocele. J Urol 1989;142(3):743–745.

38. Peng BC, Tomashefsky P, Nagler HM. The cofactor effect: varicocele and infertility. Fertil Steril 1990; 54(1):143–148.

39. Klaiker EL, Broverman DM, Pokoly TB, et al. Interrelationships of cigarette smoking, testicular varicosities and seminal fluid indices. Fertil Steril 1987;47:481.

40. Zargniotti AW, McCloud J. Studies in temperature, human semen quality and varicocele. Fertil Steril 1973;24:854.

41. Ashkenazi J, Dicker D, Feldberg D, et al. The impact of spermatic vein ligation on the male factor in IVF embryo transfer and its relation to testosterone levels before and after operation. Fertil Steril 1989;51(3):471–474.

42. Sieber A, Coburn M, Lipshultz LI. Effect of varicocele repair on sperm function. Presented at the American Urological Association Annual Meeting, New Orleans, La., May 1990.

43. Pryor JL, Howards SS. Varicocele. Urol Clin North Am 1987;14:499.

44. Jarow JP, Budin RE, Dym M, et al. Cumulative pathologic changes in human testes after vasectomy. N Engl J Med 1985;313:1252–1256.

45. Belker AM, Fuchs EF, Konnak JW, et al. Results of 1200 first vasectomy reversals by the vasovasostomy study group. Presented at the American Urological Association Annual Meeting, New Orleans, La., May 1990.

46. Thomas AJ. Vasoepididymostomy: a modified macrosurgical technique [abstract]. Presented at the 6th Forum of International Andrology, Paris, France, May 1988.

47. Wagenknect LV. Ten years experience with microsurgical epididymovasostomy: results and proposition of a new technique. J Androl 1985;6:26.

48. Meinertz H, Linnett L, Fogh-Anderson P, Hjort T. Antisperm antibodies and fertility after vasovasostomy: a follow-up study of 216 men. Fertil Steril 1990;54(2):315–321.

49. Schoysman R. Surgical treatments in male sterility. Andrologia 1969;1:33.

50. Ludvik W. Artificial spermatocele persisting for 14 years. J Urol 1990;144(4):992–994.

51. Gimenez-Cruz JF. Artificial spermatocele. J Urol 1980;123:885.

52. Ross LS, Prins GS. Alloplastic spermatoceles: 5 year experience. J Androl 1985;6:102.

53. Belker AM, Jiminez-Crus DJ, Kelami A, Wegenknect LV. Alloplastic spermatocele: poor motility in intraoperative epididymal fluid contraindicates prosthesis implantation. J Urol 1986; 136(2):408–409.

54. Muller TE, Dentinger J, Reinthaller A, et al. IVF with spermatozoa from alloplastic spermatocele. Fertil Steril 1990; 53(4):744–746.

55. Brindley GS. Deep scrotal temperature and effect on it of clothing, air, temperature, activity, posture and paraplegia. Br J Urol 1982;54:49.

56. Charny CW. Treatment of male infertility. In: Behrman SJ, Kistner RW, eds. Progress in infertility. Boston: Little, Brown, 1968:649.

57. Shill WB, Michalopoulous M. Treatment of male fertility disturbances: current concepts. Drugs 1984;28:263.

58. Sherins RJ, Howards SS. Male infertility. In: Walsh PC, Gittes RF, Perlmutter AD, et al. eds. Campbell's urology, 5th ed. Philadelphia: WB Saunders, 1986:186.

59. Crowley WF Jr. An overview of LH-RH analogues: clinical uses. Ups J Med Sci 1984;89:3.

60. Liu L, Chandhari N, Cork D, et al. Comparison of pulsatile subcutaneous gonadotropin-releasing hormone and exogenous gonadotropins in the treatment of men with isolated hypogonadotrophic hypogonadism. Fertil Steril 1988; 49:302–308.

61. Berrezin M, Weissenberg R, Rabinvitch O, Lunenfeld B. Successful GnRH treatment in a patient with Kallmann's syndrome who had failed previous HMG/HCG treatment. Andrologia 1988;20(4):285–288.

62. Haas GG. Antibody mediated causes of male infertility. Urol Clin North Am 1987;14(4):539.

63. Rumke P, Heekman A. Sterility: an immunological disorder? Clin Obstet Gynecol 1977;20:691.

64. Shulman JF, Schulman S. Methylprednisolone treatment of immunologic infertility in the male. Fertil Steril 1982;38:591.

65. Hendry WF, Treehuba K, Huges L, et al. Cyclic prednisone therapy for male infertility associated with autoantibodies to spermatozoa. Fertil Steril 1986;45:249.

66. Hendry WF. Bilateral aseptic necrosis of femoral heads following intermittent high-dose steroid therapy [letter]. Fertil Steril 1982;38:120.

67. Haas JG. Male fertility and immunity. In: Lipshultz LI, Howards SS, eds. Infertility in the male. St. Louis: Mosby–Year Book, 1991:287, 290.

68. Kropfl D, Meyer-Schwickerath M, Plewa G, et al. Restoration of antegrade ejaculation following retroperitoneal lymph node dissection. In: Thompson W, Harrison RO, Bonnar J, eds. The male factor in human fertility disorders and treatment. Lancaster: MTP Press, 1983.

69. Templeton A, Mortimer D. Successful circumvention of retrograde ejaculation in an infertile diabetic man. Case report. Br J Obstet Gynaecol 1982;89:1064.

70. Oschner MG, Burns E, Henry HH. Incidence of retrograde ejaculation following bladder neck revision as a child. J Urol 1970;104:496.

71. Murphy JB, Lipshultz LI. Abnormalities of ejaculation. Urol Clin North Am 1987;7(Suppl):109.

72. Goldwasser B, Madgar I, Jonas P, et al. Imipramine for the treatment of sterility in patients following retroperitoneal lymph node dissection. Andrologia 1983;15:588.

73. Paulson JD, Polakoski KL. Isolation of spermatozoa immobilization factor from Escherichia filtrates. Fertil Steril 1977;28:182.

74. Teague NS, Boyarsky S, Glenn JF. Interference of human spermatozoa motility by Escherichia coli. Fertil Steril 1971;22:281.

75. Fair WR, Cordonnier JJ. The pH of prostatic fluid: a reappraisal and therapeutic implications. J Urol 1978;120:695.

76. Marmar JL, Katz S, Praiss, RE, et al. Semen zinc levels in infertile and postvasectomy patients and with prostatitis. Fertil Steril 1975;26:1057.

77. Colleen S, Mardh PA. Studies on nonacute prostatitis. Clinical and laboratory findings in patients with symp-

toms of nonacute prostatitis. In: Danielsson D, Juhlin L, Mardh PA, eds. Genital infections and their complications. Stockholm: Almquist and Wiksell International, 1975:121.

78. Furr PM, Taylor-Robinson D. Prevalence and significance of *Mycoplasma hominis* and *Ureaplasma urealyticum* in the urines of a nonvenereal disease population. Epidemiol Infect 1987;98:353.

79. Friberg J, Gnarpe H. *Mycoplasma* and human reproductive failure. III. Pregnancies in "infertile" couples treated with doxycycline for *T-mycoplasma*. Am J Obstet Gynecol 1973;116:23.

80. Harrison RF, deLouvois J, Blades M, et al. Doxycycline treatment and human infertility. Lancet 1975;1:605.

81. Fowlkes DM, McCloud J, O'Leary WM. *T-mycoplasmas* and human infertility: correlation of infection with alterations in seminal parameters. Fertil Steril 1975;26:1212.

82. Swenson CE, Toth A, O'Leary WM. *Ureaplasma urealyticum* and human infertility: the effect of antibiotic therapy on semen quality. Infertil Steril 1979;31:660.

83. Uehling DT. Low dose cortisone for male infertility. Fertil Steril 1978;29:220–221.

84. Horatta O, Koskimes AI, Rauta T, et al. Bromocriptine treatment of oligospermia, a double blind study. Clin Endocrinol 1979;11:377–382.

85. Turner TT, Jones CE, Howards SS, et al. On the androgen micro-environment of maturing spermatozoa. Endocrinology 1984;115:1925–1932.

86. Wang C, Dahl KD, Leung A, et al. Serum bioactive follicle stimulating hormone in men with idiopathic azoospermia and oligospermia. J Clin Endocrinol Metab 1987;65:629–633.

87. Sherins RJ, Loriaux DL. Studies on the role of sex steroids in the feedback control of FSH concentrations in men. J Clin Endocrinol Metab 1973;36:886–893.

88. Paulson DF. Clomiphene citrate in the management of male hypofertility: predictors for treatment selection. Fertil Steril 1977;28:1226–1229.

89. Wang C, Chan C-W, Wong K-K, et al. Comparison of the effectiveness of placebo, clomiphene citrate, mesterolone, pentoxifylline and testosterone rebound therapy for the treatment of idiopathic oligospermia. Fertil Steril 1983;40:358–365.

90. Paulson DF. Cortisone acetate versus clomiphene citrate in pre-germinal idiopathic oligospermia. J Urol 1979;121:432–434.

91. Sokol RZ, Peterson G, Steiner BS, et al. A controlled comparison of the efficacy of clomiphene citrate in male infertility. Infertil Steril 1988;49:865–870.

92. Torok L. Treatment of oligospermia with tamoxifen (open and controlled studies). Andrologia 1985;17:497–501.

93. AinMelk Y, Belisle S, Carmel M, et al. Tamoxifen citrate therapy in male infertility. Fertil Steril 1987;48:113–117.

94. Mehan DJ, Chehval MJ. Human chorionic gonadotropin in the treatment of the infertile man. J Urol 1982;128:60–63.

95. Danezis JM, Batrinos ML. The effect of human postmenopausal gonadotropins in infertile men with severe oligospermia. Fertil Steril 1967;18:788–800.

96. Lunenfeld B, Mor A, Marie M. Treatment of male infertility. I. Human gonadotropins. Fertil Steril 1967;18:581–592.

97. Homonnai ZT, Peled M, Paz GF. Changes in semen quality of fertility in response to endocrine treatment of subfertile men. Gynecol Obstet Invest 1978;9:244–255.

98. Knauth UA, Honigal W, Bals-Pratsch M, et al. Treatment of severe oligospermia with human chorionic gonadotropin/human menopausal gonadotropin. A placebo-controlled, double blind trial. J Clin Endocrinol Metab 1987;65:1081–1087.

99. Badenoch DF, Waxman J, Boorman L, et al. Administration of gonadotropin: a releasing hormone analog in oligospermic infertile males. Acta Endocrinol 1988;117:265–267.

100. Aparicio NJ, Schwarzstein L, Turner EA, et al. Treatment of idiopathic normogonadotropic oligoasthenospermia with synthetic luteinizing hormone-releasing hormone. Fertil Steril 1976;27:549–555.

101. Aafjes JH, van der Vijver JC, Brugman FW, et al. Double blind crossover treatment with mesterolone and placebo of subfertile oligospermic men: value of testicular biopsy. Andrologia 1983;15:531–535.

102. Schill W-B. Improvement in sperm motility in patients with asthenozoospermia by kallikrein treatment. Int J Fertil 1975;20:61–63.

103. Schill W-B, Braun-Falco O, Haberland GL. The possible role of kallikreins in sperm motility. Int J Fertil 1974;19:163–167.

104. Schill W-B. Treatment of idiopathic oligospermia by kallikrein: results of a double blind study. Arch Androl 1979:2:163–170.

105. Homonnai ZT, Shilon M, Paz G. Evaluation of semen quality following kallikrein treatment. Gynecol Obstet Invest 1978;9:132–138.

106. Micic S. Kallikrein and antibiotics in the treatment of infertile men with genital tract infections. Andrologia 1988;20(1):55–59.

107. Cohen MS, Colin MJ, Golambu M, et al. The effects of prostaglandins on sperm motility. Fertil Steril 1977;28:78–85.

108. Barkay J, Harpaz-Kerpel S, Ben-Ezra S, et al. The prostaglandin inhibitor effect of antiinflammatory drugs in the therapy of male infertility. Fertil Steril 1984;42:406–411.

3

Indications for In Vitro Fertilization and Embryo Transfer

Gad Lavy
Alan DeCherney

Introduction

In vitro fertilization and embryo transfer (IVF-ET) has been used successfully in the treatment of human infertility for just over 10 years. This first decade can be characterized by rapid technological developments and by fierce debates over ethical issues relating to this revolutionary procedure. The initial responses of members of the scientific community and the general public to the introduction of this new technique were guarded. There was skepticism regarding its efficiency and caution as its potential for creating congenital anomalies was unknown. Following the early success, caution was quickly replaced with enthusiasm almost to the point of euphoria. At one point it appeared that the ultimate therapy for infertility had been discovered and that all other infertility therapies such as tubal surgery would eventually fall by the wayside. The pendulum now seems to be swinging yet again as the real potential of IVF is gradually being realized along with a better definition of its position among the various techniques currently available for treatment of male and female infertility.

During the first decade of its existence, some major developments in technique have resulted in simpler, more efficient IVF procedures, and overall in higher rates of success. Critical advances have been made in the areas of ovarian stimulation, ultrasound technology, and in vitro embryo culture.

Ovulation induction has received a major boost as a result of IVF. The endless manipulation required for optimal ovarian stimulation during IVF cycles has added to our understanding of ovarian function. Ovarian stimulation drug protocols have been modified and remodified over the past decade. Human menopausal gonadotropin (hMG), human follicle-stimulating hormone (FSH), and clomiphene citrate, alone and in combination, continue to be used in various regimens. The recent addition of gonadotropin-releasing hormone agonist (GnRHa) to the drug arsenal has made a significant impact on the outcome of IVF-ET. GnRHa is used to down-regulate and thus suppress pituitary function prior to initiation of gonadotropin stimulation. By suppressing pituitary gonadotropin secretion, an untimely surge of luteinizing hormone (LH) can be prevented. GnRHa has increased the predictability and efficiency of ovarian stimulation and egg retrieval. The use of GnRHa has resulted in an increase in the number of ova retrieved and in pregnancy rate per stimulation cycle (1). In addition, the ability to "program" stimulation cycles using GnRHa has allowed for increased efficiency and better utilization of resources. As a result regimens that incorporate GnRHa have become routine in most IVF programs (2).

Advances in ultrasound technology, primarily the development of transvaginal (TV) ultrasound, have had a dramatic impact on IVF. Transvaginal ultrasound was initially utilized to monitor ovarian response to stimulation. This technique allows for greater accuracy of follicular measurements and is associated with significantly less discomfort than the transabdominal scanning technique. More recently TV ultrasound has been used to guide transvaginal egg retrieval, thus eliminating the need for laparoscopy in most patients. It has become commonplace for egg retrieval procedures to be performed with local anesthesia and minimal sedation on an ambulatory basis. TV ultrasound has contributed greatly to simplification of the entire IVF procedure, reduction of the risk of anesthesia, and reduction in the cost of the procedure.

Last but not least, improvements in *embryo culture* conditions have been achieved through a better understanding of embryo metabolic and nutritional requirements and have resulted in "better" embryos and higher success rates.

The advances in IVF technology, the improved pregnancy rates, and the simplification of methods have resulted in an expansion in the primary indications for the procedure. Originally advocated for patients with missing or abnormal fallopian tubes (3), IVF-ET is now being offered for a wide range of indications such as male infertility, endometriosis, idiopathic infertility, and others (4–6).

What have we learned from IVF?

Attempts at improving success in human IVF have led to massive redirection of resources toward the study of events related to ovarian function, the fertilization process, embryo development and culture, endometrial receptivity, and reproductive aging. It should be emphasized that IVF offers an alternative form of reproduction and is not, in most cases, a specific treatment for an underlying disorder. Diseased fallopian tubes are bypassed, sperm is placed close to the eggs in couples suffering from male factor infertility, and an empirical approach is used for patients with idiopathic infertility. So, despite major advancements and improved success in some areas of the IVF-ET technology, our knowledge in many areas covered by the IVF-ET technology remains incomplete. This is underscored by the frequent IVF failures.

What are the indications for IVF-ET today? What are the factors associated with successful and unsuccessful outcome? What are the success rates of the procedure in the various indications for which it is used? These topics will be reviewed in this chapter, and the true place of IVF-ET among the various therapies for infertility in the next decade will be examined. The achievement of pregnancy continues to be the yardstick by which the success of IVF programs is measured. However, what may appear as a simple endpoint is in reality a result of multiple variables and does not always reflect the "quality" of the program. Questions regarding criteria for patient selection continue to cloud the issue of the assessment of IVF success.

Indications for IVF

The only absolute indication for this technique is the absence or complete and irreparable blockage of the fallopian tubes. All other indications are only relative. When considering IVF-ET for a patient with a specific infertility disorder, one must be familiar with the likelihood of achieving pregnancy without therapy or with alternative forms of therapy (medical or surgical). In addition, for proper counseling one should be aware of the different success rates for IVF-ET when applied to patients with different infertility disorders. With this information, the counseling physician should be able to make a more educated recommendation regarding the the applicability of IVF-ET to the individual couple's particular situation.

Tubal infertility

IVF-ET was originally advocated for patients with missing or abnormal fallopian tubes (3). It is this group, for whom IVF-ET is in many cases the only viable alternative, in which the concept of replacing the fallopian tubes as the site of oocyte fertilization and early embryo development with in vitro culture techniques was to be tested. Only after success had been achieved in these "tubal factor" patients was IVF-ET attempted in other infertility categories. Tubal infertility patients still constitute the largest single group treated with IVF-ET and still enjoy a high rate of success. In the 1989 national IVF-ET registry, tubal infertility accounted for 38% of patients entered—more than any other category. The clinical pregnancy success in this group was 20% (7). These results are in agreement with other collaborative reports.

Despite variability in response to ovarian stimula-

tion and differences in success within the group of tubal infertility patients, no correlation could be demonstrated consistently between outcome and the extent of pelvic and periovarian adhesions. Most investigators have concentrated on the potential effect of ovarian or tubal surgery and of pelvic adhesions on the response to ovarian stimulation.

Mahadaven et al. have reported on a reduction in the number of ova recovered in patients with periovarian and peritubal adhesions, suggesting that such adhesions could impair follicular development and ovarian function. These findings could not, however, be confirmed by most other studies (8).

Oehninger et al. (9) have studied 549 patients in 1031 cycles. No differences were found between the number of preovulatory oocytes, fertilization rates, or serum estradiol levels in the follicular phase between classes of tubo-ovarian disease. However, patients with previous bilateral tubal ligation had higher pregnancy rates than those with severe tubo-ovarian abscess. The type of prior pelvic surgery had no effect on IVF-ET outcome. Similarly Cooperman et al. (10) have examined the effect of tubal and ovarian surgery on the response to ovarian stimulation in patients undergoing IVF. A number of groups were studied, and their IVF-ET outcomes were compared. The oocyte yield and quality from the left ovary versus the right ovary were compared in women who had undergone unilateral cystectomy, unilateral salpingectomy, or tuboplasty. In the same study, IVF-ET outcome was compared in women with different surgical histories. Overall no differences were found between the groups in several variables related to ovarian function and oocyte development. Thus no differences were noted in folliculogenesis, estradiol levels, or quantity and maturity of the ova recovered between any of the groups.

It appears therefore that previous ovarian or tubal surgery or the extent of pelvic adhesive disease does not affect the success of ovarian stimulation or that of IVF-ET.

IVF or tubal surgery: While IVF-ET is the only treatment option for couples with absent fallopian tubes and for those with irreparably damaged tubes, many patients become candidates for IVF with only a relative indication. In these patients the tubes are normal but patent, and in some tubal surgery has not been attempted. In these situations one is often faced with the difficult task of directing the couple toward IVF or tubal surgery. Clearly, the decision between IVF and tubal surgery is relatively simple in the extreme cases—that is, those with mechanical infertility who have no real chance of success, such as those who have undergone salpingectomies or have multisite tubal occlusion or severe pelvic adhesive disease. On the other hand, those patients who need a simple reversal of tubal sterilization have a high chance of successful outcome following surgery (11). The final decision needs to rely on the chance of success with either method, the associated morbidity of the technique, and financial considerations.

The prognosis for surgery depends on a variety of factors such as the nature of the underlying disease process, the site(s) and extent of involvement, and the presence of other factors such as advanced age. Thus, the prognosis for surgery is best when the disease process involves exclusively the proximal or distal tubal segment. Unfortunately, such "pure" involvement is found in only 10% of patients with tubal disease. In most cases the prognosis for tubal surgery is much worse, and it is reasonable to ask whether it is justified in cases of severe tubal disease to use IVF as first-line therapy.

If one considers the cumulative pregnancy rate achieved with repeat IVF cycles, the success of this procedure appears to be higher than that for most cases of tubal disease. The success rate quoted for IVF-ET represents the results of a single treatment cycle. Repeat cycles increase the overall (cumulative) success. In most studies the cumulative pregnancy rates following four cycles of IVF-ET in patients with tubal infertility approaches 40% to 50%. This is clearly higher than for most cases of tubal surgery (12).

The risks of surgery, which include the potential complications of general anesthesia, are higher than those associated with IVF, although both procedures are quite safe. The higher risk of multiple pregnancy following IVF is being curbed with the increasing success and thus greater utilization of embryo cryopreservation and selective reduction of multiple gestations.

The cost of a single cycle of IVF is comparable to that of tubal surgery. The cost-effectiveness of the two procedures has been calculated to be similar (11). All these arguments seem to favor IVF-ET over tubal surgery in all but mild cases of tubal disease. On the other hand, recent developments in operative laparoscopy are making tubal surgery less invasive and less costly. Advancements in endoscopic surgical techniques now allow for many procedures to be performed laparoscopically, thus reducing cost and morbidity. The success rates of these new procedures are not yet well documented but appear in many cases to be similar to those of traditional surgery. Lower cost and morbidity in conjunction with an equal rate of success will mandate a revision of the role of tubal surgery versus IVF-ET in patients with tubal disease. At present, individualization is important in selecting the procedure of choice for each couple.

Endometriosis

As a cause of infertility, endometriosis presents a spectrum of disorders. In the most severe cases (stage III and IV), mechanical infertility is evident with severe periovarian and peritubal adhesions. In the mild forms, the association with infertility is not entirely clear.

Infertility in these cases has been linked to increased peritoneal prostaglandin concentration and abnormalities in the immune system leading to abnormal oocyte development and ovulatory defects. The treatment of infertility associated endometriosis can be medical or surgical or a combination thereof. The success of treatment of endometriosis in achieving pregnancy is clearly related to the stage of the disease. In the more advanced cases the pregnancy rates following therapy are markedly reduced, but in the minimal and mild cases the association with infertility has been questioned by some.

Not unlike those in other infertility categories, patients with endometriosis are usually referred for IVF after failure of the conventional methods of therapy. Not unlike other methods, IVF presents a somewhat nonspecific approach to therapy, as the exact nature of the factors leading to infertility in patients with endometriosis is not known.

Endometriosis and IVF results: The success of IVF-ET in patients with endometriosis is related to the stage of the disease. In a review of more than 2000 IVF-ET patients, Sharma et al. reported a high pregnancy rate in patients with mild endometriosis and markedly reduced success in patients with severe disease (13). Confirmation of the relationship of the stage of endometriosis and success in IVF-ET has been provided by Matson and Yovitch (14). Pregnancy rates of 13% and 14% were reported in stage I and II while the results in stages III and IV were only 6% and 2%, respectively. The mechanism of reduced pregnancy success in the severe cases is not entirely clear. While some have suggested impairment in oocyte fertilization parameters in cases of untreated endometriosis with persistent disease present at the time of IVF (15), others have reported fertilization rates similar to those found in patients with tubal disease (13).

It has been suggested that patients with endometriosis be referred for IVF-ET only after conservative surgery or medical therapy has been unsuccessful in achieving pregnancy. Damewood and Rock suggested a laparoscopic approach to egg retrieval in endometriosis cases to allow for surgical therapy at the time of egg recovery (16). In their study, 39 patients with mild endometriosis were treated according to this protocol during their IVF cycle. None conceived during the treatment cycle, but 12 (28%) did within 10 months of their laparoscopy. Caution should be used in applying these recommendations. The absence of pregnancy following IVF-ET may be related to the fact that laparoscopic therapy of endometriosis was performed at the time of ova retrieval. Other authors have suggested that treatment of endometriosis in preparation for IVF may have a positive effect on cycle outcome (17).

In summary IVF-ET can certainly be viewed as an alternative treatment modality for patients with endometriosis, but the success of IVF-ET in the advanced forms is reduced. IVF-ET should be offered only after other causes of infertility have been ruled out. It should also be kept in mind that medical or surgical "debulking" of endometriosis prior to ovarian stimulation and egg retrieval may improve the chances of success.

Male infertility

The initial success of IVF-ET in patients with tubal infertility, and the observation that fertilization in vitro can be achieved with relatively few sperm (18), prompted attempts to apply this new technique to couples with male subfertility.

Mahadevan et al. first reported the use of IVF-ET for male factor infertility. The authors reported significantly reduced fertilization rates of 57% in the male factor groups as compared to 80% in the tubal factor control group (19). On the other hand, rates of fertilization in males with sperm concentration as low as 0.5×10^6/ml have been reported (20). Review of the literature clearly shows that the limiting factor in achieving successful pregnancy in patients with male infertility is the rate of fertilization. Once pregnant, the pregnancy outcome is no different in male-factor and non–male-factor couples. It is clear that the fertilization rates are lower in couples with male infertility as compared to control subjects. Quantitative assessment of the success of IVF-ET in couples with male infertility is difficult, however, owing to the lack of standardization in the definition of male infertility and to the fact that different sperm preparation techniques are used in different programs.

This confusion stems from the fact that, although there seems to be an agreement regarding the values of semen parameters below which a male is considered subfertile, these values are not absolute, and fertilization and pregnancy can occur with lower values. Soon after IVF was attempted in couples with male infertility, it became clear that new definitions of this condition were needed. Unfortunately, to date no such standards have been applied.

All investigators working with male infertility patients in IVF-ET have noted a marked effect of preparation technique on fertilization success. We have recently reported high rates of fertilization in patients with male infertility with the use of discontinuous Percoll gradient centrifugation in conjunction with the "microdrop" culture method. The pregnancy rate for the entire male factor group in this and other studies was not significantly lower than that of the entire IVF-ET population, confirming the role of IVF-ET in the treatment of male infertility.

Success of IVF-ET in patients with male infertility needs to be contrasted with other treatment modalities. The success of treatment of male infertility is notoriously low, and intrauterine insemination is considered one of the accepted therapies that carries a notoriously low rate of success.

Comparison of artificial insemination with husband's semen (AIH) with IVF-ET for patients with male infertility showed IVF-ET to be significantly more effective than AIH. The incidence of pregnancy in the male infertility group was significantly higher following IVF-ET than following AIH (21% vs. 5%, $p < 0.01$) (21).

Predictors of success with male infertility: Since the various parameters used to evaluate sperm are thought to reflect its quality, several attempts have been made to determine the predictive value of the different parameters (motility, concentration, and morphology) on the success of IVF-ET (22). A fertilization rate of 55% was reported in patients in whom only one of the three semen parameters was abnormal, 50% when two were abnormal, and 20% when all three were low. Rogers has examined in detail the different semen parameters in an attempt to define threshold levels (23). A marked decrease in fertilization failures was observed when sperm motility was less than 20%. Similarly the rate of fertilization failure was higher in the abnormal morphology group than in those with normal morphology (18% vs. 12%). In the same study, the sperm concentration was found to be a relatively poor predictor of fertilization success. When a comparison of seminal parameters was made between the successful and unsuccessful IVF-ET cycles, the motility appeared to be a better predictor than concentration (23).

In addition to the traditional semen characteristics, other prognostic tests have been utilized to define sperm quality. These include the sperm penetration assay (SPA), determinations of acrosome reaction, and motility parameters such as velocity, linearity, and lateral head displacement.

Using multiple regression we have recently constructed a model to predict fertilization in vitro utilizing various semen parameters. When concentration, motility, and migrated linear velocity were entered into the model, the ability to predict outcome (fertilization) was particularly high ($R = 0.83$, $p < 0.001$) (Shamma F, Lavy G, Gutman J, unpublished data).

We have also examined the value of the hypoosmotic swelling (HOS) test as a predictor of fertilization. In a group of male infertility patients, tail curling in less than 50% of cells was associated with fertilization failure in 15 of 18 patients, and a low fertilization rate was found in the remaining three patients. In this group a regression model was constructed. Utilizing the percentage of curling and type A forward progression yielded a significant multiple correlation ($r^2 = 0.8$, $p < 0.0001$) (F.R. Parikh, P. Nadkarni, A.H. DeCherney, G. Lavy, manuscript in preparation).

One of the most popular and widely studied tests is the sperm penetration assay, in which penetration of prepared sperm into zona-free hamster eggs is evaluated. Several investigators have examined the correlation between the SPA and in vitro fertilization of human ova. The concordance described varied between 77% and 100% and appears to be related to modification of the original technique. The use of swim–up separation enhances the penetration rate significantly compared with standard SPA and reduces false-negative results (24,25). The use of test-yolk buffer appears to reduce significantly the false-negative rate and is recommended. It appears that no sperm penetration on a standard or test-yolk buffer SPA is highly indicative of fertilization failure (23).

One can therefore conclude that IVF-ET is a nonspecific therapy of male infertility in that it does not address the basic cause of the poor sperm quality. Despite successful fertilization achieved through IVF in these couples, the promise of gaining better insight into mechanisms of fertilization by observing the process in vitro has not been fulfilled. Egg-sperm interaction and the cause of its failure in these couples remains elusive.

Nonetheless, IVF-ET can be used successfully in patients with male infertility. Improved sperm preparations have increased the success of fertilization even in the most difficult cases.

Fertilization outcome can be predicted using one of the semen variables or by applying the HOS test or the SPA. The true success of IVF-ET in this group is difficult to assess owing to the lack of standardization in the definition of male infertility.

Unexplained infertility

The proper diagnosis of unexplained infertility requires a complete and meticulous infertility evaluation. Critical assessment of patients who are referred with the diagnosis of unexplained infertility often reveals identifiable causes that have not been investigated or have been missed in the previous evaluation. Evaluation of the role of IVF-ET in unexplained infertility requires the separation of those patients from the group that is truly unexplained—that is, those infertile couples in whom modern technology is not able to uncover a defect.

Thus, the assessment of patients carrying the label of infertility of undetermined origin may reveal tuboperitoneal disease or endometriosis that was missed on previous examination or some subtle abnormalities in follicular development and hormonal pattern (25).

As with other indications for IVF, the success of the procedure needs to be compared with that of other treatment modalities or with that of no therapy at all. Several studies utilizing life table analysis demonstrated that patients with unexplained infertility had a good prognosis for pregnancy without any form of therapy (27,28).

An alternative approach prior to IVF-ET includes the use of ovarian stimulation in patients with unexplained infertility. This "empirical" approach has yielded good results in a group of patients with unexplained infertility waiting for IVF-ET (29). Other studies have also shown that the combination of ovarian stimulation and intrauterine insemination yielded success comparable to IVF-ET or gamete intrafallopian transfer (30,31).

The value of IVF-ET in unexplained infertility: The success of IVF-ET in patients with unexplained infertility appears to be comparable to that of patients with tubal disease. Although Mahadevan et al. in an early study reported reduced fertilization in patients with unexplained infertility (18), most other authors describe excellent results in this group of patients.

In a group of 26 patients with unexplained infertility by strict criteria studied by Navot et al., the number of oocytes retrieved and successfully fertilized was lower than that of a control population consisting of tubal disease patients (32). However, the pregnancy rates and the miscarriage rates in the strict unexplained infertility group (32% and 12%, respectively) were not different from those of the control group (24% and 25%).

In conclusion, it appears that patients with unexplained infertility constitute a favorable group for IVF-ET. A trial of superovulation with or without intraueterine insemination prior to IVF-ET should be considered.

Immunologic infertility

The evidence that antisperm antibodies in the female or the male may interfere with the fertilization process seems conclusive. Fertilization failure may result from agglutination or immobilization of spermatozoa in the female reproductive tract or from specific interruption of the egg-sperm interaction. Antibodies have been shown to affect different stages of the fertilization process including the acrosome reaction, zona pellucida recognition and penetration, and sperm-vitellus interaction.

The early evidence of an effect of antisperm antibody on fertilization was derived from the zona-free hamster oocyte model. A significant reduction in fertilization resulted from exposure of spermatozoa to antisperm antibodies (33). Despite the limitations of this model, these findings suggest that antisperm antibodies can interfere with the process of sperm-vitellus binding. This observation does not, however, provide information on the effect of antibodies on sperm penetration through the cumulus oophorus, zona binding, and zona penetration. That information had to be obtained directly from observation in human IVF-ET systems.

Sperm antibody in IVF: In 1984 Yovich et al. reported their experience with IVF-ET treatment of five women whose infertility was attributed to the presence of circulating antisperm antibodies and whose ova were incubated and inseminated with donor serum. Normal fertilization rates and viable pregnancies were achieved in this group of women (34). The establishment of ongoing pregnancies in these patients implied that the antibodies did not affect the embryo or the implantation process in the same manner in which they affected the spermatozoa. Clarke et al. have reported on the result of IVF-ET treatment in 20 patients in whom circulating antibodies were detected in serum using the indirect immunobead test. Patients whose titer of antibody of the IgA and IgG class was less than 1:10 demonstrated normal fertilization rates. Higher antibody levels were associated with a marked reduction in fertilization rates. In this group the presence of antibodies from the IgG class alone was not associated with abnormal fertilization rates (35). Mandelbaum et al. have reported the result of IVF in 40 patients. In this study, the presence of sperm antibodies directed against the sperm head was associated with poor fertilization (36).

The effect of sperm autoantibodies in semen has also been investigated. Clarke et al. reported low fertilization rates when at least 80% of the spermatozoa were coated with antibody of the IgA or IgG classes (37). Junk et al. reported similar findings. In their study the presence of more than 20% antibody-coated spermatozoa in seminal fluid was associated with adversely affected fertilization (38).

Modifications in the IVF-ET system are required to increase the rate of fertilization when antisperm antibodies are present in female serum. Substituting the woman's serum as a medium supplement results in fertilization rates that are indistinguishable from control rates. On the other hand, no simple remedy exists when the antibodies are present in seminal plasma. Repeated washings and ejaculation into medium have been suggested, but no evidence exists as to their effect on improving fertilization rates.

The study of the effect of antisperm antibody on IVF-ET success has been limited by the small numbers of patients available for study and by the use of a variety of detection assays. The immunobead binding assay is now considered the gold standard, and its universal use allows for comparison of results from different centers.

In summary, the effect of antisperm antibodies on in vitro fertilization is well documented. It does not appear that the presence of these antibodies has an effect on implantation or on pregnancy maintenance. A clear distinction needs to made between antibodies detected in the male and those detected in the female. In the female, head directed IgA and IgG appear to have an adverse effect on fertilization. This can be averted by the use of a substitute to patient sperm as medium supplement. When the system is thus modified, the fertilization and pregnancy rates in these couples following IVF-ET do not differ from control rates. Antibodies in seminal plasma of the IgG and IgA variety also affect fertilization. For this condition, no simple remedy is available, and low or absent fertilization can be expected in these couples.

Diethylstilbestrol

Exposure to diethylstilbestrol (DES) in utero is associated with abnormalities in the paramesonephric system (39,40) and with adverse reproductive outcome (41–43). An increased incidence of spontaneous abortion, ectopic pregnancy, and premature labor has been reported in this population of women. The effect of DES exposure on fertility, however, remains controversial.

IVF-ET is occasionally used in DES-exposed patients. In most cases the indication for IVF-ET is not related to DES-associated abnormalities. However, as this condition affects the morphology and function of the reproductive tract, concern regarding the results of in vitro fertilization and pregnancy outcome in this group of patients has been expressed.

Early results in 33 DES-exposed women undergoing IVF-ET were reported by Muasher et al. (44). The incidence of successful pregnancy in the DES-exposed women did not differ from that in the general IVF-ET population. More recently the same group has reviewed the IVF-ET outcome of 46 DES-exposed women who have undergone 149 stimulation cycles (45). The numbers of ova recovered and embryos transferred were not different when compared with a control group of patients with tubal infertility. The term/ongoing pregnancy rate, however, was reduced in the DES group as compared with controls (8% vs. 16%). Closer examination of the pregnancy failures suggests that uterine anomalies such as constrictions and T-shaped uterus are associated with a worse prognosis.

In summary, it appears that a history of DES exposure in women undergoing IVF-ET does not affect fertilization or pregnancy rates but, similar to non-IVF cycles, is associated with increased pregnancy wastage.

Future indications for IVF

The future of IVF-ET is closely linked to improved pregnancy rates. Higher success rates will widen the scope of this method and will make it a more attractive alternative to be used for the existing indications. Couples with tubal, male, and immune infertility and those with endometriosis will be directed to IVF-ET earlier in the course of the therapeutic intervention before surgery, repeated inseminations, or medical therapy are attempted.

In addition, some novel indications are being developed. Over the past several years, intense research has been focused on combining the techniques of IVF-ET with micromanipulation of cells and embryos to provide powerful diagnostic and therapeutic tools. The new technology may be applied therapeutically in assisting the process of fertilization in patients with male infertility, in removing "excess" pronuclei from polyploid embryos, or diagnostically in obtaining "tissue" for genetic diagnosis.

Micromanipulation

The ability to manipulate individual cells has been refined over a century of experimentation, first with lower animals and later in mammalian species. Improvements in equipment and culture conditions have permitted the manipulation of smaller cells with high rates of survival. The technique has been used to study mechanisms of differentiation and cell lineage in early embryos, as well as the effects of nuclear transplantation and of gene insertion into somatic cells and embryos (46). Attempts at microinjection of sperm heads into oocytes were used to study the process of fertilization (47).

With the establishment of human IVF, it became clear that, ethical issues aside, the two techniques could be successfully combined. The initial attempts at micromanipulation in the human focused on couples with male infertility in whom sperm penetration into the ooplasm appeared to be the limiting factor in achieving success.

To overcome this limitation, three approaches have been developed and tried. The first methods involved partial disruption of the zona pellucida by chemical or mechanical means (48). Alternatively, sperm cells were injected into the perivitelline space or directly into the ooplasm (49). The impact of micromanipulation on male factor infertility is still being evaluated. Of the methods described, the mechanical dissection of the zona appears to provide the best fertilization results. Some success has been reported with the perivitelline space sperm insertion. Direct injection appears to be too disruptive to the egg, and no viable embryos have resulted.

Some of the undesirable effects of this method are the creation of polyploid embryos by disruption of the zona pellucida, or by the injection of multiple spermatozoa into the perivitelline space, and damage to the developmental program of the embryo. Malter and Cohen reported a 26% incidence of polyspermy following mechanical zona dissection (50).

The developmental potential of manipulated embryos was studied by J. Garrissi and associates. Only 61% of the diploid embryos obtained following mechanical zona dissection were found to cleave. Although the morphology of these embryos was comparable to that of controls, the cleavage rates of unmanipulated embryos are substantially higher (G.J. Garrissi 1990, #78).

Another therapeutic application of embryo micromanipulation has been attempted with the removal of "extra" pronuclei from polyploid embryos (51). Chromosomal studies of tripronuclear embryos demonstrated that after the first cell division the majority will cleave into three cells and contain aneuploid components (52). The technique of pronuclear removal was developed in the mouse model by McGrath and Solter (53). The male pronucleus can be identified and removed. In a preliminary report on manipulation of three zygotes, one of three zygotes survived the procedure, and no cleavage was observed (51).

Concerns have been expressed regarding the performance of this procedure in humans. The procedure requires the use of substances to stabilize the cytoskeleton such as colcemid and cytochalasin B or D; the potential of these agents to produce a chromosomal abnormality is not known. Another potential complication is the possibility of removing a female pronucleus instead of the excess male pronucleus. These androgenomes have a limited developmental capability but may reach the blastocyst stage.

Perhaps the most dramatic application of IVF in the future will be for genetic analysis of preimplantation embryos (preimplantation diagnosis). Using micromanipulation technology, a sample of the embryo may be removed without altering developmental potential. The separated blastomeres can then be cultured and allowed to divide and multiply or used immediately. Biochemical techniques have been utilized to detect hypoxanthine phosphoribosyltransferase (HPRT) deficiency in separated mouse blastocyst. Recently the successful use of polymerase chain reaction technology has allowed for rapid amplification of DNA segments, permitting quick diagnosis using a small amount of material. DNA probes are already available for a variety of genetic disorders, and new probes are being developed. An efficient system of preimplantation embryo biopsy and genetic analysis will allow the diagnosis to be made within hours and the decision regarding the normality of the embryo and its fate to be made rapidly.

Both ethical and practical issues relating to this application of micromanipulation have been raised; potential damage to the developmental program of the embryo caused by the removal of blastomeres is of concern but appears not to be significant. In the mouse, normal development can be expected despite the reduction of the number of blastomeres to half (54). To circumvent this problem, some have proposed obtaining biopsy specimens from late developmental stage embryos, after the trophectoderm has differentiated, and thus avoiding direct damage to the embryo proper (55).

Many ethical issues related to preimplantation diagnosis have been raised and cannot be addressed in this review. However, the major obstacle for the introduction of routine preimplantation diagnosis as an accepted indication for IVF is and will continue to be the low implantation rate per embryo currently obtained with human IVF. Implantation rates of less than 10% will dramatically reduce the efficiency of this highly advanced system.

The final frontier of IVF appears to be the possibility of gene therapy, which seems quite remote at present. Although dramatic growth of mice was obtained by microinjection of oocytes with growth-hormone gene (56), application of gene therapy to the preimplantation embryo to correct for various gene defects remains elusive. The promise of IVF in this area remains to be realized. Here too the technique can only be as successful as the implantation rate per embryo. Unless dramatic improvements are made in this area, it does not appear to be a viable method. However, the drama associated with the technical ability to correct gene defects in eggs or embryos obscures the real issue, which is the fact that the major impact of gene therapy will be found in treatment of adults and children with defective genes. In these cases the gene therapy could be applied to a sample of bone marrow, and the cells returned to the individual. No doubt, the new genetics holds great promise with regard to research into human embryo development.

Predictors of success

Individualization is key in planning the treatment strategy of the infertile couple. In counseling a couple for IVF, available information should be utilized to predict the likelihood of successful outcome. Defining a profile of the couple that is more likely to succeed in IVF-ET is helpful in counseling the couple prior to embarking on an IVF cycle. Various parameters have been examined with regard to their ability to predict success in IVF-ET cycles.

One of the most obvious parameters is the indication for which IVF-ET is performed. As discussed above, the success of IVF-ET differs among the various infertility categories. For each couple one has to compare the success of IVF-ET in their infertility category with that which can be achieved with other forms of therapy for that condition. One should also keep in mind that when more than one indication exists (e.g., male factor infertility and endometriosis), the prognosis worsens significantly. No specific information, however, is available in the literature to account for the many possible permutations.

Categorizing patients on the basis of their infertility diagnosis is often insufficient. It is clear that within each infertility category the chances of success also vary widely. Extrapolation of findings in other forms of infertility therapy has led to examination of variables such as patient age, serum FSH levels, and performance on previous cycles. Those variables have been found to be highly predictive of IVF outcome.

Age

The effect of age on female fecundity is more relevant today than ever before because of the continuing rise in the age at which women first attempt conception. Changes in lifestyle have resulted in delay of childbirth into the mid and late thirties. This trend has resulted in the resurgence of the well-documented phenomenon of declining female fecundity with age. When considering the effectiveness of any of the new therapeutic modalities, one has to account for this social trend as it adversely affects the overall outcome. This is particu-

larly relevant in IVF-ET, which is often used as the last resort in the path of infertility therapy and is thus associated with higher mean age than other treatment modalities.

A general decrease in female fecundity with increasing age has been well documented. Tietze described a decline in fecundity with age in Hutterite women who did not practice contraception (57). This early report was criticized for the presence of various confounding variables such as decreased coital frequency, male infertility, and endometriosis, which also may increase in significance with age. More recent studies in a population of women undergoing donor insemination were undertaken to attempt to minimize these confounding variables. A study by Stovall et al. has demonstrated a significant decline in fecundity with age in women undergoing donor insemination after proper infertility evaluation (58). Similar observations have been made in women following various forms of infertility therapy such as tubal surgery or the application of assisted reproductive techniques. A report by Penzias et al. indicated a threefold decline between pregnancy rates in women undergoing gamete intrafallopian transfers under age 35 and those in women over 40 (59). Similar findings have been reported by other investigators (60). Cittadini and Palermo have addressed the potential cause of infertility in advanced reproductive age and the most effective therapeutic approach. They conclude that the more advanced conception techniques such as IVF-ET and gamete and zygote intrafallopian transfer should be preferred over surgery in women over a certain age, especially if the infertility problem is of more than 5 years' standing (61).

This notable decline in fecundity and in success of infertility therapy with advancing age is probably multifactorial. The response to ovarian stimulation decreases and the rate of cancellation increases with age. Sharma et al. have reported a cancellation rate of 64% in women over age 40, and the cancellation rate in women aged 36 to 40 was twice that of those 26 to 30 years of age (12). Once ovulation occurs the rates of fertilization appear to be similar in the "older" and "younger" patients.

In addition to poor response to ovarian stimulation, a higher rate of pregnancy wastage characterizes the older age group. This phenomenon probably reflects poor egg quality or decreased endometrial receptivity or both. This is further supported by reports of a high rate of success following IVF-ET in cycles where donor eggs and exogenous hormones were used in women over age 40. It therefore appears that endometrial receptivity and egg quality are contributing to the decline in success in the "older" woman (62,63).

Review of a recent series of patients undergoing IVF-ET at Yale demonstrates similar findings. The mean number of ova recovered per patient was significantly lower in women over 39 (4.5 ± 1.2) than in women 38 or younger (9.4 ± 2.1). The fertilization rates were not different between the groups, and consequently the number of embryos transferred was higher in the younger group (3.5 ± 0.4 vs. 2.0 ± 0.2). The pregnancy rate in the older age group was markedly reduced as compared to that in younger patients (8.8% versus 27.3%). The incidence of pregnancy wastage in the older group was also markedly higher (50% vs. 32%). It appears, therefore, that advancing age is associated with a decline in IVF-ET success. This decline is the result of a decrease in the number of embryos transferred and in the higher incidence of pregnancy wastage.

FSH levels

Although age appears to be a fairly good predictor of success, it is not uncommon to find significant variation in response to treatment and success among women of the same chronological age. The hallmark of biological aging is the slow deterioration in ovarian function. One should therefore search for markers of ovarian function and of ovarian reserve in order to improve the prediction of success.

One such marker that has been studied extensively is the serum level of FSH. Pituitary FSH secretion and subsequently serum FSH levels are under feedback control of hypothalamic and ovarian factors. Ovarian failure as occurs in menopause results in marked elevations of this peptide. Prior to frank ovarian failure, an increase in baseline FSH levels may signify a decline in ovarian reserve. Measurements of baseline (cycle day 1–5) serum levels of FSH have been explored as a potential predictor of the success of infertility therapy.

Scott et al. have grouped 758 consecutive cycles according to basal (cycle day 3) FSH levels (64). Patients with low basal FSH (< 15 mIU/ml) had higher pregnancy rates per attempt and higher ongoing pregnancy rates than those with moderate levels (15–25 mIU/ml), both of which fared better than those patients with high FSH (> 25 mIU/ml).

The process of ovarian failure appears to occur over extended periods. Elevations of baseline levels of FSH represent a marked deficiency in ovarian reserves. Prior to the elevations of baseline FSH, reduced ovarian reserve may be detected by provocative testing. Navot et al. have reported on the predictive value of a "clomiphene stimulation test" in determining the chances for conception (65). FSH levels at baseline (cycle day 2–3) and stimulated (cycle day 9–11) following administration of clomiphene citrate were evaluated in 51 women with unexplained infertility. Although all women had normal baseline FSH levels, 18 had an exaggerated response (26 mIU/ml or more) following clomiphene administration. This was regarded as diminished ovarian response. In this group, 1 of 18 conceived as compared to 14 of 33 in the normal response group.

In comparing age and FSH levels as predictors of IVF success, FSH levels rated higher. Younger women with elevated FSH levels did poorly, and older women with normal FSH levels did well (66).

In summary, elevations of baseline serum FSH levels are associated with poor reproductive performance and are more predictive of such performance than the woman's age. Basal FSH levels should be determined in any woman considering IVF, and the results should be used to counsel the couple on the chances of success. Recent reports on the high success rates in women over 40 receiving donor eggs open new avenues and opportunities for those women with failing ovaries. The full psychosocial impact of this procedure is yet to be determined.

Performance in previous cycles

The patient's performance in previous IVF cycles or in cycles of ovarian stimulation without IVF can also predict her response to ovarian stimulation during the IVF-ET cycles and thus her likelihood to achieve a successful pregnancy with IVF. As a rule, the initial response to therapy will repeat in future cycles. Therefore, the patient's past performance on hMG, non-IVF cycles can be used to gauge the likelihood of a favorable response. This information should also be used in counseling the couple regarding the likelihood of success. A "low-response" pattern in which follicular development is poor despite high doses of ovulatory drugs is likely to repeat on future attempts and, as a rule, is associated with poor prognosis. Changes in stimulation regimens in this group of poor responders may improve the response to stimulation but may not increase the rate of success. Even the use of GnRHa in this group of poor responders appears not to improve the prospects of success (67).

The etiology of low response is not always clear. In some cases baseline elevations of FSH can be docu-mented while in others stimulation tests are required to demonstrate the decreased ovarian reserve. In the majority of low responders, however, no underlying cause can be demonstrated. Recent reports on the role of growth hormone (GH) in enhancing ovarian response to hMG may suggest a role for this and other related substances in the modulation of ovarian response to therapy.

Patient selection

Pre-IVF evaluation

Prior to their IVF-ET cycle, the couple should be evaluated thoroughly to exclude conditions that may have been overlooked and can either interfere with the IVF-ET procedure or be treated by other modalities. Following the initial evaluation, a profile can be created of the individual couple that can predict their likelihood of success.

The initial visits are also used to educate patients and provide information regarding the IVF process and the details of ovarian stimulation, egg retrieval, and embryo transfer. Before being accepted into a program, the couple should be interviewed by a social worker or psychologist. For many couples IVF-ET is the final step in a long road of infertility evaluation and therapy, and thus the last hope for fertility. The psychological impact of the IVF-ET cycle can therefore be quite significant, and proper counseling should be available.

How many cycles should be attempted?

The relatively low success rate in a single cycle of IVF-ET underscores the importance of assessment of success on repeat cycles. Couples who are considering their first attempt and those who have been through several unsuccessful trials often ponder over the logic of returning for repeat cycles.

The data reported from various programs of thousands of cycles of ova retrievals clearly show that the great majority of pregnancies (more than 90%) are achieved within the first four attempts (68–71). Due to smaller numbers of patients who have undergone more than four cycles, the data to allow for assessment of success rates after the first four cycles are not available.

Life table analyses have been used in several large series to examine the success of repeat cycles. Padilla et al. (68) have reviewed records of 512 patients who underwent 1001 egg retrievals. The majority of pregnancies occurred in the first or second attempt, with 94% of the pregnancies in the first four cycles; however, the probability of pregnancy on the seventh cycle was unchanged at 23%. The authors concluded that the clinical pregnancy rates were not different after multiple attempts. Other studies using life table analysis reported similar findings.

As life table analysis may not be applicable to IVF-ET results, other models have been developed. Data from our program for 1257 IVF-ET cycles were analyzed and used to develop such a model. In our patient population, the pregnancy rate declined from 13% on the first attempt to 4.8% on the fifth attempt. No pregnancy was conceived after the fifth treatment cycle (72).

On the basis of these findings, we are currently discouraging couples from attempting more than four treatment cycles. The difference between our data and those reported from other programs, which show no change in pregnancy rate across treatment cycles, may be attributed to different practices that are used to allow patients to continue.

Setting a threshold number of allowable cycles based on this model allows one to minimize waiting time with minimal impact on the probability of achieving pregnancy. This may have significant economic impact and allow for maximal utilization of the program (71).

Alternatives

Patients about to be enrolled into IVF programs should be well informed regarding other options available to them. Those options include other assisted reproductive techniques and other forms of therapy such as insemination, ovulation induction without IVF, and surgery. A comparison between these methods and IVF with regard to morbidity, the success rates, and cost has been reviewed in other sections and should be discussed with the couple.

One of the consequences of the simplification of the IVF-ET procedure has been the tendency to use it earlier in the course of therapy. IVF-ET is no longer used as a method of last resort after all other therapies have failed but, rather, as a successful and minimally invasive method that, even if unsuccessful, can provide important information on fertilization, egg and sperm interaction, and help in planning a future approach. It is therefore not uncommon for couples with moderate tubal disease to undergo an IVF-ET cycle followed by more conventional therapy of their infertility disorder.

Adoption

In this era of almost endless variations on the theme of infertility therapy, one should not forget the couple that has reached the end of the road. The assessment of the point in time when a couple should abandon further attempts should be individualized to the couple, taking into consideration the predictive factors described above as well as assessment of their mental and emotional resources. When patients are encouraged to abandon further attempts, alternatives should be offered. Adoption or a childless relationship are offered as appropriate. The final decision will be made by the couple.

Conclusion

IVF-ET has undergone dramatic changes during the first decade of its existence. The procedure has become more successful and at the same time simpler and less invasive. These factors have greatly expanded the use of IVF-ET in the already existing indications. In addition, novel applications utilizing micromanipulation technology in conjunction with the new genetics hold great promise for IVF-ET in areas of prenatal-preimplantation diagnosis, therapy of male infertility, and probably some new and yet unforeseen indications.

References

1. Ron-El R, Herman A, Golan A, Nachum H, Soffer Y, Caspi E. Gonadotropin and combined gonadotropin-releasing hormone agonist—gonadotropin protocols in a randomized prospective study. Fertil Steril 1991;55(3):574–582.

2. Meldrum DR, Wisot A, Hamilton F, Gutlay AL, Kempton W, Huynh D. Routine pituitary suppression with luprolide before ovarian stimulation for oocyte retrieval. Fertil Steril 1989;51:455–459.

3. Edwards RG, Steptoe PC, Purdy JM. Establishing full term human pregnancies using cleaving embryos grown in vitro. Br J Obstet Gynaecol 1980;87:737–756.

4. Jones HW Jr, Acosta AA, Andrews MC, Garcia JE. Three years of in vitro fertilization at Norfolk. Fertil Steril 1984;42:826–834.

5. Lopata A, Johnston I, Spiers A. In vitro fertilization. In: Garcia CR, Mastroianni L, Amelar RD, Dubin L, eds. Current therapy of infertility. Trenton, N.J.: BC Decker, 1982.

6. Muasher SJ, Garcia JE, Jones HW Jr. Experience with diethylstilbestrol-exposed infertile women in a program of in vitro fertilization. Fertil Steril 1984;42:20–24.

7. Medical Research International, Society of Assisted Reproductive Technology, American Fertility Society. In vitro fertilization–embryo transfer (IVF-ET) in the United States: 1989 results from the IVF-ET registry. Fertil Steril 1991; 55(1):14–23.

8. Mahadevan MM, Wiseman D, Leader A, Taylor PJ. The effect of ovarian adhesive disease upon follicular development in cycles of controlled stimulation for in vitro fertilization: Fertil Steril 1985;44:469–501.

9. Oehninger S, Scott R, Muasher SJ, Acosta AA, Jones HW Jr, Rosenwaks Z. Effects of the severity of tubo-ovarian disease and previous tubal surgery on the results of in vitro fertilization and embryo transfer. Fertil Steril 1989;51(1):126–130.

10. Cooperman AB, Lavy G, DeCherney AH, Diamond MP. The effect of tubal and ovarian surgery on ovarian function in cycles of controlled ovarian stimulation in patients undergoing in vitro fertilization. J Gynecol Surg 1990; 6(4):263–268.

11. Lilford RJ, Watson AJ. Has in-vitro fertilization made salpingostomy obsolete? Br J Obstet Gynaecol 1990; 97:557–560.

12. Dubois M, Stassen M, Hircourt M. Comparison between micro-surgery and IVF in the treatment of tubal infertility. Hum Reprod 1987;2:82–83.

13. Sharma V, Riddle A, Mason BA, Pampiglione J, Campbell S. An analysis of factors influencing the establishment of a clinical pregnancy in an ultrasound-based ambulatory in vitro fertilization program. Fertil Steril 1988;49:468–478.

14. Matson PL, Yovitch JL. The treatment of infertility associated with endometriosis by in vitro fertilization and embryo transfer. Fertil Steril 1986;46:432–434.

15. Wardle PG, Mitchell JD, McLaughlin EA, Ray BD, McDermott A, Hull MGR. Endometriosis and ovulatory disorders: reduced fertilization in vitro compared with tubal and unexplained infertility. Lancet 1985;2:236–239.

16. Damewood MD, Rock JA. Treatment independent pregnancy with operative laparoscopy for endometriosis in an in vitro fertilization program. Fertil Steril 1988;50:463–465.

17. Wardle PG, Foster PA, Mitchell JD, McLaughlin EA, McDermott A. Endometriosis and IVF: effect of prior therapy. Lancet 1986;1:276–277.

18. Wolf DP, Byrd W, Dandekar P, Quigley MM. Sperm concentration and the fertilization of human eggs in vitro. Biol Reprod 1984;31:837–848.

19. Mahadevan MM, Trounson AO, Leeton JF. The relationship of tubal blockage, infertility of an unknown cause, male infertility and endometriosis to success of in vitro fertilization and embryo transfer. Fertil Steril 1984;40:755–762.

20. Cohen J, Edwards R, Fehilly C, et al. In vitro fertilization: a treatment for male infertility. Fertil Steril 1985;43:422–432.

21. Hewitt J, Cohen J. Repeated pregnancies following in vitro fertilization therapy in cases of male infertility. Br J Urol 1985;57:484–485.

22. De Krester DM, Yates CA, McDonald J, et al. The use of in vitro fertilization in the management of male infertility. Presented at the Fifth Renier de Graf Symposium, 1985.

23. Rogers BJ. Examination of data from programs of in vitro fertilization in relation to sperm integrity and reproductive success. Prog Clin Biol Res 1989;302:69–89.

24. McDowell JS, Veeck LL, Jones HW. Analysis of human spermatozoa before and after processing for in vitro fertilization. J In Vitro Fert Embryo Transf 1985;2:23–26.

25. Russell LD, Rogers BJ. Improvement in the quality and fertilization potential of a human sperm population using the rise technique. J Androl 1987;8:25–33.

26. Lewinthal D, Furman A, Blankenstein J, Coreblum B, Shavlev J, Lunenfeld B. Subtle abnormalities in follicular development and hormonal profile in women with unexplained infertility. Fertil Steril 1986;46:833–839.

27. Rosseau S, Lord J, Lepage Y, Van Campenhout JV. The expectancy for pregnancy for "normal" infertile couples. Fertil Steril 1983;40:768–772.

28. Templeton AA, Penney GC. The incidence, characteristics, and prognosis of patients whose infertility is unexplained. Fertil Steril 1982;37:175–182.

29. Welner S, DeCherney AH, Polan ML. Human menopausal gonadotropin: a justifiable therapy in ovulatory women with long standing infertility. Am J Obstet Gynecol 1988;158:111–117.

30. Serhal PF, Katz M, Little V, Woronowski H. Unexplained infertility—the value of Pergonal superovulation combined with intrauterine insemination. Fertil Steril 1988;49:602–606.

31. Dodson WC, Whitesides DR, Hughes CL, Easley HA, Haney AF. Superovulation with intrauterine insemination in the treatment of infertility: a possible alternative to gamete intrafallopian transfer and in vitro fertilization. Fertil Steril 1987;48:441–445.

32. Navot D, Muasher SJ, Oehninger S, et al. The value of in vitro fertilization for the treatment of unexplained infertility. Fertil Steril 1988;49(5):854–857.

33. Mengle AC, Black CS. The effect of antisera on human sperm penetration of zona-free hamster ova. Fertil Steril 1979;32:214–218.

34. Yovich JL, Kay D, Stranger JD, Boettcher B. In vitro fertilization in women with serum antisperm antibodies. Lancet 1984;1:369–370.

35. Clarke GN, Lopata A, Jhonston WIH. Effect of sperm antibodies in females on human in vitro fertilization. Fertil Steril 1986;46:435–441.

36. Mandelbaum SL, Diamond MP, DeCherney AH. Relationship of antisperm antibodies to oocyte fertilization in in vitro fertilization–embryo transfer. Fertil Steril 1987;47:644–651.

37. Clarke GN, Lopata A, McBain JC, Baker HWG, Jhonston WIH. Effect of antisperm antibodies in males in human in vitro fertilization (IVF). Am J Reprod Immunol Microbiol 1985;8:62–66.

38. Junk SM, Matson PL, Yovich JM, Boostma B, Yovich JL. The fertilization of human oocytes by spermatozoa from men with antispermatozoal antibodies in semen. J In Vitro Fert Embryo Transf 1986;3:350–352.

39. Kaufman RH, Binder GL, Gray PM Jr, Adam E. Upper genital tract changes associated with exposure in utero to diethylstilbestrol. Am J Obstet Gynecol 1977;128:51–59.

40. Kaufman RH, Adams E, Noller K, Irwin JF, Gray M. Upper genital tract changes and infertility in diethylstilbestrol exposed women. Am J Obstet Gynecol 1986;154:1312–1318.

41. Barnes AB, Colton T, Gunderson J, et al. Fertility and outcome of pregnancy on women exposed in utero to diethylstilbestrol. N Engl J Med 1980;302:609–613.

42. Cousins L, Karp W, Lacey C, Lucas WE. Reproductive outcome of women exposed to diethylstilbestrol in utero. Obstet Gynecol 1980;56:70–76.

43. Herbst AL, Hubby MM, Blough RR, Azizi F. A comparison of pregnancy experience in DES-exposed and DES-unexposed daughters. J Reprod Med 1980;24:62.

44. Muasher S, Garcia JE, Jones HW. Experience with diethylstilbestrol-exposed women in a program of in vitro fertilization. Fertil Steril 1984;42:20–25.

45. Krandle VC, Lester RG, Muasher SJ, Jones DL, Acosta AA, Jones HW Jr. Are implantation and pregnancy outcome impaired in diethylstilbestrol-exposed women after in vitro fertilization and embryo transfer? Fertil Steril 1990; 54(2):287–291.

46. Gordon K, Ruddle FH. Gene transfer into mouse embryos. Manipulation of Mammalian Development 1986;1.

47. Markert CL. Fertilization of mammalian eggs by sperm injection. J Exp Zool 1983;228:195–203.

48. Gordin JW, Grunfeld L, Garrissi GJ, Talansky BE, Richards C, Laufer N. Fertilization of human oocytes by sperm from infertile males after zona pellucida drilling. Fertil Steril 1988;50:68–73.

49. Ng SC, Bongso TA, Chang SI, Sathananthan AH, Ratnam SS. Transfer of human sperm into the perivitelline space of human oocytes after zona-drilling or zona-puncture. Fertil Steril 1989;52.

50. Malter HE, Cohen J. Partial zona dissection of the human oocyte: a non-traumatic method using micromanipulation to assist zona pellucida penetration. Fertil Steril 1989;51(1):139–148.

51. Rawlins RG, Binor Z, Radwanska E, Dmowski WP. Microsurgical enucleation of tripronuclear human zygotes. Fertil Steril 1988;50:266–272.

52. Kola I, Trounson A, Dawson G, Rogers P. Tripronuclear human oocytes: altered cleavage patterns and subsequent karyotypic analysis of embryos. Biol Reprod 1987;37:395–405.

53. McGrath J, Solter D. Nuclear transplantation in the mouse embryo by microsurgery and cell fusion. Science 1984;220:1300–1302.

54. Tsunoda Y, McLaren A. Effect of various procedures on the viability of mouse embryos containing half the normal number of blastomeres. J Reprod Fertil 1983;69:315–318.

55. Summers PM, Campbell JM, Miller MW. Normal in vivo development of marmoset monkey embryos after trophectoderm biopsy. Hum Reprod 1988;3:389–394.

56. Palmiter RD, Brinster RL, Hammer RE, et al. Dramatic growth of mice that develop from eggs microinjected with metallothionein–growth hormone fusion gene. Nature 1982;300:611.

57. Tietze C. Reproductive span and rate of reproduction among Hutterite women. Fertil Steril 1957;8:89–97.

58. Stovall DW, Toma SK, Hammond MG, Talbert LM. The effect of age on female fecundity. Obstet Gynecol 1991;77(1):33–36.

59. Penzias AS, Thompson IE, Alper MM, Oskowitz SP, Berger MJ. Successful use of gamete intrafallopian transfer does not reverse the decline in fertility in women over 40 years of age. Obstet Gynecol 1991;77(1):37–39.

60. Craft I, Ah-Moye M, Al-Shawaf T. Analysis of 1071 GIFT procedures: the case for a flexible approach to treatment. Lancet 1988;1:1094–1098.

61. Cittadini E, Palermo R. Infertility in advanced reproductive age. Results of in vitro fertilization and embryo transfer according to the woman's age. Acta Eur Fertil 1989;20(5):285–297.

62. Sauer M, Paulson RJ, Lobo RA. A preliminary report on oocyte donation extending reproductive potential to women over 40. N Engl J Med 1990;323(17):1157–1160.

63. Levran D, Dor J, Rudak E, Nebel L, Ben-Shlomo I, Ben-Raphael Z, Mashiach S. Pregnancy potential of human oocytes—the effect of cryopreservation. N Engl J Med 1990;323(17):1153–1156.

64. Scott RT, Toner JP, Muasher SJ, Oehninger S, Robinson S, Rosenwaks Z. Follicle-stimulating hormone levels on cycle day 3 are predictive of in vitro fertilization outcome. Fertil Steril 1989;51(4):651–654.

65. Navot D, Rosenwaks Z, Margalioth EJ. Prognostic assessment of female fecundity. Lancet 1987;2(8560): 645–647.

66. Toner JP, Karande V, Jones GS, Muasher SJ. Basal follicle stimulating hormone (FSH) levels is a better predictor of in vitro fertilization performance than age. Presented at the 46th Annual Meeting of the American Fertility Society, Washington, D.C., October 1990.

67. Lavy G, Grifo J, Im D, Comite F, Holm C. GnRH-a in low and poor responders to gonadotropin ovarian stimulation. Presented at the 45th Annual Meeting of the American Fertility Society, San Francisco, Calif., 1989.

68. Padilla SL, Garcia JE. The effect of maternal age and number of in vitro fertilization procedures on pregnancy outcome. Fertil Steril 1989;52:270–281.

69. Guzik DS, Wilkes C, Jones HW. Cumulative pregnancy rates for in vitro fertilization. Fertil Steril 1986;46: 663–667.

70. Bustillo M, Bhattarai S, Munabi AK, Bender S, Dorfman A, Schulman JD. Life table analysis of pregnancy attainment in an IVF program exclusively using ultrasound-guided follicle retrieval. Presented at the Sixth World Congress of In Vitro Fertilization and Alternate Assisted Reproduction, 1989.

71. Kaplan EH, Hershlag A, DeCherney AH, Lavy G. To be or not to be? That is conception! Managing in vitro fertilization programs. Management Sci 1991.

72. Hershlag A, Kaplan EH, Loy RA, DeCherney AH, Lavy G. Heterogeneity in patient population explains differences in in vitro fertilization programs. Fertil Steril 1991;56: 913–917.

4

Gamete Intrafallopian Transfer, Zygote Intrafallopian Transfer, Tubal Embryo Transfer, and Beyond

Louis N. Weckstein
Ricardo H. Asch

Introduction

Gamete intrafallopian transfer (GIFT) was proposed in 1984 as a new infertility treatment (1). GIFT provides a greater degree of "naturalness" than in vitro fertilization (IVF) and is also more acceptable in some religious circles. IVF was originally designed as therapy for patients with severely damaged or absent fallopian tubes (2); however, more recently its use has been extended to other etiologies of infertility. A significant number of these patients have normal tubes, theoretically capable of normal embryo transport. The GIFT technique ensures that oocytes and capacitated sperm meet at the normal site of fertilization and then allows for a favorable milieu for early embryonic development.

Advantages of tubal over uterine transfer include 1) a possible benefit to the early embryos of the tubal environment, 2) a more appropriate time of entry of the embryos into the uterine cavity (possibly of importance with regard to hyperstimulation's effect on the enometrium), and 3) avoidance of the trauma to the endometrium of a uterine transfer. Disadvantages include 1) failure to obtain knowledge regarding the sperm's ability to fertilize the egg (this knowledge would be available if there are supernumerary oocytes), and 2) possible placement of gametes in suboptimally functioning fallopian tubes. This chapter will discuss in detail all aspects of tubal transfer.

Gamete intrafallopian transfer

Research in primates

Initial attempts to achieve intrafallopian fertilization and pregnancy in nonhuman primates began in 1977 in the laboratory of Ricardo H. Asch at the Department of Obstetrics and Gynecology, University of Texas, at San Antonio. Ten regularly cycling animals underwent intrafallopian insemination using unwashed sperm within 24 hours of spontaneous ovulation. Early on only a few pregnancies occurred, and most of the initial frustrations originated in the lack of knowledge regarding preparation of the monkey's sperm specimens obtained by electroejaculation. A few cases of intratubal inseminations performed in humans during diagnostic laparoscopies at the preovulary stage in 1977 resulted in no pregnancies; however, they showed how simple the technique of catheterizing the fallopian tube was (R. H. Asch and J. E. Martin, unpublished data). Major progress was slow until 1984, when insight was gained from in vitro fertilization techniques. Using a stimulated cycle and a human chorionic gonadotropin (hCG) trigger, laparotomy, follicular aspiration, and GIFT were carried out in rhesus monkeys. Semen was prepared with an in vitro technique. Pregnancy occurred in 40% of this group, although there was a high rate of spontaneous miscarriage (3). These initial encouraging results paved the way for GIFT attempts in humans, culminating in the initial report in 1984 (1).

Patient selection

The GIFT technique was initially proposed for patients with idiopathic infertility. Indications for its use have, however, been extended to include almost every etiology for infertility other than complete tubal obstruction. All patients considered for GIFT must have demonstration of tubal patency either by hysterosalpingogram or laparoscopy. Some authors have advocated using a laparoscopic GIFT cycle for diagnostic as well as therapeutic purposes (4,5). Patients with a history of more than 2 years of infertility, with a normal semen analysis, and with a previous hysterosalpingogram demonstrating at least one patent tube were offered a stimulation cycle combined with laparoscopy and GIFT. Pregnancy rates of 24% and 32% were reported.

Evaluation of the male factor is critical prior to accepting a couple for GIFT. In our center, if the following basic criteria are met following preparation of a semen sample, the male factor is deemed appropriate for GIFT: 1) recovery of more than 1.5 million total motile sperm, 2) a sperm motility progression of at least 2–3, and 3) at least 30% normal sperm morphology. We do not require a hamster sperm penetration assay (SPA) in our patients; however, if they have failed an SPA, we do not recommend GIFT initially.

In our center, couples with recalcitrant infertility who have failed to conceive after three to four cycles of controlled ovarian hyperstimulation and intrauterine insemination, with at least one normal fallopian tube and sperm criteria as outlined above, are appropriate GIFT candidates.

Chronology of a GIFT cycle

Once a couple's fertility status has been evaluated and they are deemed appropriate candidates for GIFT, a series of steps are carried out for the GIFT cycle.

Controlled ovarian hyperstimulation: A number of different treatment regimens may be used to recruit multiple follicles (see Chapter 1, Controlled Ovarian Hyperstimulation: Physiology, Techniques, and Controversy). Most commonly in our institution we utilize a combination of gonadotropin-releasing hormone agonist (GnRHa), begun in the luteal phase, and human menopausal gonadotropins (hMG), or a combination of clomiphene citrate (CC) and hMG. Follicular maturation is assessed by periodic vaginal ultrasounds and serum estradiol (E_2) levels. Human chorionic gonadotropin at 10,000 IU is given when a minimum of two or three follicles have a maximal diameter of at least 20 mm when utilizing the GnRHa-hMG protocol, and when the lending follicle has a maximum diameter of 18 mm with the CC-hMG protocol. Oocyte retrieval is carried out 34 to 36 hours after hCG injection. If a GIFT cycle is cancelled (endogenous luteinizing hormone surge), intrauterine insemination is performed (6).

Oocyte retrieval: Oocyte retrieval may be carried out by transvaginal ultrasound guidance, laparoscopy, or minilaparotomy. We routinely aspirate oocytes by transvaginal ultrasound guidance even though GIFT requires a laparoscopy or minilaparotomy. We do this for a number of reasons. First, we are able to assess oocyte maturity before committing the patient to a more major surgical procedure. If oocytes are immature, GIFT is not carried out, and the oocytes are later fertilized, and if good quality embryos develop, tubal embryo transfer (TET) is subsequently carried out (7). This policy is based on data demonstrating that the pregnancy rate is higher in GIFT cycles when only mature oocytes are used (8). Retrieval of oocytes in this way spares the patient an unnecessary surgical procedure with minimal chance of success. Second, we obtain a higher number of oocytes by transvaginal ultrasound retrieval. Third, the oocytes are exposed to the potential deleterious effects of carbon dioxide during laparoscopy for a shorter period of time utilizing transvaginal retrieval. Last, during transvaginal ultrasound-guided aspiration, usually only one puncture is performed within the surface of the ovary, reducing the amount of hemoperitoneum.

Sperm preparation: Semen is obtained by masturbation 2 hours prior to the procedure. Samples are prepared by a swim-up (9) or Percoll sedimentation technique (10). Prior to acceptance of the couple for the GIFT procedure, a semen sample is analyzed and prepared in order to determine which technique is most suitable for the sample. Some authors have suggested the use of follicular fluid to capacitate the semen (11,12). If at least 1.5 million total motile sperm with a progression of 2–3 or greater and at least 30% normal morphology are not recovered, we feel TET is a more appropriate procedure than GIFT (13). Once the sperm are prepared, 100,000 to 500,000 motile sperm are utilized for the GIFT procedure.

GIFT procedure: The actual GIFT procedure is carried out by either laparoscopy or minilaparotomy. Though we initially described the procedure by laparoscopy, and this is the technique most commonly utilized worldwide, many GIFT procedures are still performed in our center by minilaparotomy via a 3 cm suprapubic incision. It is often easier to deliver the gametes deep into the tube in a quick, atraumatic fashion via minilaparotomy. Some clinicians have suggested that performing GIFT via laparoscopy allows concomitant laparoscopic treatment of endometriosis or adhesions without affecting the pregnancy rate. Rodriquez-Rigau et al. reported on a series of 324 GIFT cycles in which 157 underwent laparoscopic laser treatment for adhesions or endometriosis at the time of GIFT (14). There was no difference in pregnancy rates or ectopic pregnancy rates between GIFT cases with and those without laser treatment. Corson et al. reported similar results in 92 GIFT cycles (15). A Tomcat catheter (Sovereign Tomcat 8890-704003; Monoject Division, Sherwood Medical, St. Louis, Mo.) with a 1 cc Hamilton syringe is used for minilaparotomy transfer. A Marrs GIFT catheter with a 1 cc Hamilton syringe is used for laparoscopic transfer. The catheter is loaded with two to four oocytes and at least 100,000 sperm in a total volume of 50 μl or less. If both tubes appear normal, transfer is carried out to each tube. If one tube is difficult to cannulate, transfer is made to the good tube only. Generally, three to five oocytes in total are transferred depending on the patient's age, oocyte maturity, and so forth. If possible, gametes are transferred at least 3 to 4 cm into the fimbriated end of the tube (16). It is important to maintain good temperature control of the oocytes while awaiting transfer to the fallopian tube. Oocytes should not be removed from the incubator until it is ensured that rapid cannulation of the fallopian tubes will be possible. A study reported by Pickering et al. noted a significant disruption of oocyte spindle structure when cooling the oocyte to room temperature for as little as 10 minutes (17).

Follow-up after transfer: Patients are discharged the day of the procedure. The luteal phase is supported with 50 mg of progesterone intramuscularly daily. Serum βhCG beta human chorionic gonadrotropin is obtained 14 days after transfer, and if pregnancy occurs progesterone is continued until 6 weeks after transfer.

Results

The United States In Vitro Fertilization–Embryo Transfer (IVF-ET) Registry recently reported results for 1989 as a clinical pregnancy rate of 30% per GIFT cycle and a live delivery rate of 23% per GIFT cycle (18). Reported rates for IVF for the same time were an 18% clinical pregnancy rate per retrieval and a 14% live delivery rate per retrieval. These differences are highly significant in favor of GIFT, although the patient populations may be slightly different. However, recent information showed no difference in success rates when assisted reproductive technology (ART) procedures are performed in women with different etiologies of infertility.

The Multinational Cooperative Study (MCS) on GIFT reported on 2092 GIFT cycles with a 28.7% clinical pregnancy rate (19). There was a 16.8% miscarriage rate, a 3.9% ectopic pregnancy rate, and a 15.4% multiple birth rate. Results by etiology are listed in Table 4.1.

Unexplained infertility: GIFT was originally proposed as a treatment for cases of idiopathic infertility. Possible factors involved in idiopathic infertility include failure of

tubal pick-up of the oocyte after ovulation, luteinization of follicles without extrusion of the oocyte, and alteration in sperm transport. The GIFT technique overcomes all these potential factors, delivering a high number of capacitated sperm and oocytes to the site of fertilization, the midampullary portion of the fallopian tube. Pregnancy rates for unexplained infertility in large series have been reported as 31% to 36% (18–20). The MCS reported a 31% pregnancy rate for 796 cases of unexplained infertility (19).

Endometriosis: The second most common indication for GIFT is endometriosis. This is, of course, only applicable if there is access to at least one patent fallopian tube. Some theories for the effect of endometriosis on fertility include failure of tubal oocyte pick-up and phagocytosis of sperm, both of which may be overcome with GIFT. Pregnancy rates for endometriosis range from 20% to 33% (18–20).

Male factor: Results of GIFT in male factor patients vary widely, based on a varying definition of male

Table 4.1 Multinational Cooperative Study on GIFT: results by etiology

Etiology	No. of cases	No. of pregnancies	Success (%)
1. Unexplained infertility	796	247	31
2. Male factor	397	61	15
3 Endometriosis	413	132	32
4. Failed AID	160	66	41
5. Tubal peritoneal	210	61	29
6. Cervical	68	19	28
7. Immunologic	30	5	16
8. Premature ovarian failure	18	10	56
Total	2092	601	28.7

factor. Results reported from large studies range from 15% to 33% (18–20). If male factor is considered to be anything below the normal semen parameters according to the World Health Organization (count $> 20 \times 10^6$/ml, motility $> 60\%$, morphology $> 70\%$ normal), then GIFT may have a very high success rate. Wiedemann et al. reported on 65 cases of GIFT in male subfertility (21). They found that male factor only became significant with GIFT below a sperm density of 10×10^6/ml, and/or less than 30% motility, and/or less than 30% normal morphology. Males with semen parameters above these levels had pregnancy rates equal to those of couples with unexplained infertility.

Cittadini et al. have proposed the criterion for acceptance for GIFT of 1.5×10^6/ml spermatozoa with grade 3–4 motility after a 30 minute swim-up (22). This was based on observations of subfertile males in IVF programs and on the lack of GIFT pregnancies in patients with semen parameters below these levels (small numbers). Even above this cutoff, they found a significant difference in pregnancy rate between oligoasthenospermic and normospermic men (19.7% vs. 35.2%) (23). They further analyzed their data and found that two groups emerged. Men with fewer than 8×10^6/ml sperm with forward progressive motility in an untreated ejaculate had a significantly lower pregnancy rate with GIFT (15.3% vs. 26.2%).

Matson et al. noted poor initial results with GIFT and oligospermia infertility when transferring 100,000 motile sperm per tube (24). They therefore proposed a modified GIFT technique, transferring a minimum of 325,000 motile sperm in cases of oligospermia infertility. They have since recommended pronuclear stage tubal transfer (PROST) or tubal embryo transfer (TET) in cases of significant male factor.

Contradictory data have been reported by Khan et al. (25). They varied sperm concentration transferred with GIFT from 100,000/ml to 2500/ml and found no significant difference in pregnancy rates. Even couples with so-called andrologic infertility (not defined) did not have a lower pregnancy rate until a concentration of 2500/ml was reached. This may be because these cases did not represent a severe male factor.

In an analysis of our first 218 GIFT cycles, we found that sperm and egg factors were the main variables having a strong association with pregnancy (8). Sperm motility of 50% or less was associated with significantly lower pregnancy rates. GIFT seems to be an appropriate treatment for mild cases of male subfertility. These couples appear to have a pregnancy rate equivalent to that of couples with unexplained infertility. We use a cutoff of 1.5 million total motile sperm with a progression of 2–3 and more than 30% normal morphology to choose appropriate GIFT candidates. Below these criteria we prefer to do TET to evaluate fertilization prior to tubal transfer.

Rodriquez-Rigau et al. reported that no clinical pregnancies were achieved if GIFT was performed with a total motile sperm count below 5 million, while chemical pregnancies occurred with total motile sperm counts of 1.3 million (26). Sperm counts were directly correlated with incidence of pregnancy, this being almost doubled when counts were above 30×10^6/ml as compared with those below 10×10^6/ml. Interestingly, percentage of motility and morphology were not correlated with occurrence of pregnancy.

Al-Shawaf et al. reported three cases in which cryopreserved spermatozoa from men having been treated for lymphomas or testicular tumors were used for GIFT (27). Three pregnancies were obtained out of four cycles of GIFT. Their conclusion was that men with malignant tumors that require intensive chemotherapy or radiotherapy should be counseled regarding cryopreservation of sperm for future use, and that GIFT should be a treatment of choice due to the high success rate.

Immunologic infertility: Most early reports of GIFT in couples with antisperm antibodies were disappointing. The MCS reported a 16% pregnancy rate for 30 GIFT cycles with immunological infertility (19). Cittadini and Cimino reported one pregnancy in 22 GIFT cycles (4.5%) with female antisperm antibodies and five pregnancies in 25 GIFT cycles (20%) pretreated with steroids (28). No pregnancies were obtained in 15 GIFT cycles with male antisperm antibodies, and four pregnancies were reported in 23 GIFT cycles (17%) pretreated with steroids.

It seems logical that GIFT would have a poor success rate in cases of female antisperm antibodies. These antibodies are probably not only in the serum but also in the fallopian tube fluid, and therefore may affect fertilization in a GIFT cycle. It seems less likely that male antisperm antibodies should negatively affect GIFT success even if the semen is quickly and thoroughly washed. Van der Merwe et al. have reported a 41% pregnancy rate (12 of 29 GIFT cycles) in cases of male sperm autoimmunity (29). Most of these male patients had otherwise completely normal semen parameters.

Currently we recommend TET in cases of female immunologic infertility in order to achieve fertilization outside the antibody environment. Further studies are needed to confirm the results of van der Merwe with GIFT and male autoimmunity.

Tubal/pelvic factor: One of the originally described prerequisites for a GIFT cycle has been at least one patent fallopian tube. Most clinicians will not perform GIFT in a patent tube that appears abnormal. Similarly most clinicians feel that previous surgery on a fallopian tube, such as for an ectopic pregnancy or neosalpingostomy and even tubal reanastamosis, is a contraindication to GIFT. The fear in these cases is that either the tube will not function normally for gamete transport and the procedure will be unsuccessful or an ectopic pregnancy will result.

Smith et al. reported a study comparing outcome of gamete or embryo transfer in patients with normal tubes with that in patients with severely damaged but patent tubes (30). Patients with damaged fallopian tubes had previous salpingitis, pelvic adhesive disease, or surgically repaired tubes. They found no significant difference in the overall pregnancy rate between the two groups (39% for normal tubes and 46% for damaged tubes), but a higher delivery rate in patients with normal tubes (25% vs. 11%). They stated no significant difference in ectopic pregnancies (9% vs. 15%), but one may wonder whether some pregnancies termed miscarriages may have been undiscovered ectopic pregnancies. This uncertainty aside, an 11% live birth rate from GIFT cycles in patients with damaged fallopian tubes is no better than pregnancy rates with IVF, and until further data to the contrary are available, tubal transfer should not be performed routinely in patients with abnormal tubes.

Limited data also exist in cases where fallopian tubes are normal, but there is a significant amount of pelvic adhesions or endometriosis or both. Rodriquez-Rigau et al. reported on a series of 324 GIFT procedures and compared pregnancy rates in patients with pelvic adhesions, endometriosis, or a normal pelvis (14). They found no significant difference in pregnancy rates between the three groups. However, the incidence of ectopic pregnancy was higher in both the pelvic adhesion and the endometriosis groups and was much higher in patients with both endometriosis and pelvic adhesions. Also pregnancy rates were no different for severe versus mild endometriosis. Holtz et al. recently reported performing GIFT in patients at risk for ectopic pregnancies (31). Patients at risk included those with a prior history of an ectopic pregnancy and those who had undergone previous tubal surgery (reanastamosis, salpingostomy) with excellent postoperative tubal status. Eight pregnancies resulted from 24 GIFT cycles in these patients (33%). The authors state that only one pregnancy was an ectopic pregnancy; however, there were also three "biochemical pregnancies" (hCG titers < 500 mIU/ml). The live birth rate was 17% per transfer. Once again one has to wonder whether some of the "biochemical pregnancies" were actually aborting ectopic pregnancies. Also a 17% live birth rate is not much better than that achieved with IVF in many centers worldwide.

Similarly Fakih and Harris reported on the efficiency of GIFT in the treatment of advanced periadnexal disease due to endometriosis when at least one fallopian tube is accessible for cannulation (32). In 152 GIFT procedures, they found excellent pregnancy rates in all stages of endometriosis with no significant difference when comparing stages. In addition, they did not find an increased incidence of ectopic pregnancy. It therefore seems reasonable to perform GIFT in cases of endometriosis or pelvic adhesions in which the fallopian tubes appear normal. These patients may, however, be at increased risk for developing an ectopic pregnancy.

GIFT and artificial insemination with donor semen: Many women are requesting artificial insemination with donor semen (AID). Success rates with cryopreserved donor semen are approximately 10% per cycle. A significant number of women, however, will not conceive after multiple cycles (20%–25%). Some of these patients may not conceive because of a defect in sperm transport to the site of fertilization, or because of a defect in oocyte expulsion or oocyte tubal pick-up. GIFT has been proposed as a method to circumvent these defects in gamete transport in women with multiple failed AID cycles (33). In our initial report, 48 women who had undergone multiple (9–24) cycles of AID without success underwent GIFT cycles with donor sperm. Of

the 48 women, 27 (56%) conceived in just one single GIFT attempt. Since that report we have continued to have a 50% clinical pregnancy rate with GIFT in women with failed AID.

Pilikian et al. reported that when using GIFT after failed AID with cryopreserved donor sperm, the overall pregnancy rate was 26.8% per cycle (34). Of interest, 64% of all the pregnancies occurred during the first GIFT attempt.

Fromigli et al. showed that in a group of 106 women undergoing GIFT with donor sperm, after failure of conception with conventional AID for an average of 11 cycles, the pregnancy rate was 52% per each single GIFT attempt (35).

Kirby et al. demonstrated that pregnancy rates in similar groups of patients that previously failed to conceive with donor insemination was 66% with GIFT using donor sperm (36).

Because success with cryopreserved donor semen is somewhat less over a long period of time as compared with statistics with fresh donor semen, many would argue to use a more aggressive approach in these couples. We are currently using clomiphene citrate and washed intrauterine insemination (IUI) with the cryopreserved donor sperm for three to six cycles (depending on the patient's age and other factors). If the patient fails to conceive, we will then use hMG and IUI AID for an additional three cycles. In patients who still have not conceived, GIFT AID is considered. Because of the low cycle fecundity with cryopreserved donor sperm and the increasingly high cost of cryopreserved semen, we feel that an aggressive approach is reasonable.

GIFT in women age 40 and older: It is clear that in women reproductive efficiency decreases with age. Cycle fecundity in women 40 years of age and older is markedly decreased. It is important to know how best to counsel these infertile women with regard to the best approach in ART. In 1987, the Norfolk group reported on 29 women age 40 and older who underwent IVF with a pregnancy rate of 23% per cycle, but an ongoing pregnancy rate of 12% per cycle (37). Most investigators, however, have found poorer overall pregnancy rates in IVF cycles in this age group. Statistics from the 1989 IVF-ET Registry in the United States reported a 12% clinical pregnancy rate and a 6% live birth rate in women age 40 and older (18). A 20% clinical pregnancy rate and an 8% live birth rate were reported for GIFT.

Kerin et al. reported on the effect of maternal age on results of IVF and GIFT cycles in 1987 (38). They found a 17% clinical pregnancy rate (13% live birth rate) in GIFT cycles and a 5% clinical pregnancy rate (5% live birth rate) in IVF cycles in women 40 and older. In more than 190 GIFT procedures performed on women 40 and above, Craft and Brisden reported a 19% clinical pregnancy rate with a 10% live birth rate (20). Penzias et al. reported a 9.6% clinical pregnancy rate in 73 GIFT cycles in women 40 and older (39). Their pregnancy rate for GIFT in women under 40, however, was only 27.3%.

Our own results with ART for women aged 40 and above support the efficacy of GIFT over IVF in this age group (40). We analyzed the results of 136 transfer cycles in women aged 40 and older. Clinical pregnancy rates were 31% for GIFT cycles, 45% for TET cycles, and 9% for IVF transfers. The abortion rate in this age group was 48% and 60% for tubal and uterine transfers, respectively. The "take home baby" rate for tubal transfers (19.7%) versus uterine transfers (3.6%) was statistically significantly different ($p < 0.01$).

In women 40 years of age and older who have normal fallopian tubes, tubal gamete or embryo transfer appears to be advantageous over uterine transfer. These women need to be aware, however, of the high rate of abortion in their age group. Because of the high success rate with oocyte donation, these women should be counseled as to that possibility, and if they are repeatedly unsuccessful with their own oocytes, consideration should be given to oocyte donation.

Unilateral versus bilateral GIFT: The initial protocol for the GIFT procedure described transfer of gametes to both fallopian tubes. This is the method most commonly used; however, recent reports in the literature suggest that unilateral gamete transfer is at least as good as bilateral gamete transfer (31). Haines and O'Shea compared results from unilateral versus bilateral tubal transfer (41). Unilateral transfer was performed because one tube was absent, was difficult to cannulate, or was felt to be abnormal. The pregnancy rate was 25% in 110 bilateral GIFT transfers of three or four oocytes compared with a pregnancy rate of 57% in 14 cases of unilateral GIFT transfers using three or four oocytes. Though numbers were small, this was still statistically significant. A more recent follow-up report from the same authors compared the pregnancy rate in 142 bilateral GIFT transfers with that in 112 unilateral GIFT transfers (42). There was no statistically significant difference in pregnancy rates with unilateral versus bilateral transfer. The authors state that unilateral GIFT may be preferable because it decreases operating and anesthetic time and reduces chances of fimbrial damage that may influence future GIFT attempts.

Yee et al. also compared results from unilateral and bilateral GIFT (16). The pregnancy rate was 38% in 101 unilateral GIFT transfers versus 26% in 145 bilateral GIFT transfers. These results were not, however, statistically significant.

Similarly we have found no difference in pregnancy rates when transferring gametes to one versus two fallopian tubes. If both tubes appear normal and are easily cannulated, we routinely transfer to both tubes. If one tube is abnormal or difficult to cannulate, we transfer only to the contralateral tube. One would think that if both tubes are normal and easy to cannulate, it would be preferable to transfer to both tubes in case some mechanical error occurred. However, if one tube appears to be much better than the other, gametes transferred to the abnormal tube may have little chance to reach the uterus, and hence unilateral transfer would be preferred.

Influence of intercourse/insemination: Marconi et al. reported on the effect of sexual intercourse on pregnancy rates in GIFT cycles (43). They performed a prospective randomized study in which one group was asked to have intercourse close to the time of hCG administration and the other group was asked to abstain. There were 13 clinical pregnancies in 16 patients in the intercourse group (81%) and five clinical pregnancies in 16 patients in the abstaining group (31%). Unfortunately little information was available in the patient population, and a control group of just ovarian stimulation and intercourse was lacking.

Tucker et al. compared pregnancy rates in GIFT cycles with and without postoperative intrauterine and intracervical insemination (postoperative IUI/ICI) (44). There were 38 clinical pregnancies in 102 standard GIFT cycles (37%) and 48 clinical pregnancies in 92 cycles with GIFT and postoperative IUI/ICI (52%).

Allowing sperm migration through the female reproductive tract may be important in two ways. First, it is reasonable to suspect that sperm capacitation is better accomplished within the female reproductive tract than in a test tube. These sperm may provide a reservoir of "back-up" spermatozoa that can, over time, reach any eggs placed by GIFT remaining unfertilized in the tubes. Second, there may be a "priming" effect on the endometrium of these extra migrating sperm that may enhance the chances of implantation.

It seems from these two reports that some additional sperm migration throughout the female reproductive tract is beneficial at the time of GIFT. However, whether intercourse or postoperative IUI/ICI is preferable remains unproved. It would seem logical that in couples with a normal postcoital test (sperm-mucus interaction), sexual intercourse may suffice, but in couples with a poor postcoital test, postoperative IUI/ICI may be preferable. Our present policy is to perform intraoperative ICI in all GIFT cycles.

Influence of egg maturity/number on success: Our first 218 GIFT cycles were analyzed to determine the relative contribution of different factors in predicting the likelihood of pregnancy from GIFT (8). The main variables having a strong association with pregnancy were sperm and egg parameters. Transfer of mature eggs is critical. In our laboratory egg maturity is classified on a 1 to 5 scale. Mature eggs with an expanded cumulus are given a grade 4, and those with an extruded polar body a grade 5. Eggs with a fully radiant corona are given a grade of 4+. When only eggs of grade 4+ or 5 were transferred, there was a significant direct association between number of eggs transferred and pregnancy rate. When no eggs of grade 4+ or 5 were transferred, the pregnancy rate was 16%. This increased to 25% when two eggs of grade 4+ or 5 were transferred and to 50% when three or more such eggs were transferred. Based on adds ratios calculated from multiple logistic analysis, pregnancy was 3.80 times more likely to occur if three or more fully mature eggs were transferred.

Penzias et al. assessed the optimal number of oocytes to transfer in a GIFT cycle (45). Their results did not take into account egg maturity. They reported that women who received four or more oocytes were three times more likely to achieve a clinical pregnancy than women receiving fewer than four oocytes. Transfer of five oocytes was superior to four oocytes, but there did not appear to be any advantage to transferring six or more eggs.

Because of the above data, we recommend transvaginal oocyte retrieval and then GIFT only if three or more mature eggs are obtained. If fewer than three mature eggs are retrieved, fertilization in vitro and subsequent IVF or TET is performed depending on the number and quality of embryos. We generally transfer three to five oocytes, but this is somewhat dependent on maturity of oocytes and the age of the patient.

Fertilization of supernumerary oocytes in GIFT cycles

Some controversy exists regarding the value of GIFT in the management of infertility because of its failure to provide information about fertilization. Some clinicians feel that a cycle of in vitro fertilization should precede a GIFT cycle to determine if, in fact, fertilization can occur. Others have suggested that since it is common to obtain more than four oocytes from a GIFT cycle, information could be obtained from attempted fertilization of supernumerary oocytes. A number of studies have now addressed this issue. In 1987 Quigley et al. reported on a small study of 16 patients who underwent a GIFT cycle with at least two oocytes transferred for GIFT and at least two oocytes inseminated in vitro (46). Of the 16 couples, only one achieved a pregnancy, and 50% of the couples had no oocytes fertilized in vitro. They concluded that the failure of fertilization of oocytes not used in GIFT allows "appropriate recommendations concerning future fertility management." It seems likely, however, that their poor results may have been due to the small number of oocytes used for the GIFT procedure and left for fertilization in vitro. Most other investigators disagree with their conclusion.

Matson et al. evaluated the value of fertilization in vitro of supernumerary oocytes to predict outcome of GIFT cycles (47). They found no correlation between fertilization of supernumerary oocytes and the likelihood of pregnancy from the GIFT cycle. They felt that

this was partly attributable to a low number of supernumerary oocytes. Similarly, McKenna et al. found that failure of fertilization of supernumerary oocytes is not crucial as a diagnostic procedure for male fertility (48). They suggested that the reason for this is the poorer quality of oocytes left for insemination. Their data demonstrated that the best oocytes are typically used for the GIFT procedure, and that "the proportion of oocytes graded as good in the supernumerary oocyte group is much decreased from that in pure IVF cases" (9% vs. 34%). This in turn dramatically influenced fertilization rates. Al-Shawaf et al. found that, although the overall fertilization rate of supernumerary oocytes was significantly higher in patients who became pregnant from GIFT, the failure to fertilize any supernumerary oocytes was not significantly different between those who did and did not become pregnant from the GIFT cycle (49).

Carrying this one step further, Curole et al. found that the chance of pregnancy from a GIFT cycle was correlated with development of supernumerary oocytes fertilized to the blastocyst stage (50). They also found, however, that there was no relationship between fertilization of the supernumerary oocytes and pregnancy.

We feel that in most cases since the pregnancy rate with GIFT is superior to that with IVF, proven fertilization with IVF prior to a GIFT cycle is not necessary. If there is a significant male factor involved, then TET is a better alternative (see below). In our program, however, if a couple fails to achieve a pregnancy with a "perfect" GIFT, we recommend TET for their next attempt. In this way we rule out an occult male factor and transfer only fertilized oocytes.

Since the upsurge in use of GnRHa for stimulation protocols, it is very common to obtain supernumerary oocytes in GIFT cycles. Approximately 60% of patients undergoing a GIFT transfer will have a surplus of embryos for cryopreservation in our center. These embryos are then available for transfer in subsequent unstimulated cycles should the patient not conceive from her GIFT cycle or should the couple desire another child. We recently evaluated the cumulative pregnancy rate from one GIFT cycle and subsequent transfer of cryopreserved embryos (Table 4.2) (51).

From January 1989 through December 1990, we evaluated the cumulative pregnancy rate of patients having their first GIFT cycle and subsequent cycles of frozen-thawed embryos from the original GIFT (52). Ovarian stimulation was accomplished with regimens of clomiphene and human menopausal gonadotropins (CC-hMG) or leuprolide luteal phase, pure follicle-stimulating hormone, and human menopausal gonadotropins (LLPh-FSH-hMG). GIFT was performed with three to five oocytes and supernumerary oocytes were then inseminated. Embryos of good quality were cryopreserved at the two-to-four-cell stage with 1–2 propanediol. When the GIFT cycle did not result in a pregnancy, thaw and uterine transfers were carried out during unstimulated cycles.

Table 4.2 Cumulative pregnancy rate from one GIFT cycle with cryopreservation of supernumerary embryos

	No.	% A	% C	% E	% G
A. Began stimulation GIFT cycle	142				
B. Cancel—poor response	25	17.6			
C. Oocyte aspiration	117	82.4			
D. Switch to IVF/TET	28	19.7	24		
E. GIFT transfer	89	62.7	76		
F. Pregnant from GIFT	41	28.8	35	46	
G. Not pregnant from GIFT	48	33.8	41	54	
1. With frozen embryos	21	14.8	18	23.6	43.8

Thirteen patients have undergone a frozen–thaw embryo transfer, and two of them achieved a pregnancy. On the basis of the above-mentioned data, we project that out of 100 GIFT transfers, approximately 46 patients would achieve a pregnancy. Of those not pregnant, approximately half would have cryopreserved embryos, and according to our 15% consistent pregnancy rate in cryopreserved embryo transfer cycles, an additional four patients could expect a pregnancy. Thus, theoretically, patients having a GIFT transfer could expect a 50% cumulative pregnancy rate.

Tubal embryo transfer

GIFT was originally developed as a therapeutic alternative for patients with at least one functional fallopian tube. In most investigators' experience, it has proved more more efficacious than IVF in couples with most categories of infertility. Unfortunately success rates with GIFT in cases of significant male factor infertility are lower than with other etiologies. In these cases, IVF offers the advantage of exposing the oocytes to high concentrations of motile sperm and, diagnostically, offers the definitive answer to the question of fertilization. The implantation rate in GIFT is, however, superior to that in IVF, theoretically because of the intratubal milieu's effect on early development and the more chronologically appropriate entrance of the embryo into the uterus. The concept of tubal embryo transfer (TET) was therefore explored as a hybrid of both GIFT and IVF. In 1988 Balmaceda et al. reported on the outcome of in vitro generated embryos transferred to the fallopian tubes in nonhuman primates (53). Seven pregnancies occurred out of 18 embryo transfers performed during the first 72 hours after follicular aspiration in cynomolgus monkeys.

Subsequently, Devroey et al. reported on the first successful case of TET in a patient with antisperm antibodies in 1986 (54). They termed the procedure a zygote intrafallopian transfer (ZIFT). Transfer was performed 18 hours after insemination, hence the designation *zygote*. In 1987 Yovich et al. reported their results in a series of patients undergoing pronuclear stage tubal transfer, or PROST (55). This technique was utilized in cases of severe male factor, female antisperm antibodies, poor results from multiple previous GIFT cycles, and in women receiving donated oocytes. Results were superior to those with IVF. They commented that the diagnostic value of PROST was clearly demonstrated by the confirmation of fertilization failure in many severe male factor couples. These couples can then be counseled as to future therapy. They concluded that PROST is superior to IVF for managing cases of severe male factor and female antisperm antibodies. In their discussion they comment that in couples who have failed multiple previous GIFT cycles, use of PROST, which documents fertilization only, may be inferior to TET, which contributes further knowledge regarding cleavage and early embryo development.

In 1988 we reported our preliminary results with TET in cases of male factor infertility (56). Sixteen couples began a TET cycle. Following controlled ovarian hyperstimulation and transvaginal oocyte retrieval, insemination was performed. No fertilization occurred in six cases. In the remaining 10 patients, TET was performed 45 to 50 hours after oocyte retrieval. Six pregnancies occured, including one twin and one triplet. The implantation rate of 25.7% was superior to the 7% to 10% implantation rate expected from uterine transfer. In an article comparing the relative chance of pregnancy following tubal and uterine transfer procedures, Yovich et al. similarly reported that the pregnancy rate per transfer and the implantation rates were significantly higher for tubal transfer (57). Devroey et al. presented their data on 245 ZIFT cycles. They had a 43% pregnancy rate from transferring three or less zygotes (58).

Results of TET at our center to date are presented in Table 4.3. We have had 67 pregnancies in 126 transfers, for a 53% pregnancy rate per transfer. Of interest is the implantation rate of 18% per embryo transferred as compared with the 7% to 10% rate quoted for uterine transfer. Miscarriage and multiple birth rates are similar to those reported with IVF and GIFT. Thus TET appears quite promising in male factor and immunologic infertility when compared with GIFT (16%) and IVF (12%).

Though the pregnancy rate per transfer in our center is 53%, many severe male factor patients do not make it to transfer because of a failure of fertilization overall (pregnancy rate of 28% per cycle attempted). Methods are needed to improve sperm recovery and fertilization in severe male factor cases. Yovich et al. reported on the use of the phosphodiesterase inhibitor pentoxifyllin (PF) to enhance the number of progressively motile sperm available for insemination (59). An in vitro trial demonstrated an improvement in concentration of motile spermatozoa and progressively motile sperm in oligospermia samples after PF treatment. PF washing of sperm was then carried out in nine couples who had previously failed attempts at fertilization in vitro. Six couples achieved fertilization with PF-treated

Table 4.3 University of California, Irvine, Center for Reproductive Health tubal embryo transfer results

	No.	% of A	% of B	Other
A. Transfers	126			
B. Pregnancies	67	53		
C. Implantation rate (per embryo)				17.8%
D. Miscarriages	12		18	
E. Ectopic pregnancies	1		1.5	
F. Multiple births	16		24	
G. Take home baby rate	54	43		

sperm, and five pregnancies ensued following PROST. Further study of this promising treatment is needed.

In our center, we have obtained good sperm recovery in cases of severe male factor using the Minipercoll technique (10). Semen samples are collected and diluted 1:2 with medium and then centrifuged at $200 \times g$ for 10 minutes. Pellets are suspended in 0.3 ml of medium (human tubal fluid [HTF] and Hepes, Irvine Scientific, Irvine, Calif.) and layered on a discontinuous Percoll (Pharmacia, Sweden) gradient consisting of 0.3 ml each of 50%, 70%, and 95% isotonic Percoll (Minipercoll). The gradient is centrifuged at $300 \times g$ for 45 minutes. Following centrifugation the 95% Percoll layer is removed, washed two times, and resuspended in 1 ml of HTF and 10% human cord serum. Cumulus denuded oocytes are then added to the culture tube containing sperm. In our comparative study with a standard swim-up technique, semen samples prepared with the Minipercoll technique had better motility and progression and normal morphology. In addition, the fertilization rate and pregnancy rate were superior in the Minipercoll group. Based on our preliminary data, the Minipercoll technique for sperm preparation seems to offer significant advantages in cases of severe oligoasthenospermia.

Our present policy for triaging patients for ART cycles includes utilizing TET for four indications: 1) severe male factor, 2) immunologic infertility, 3) previous failed GIFT cycle, and 4) immature eggs obtained at the time of a GIFT cycle.

Prior to beginning a cycle, a semen analysis with preparation of the sample is obtained. If the following criteria are not met, TET rather than GIFT becomes our method of choice: 1) recovery of more than 1.5 million total motile sperm, 2) progression of 2 to 3 or greater, and 3) percentage of normal forms greater than 30%. Any sperm preparation not fulfilling these criteria is considered a male factor, and TET is recommended.

In cases of female antisperm antibodies, TET rather than GIFT is performed. In these couples female serum is not used for culture, and fertilization takes place outside the body.

Any couple who have previously undergone a GIFT cycle in our program and failed to achieve a pregnancy are also triaged to TET in the following cycle. In this way we find out about fertilization and also put back only fertilized eggs rather than some that may not fertilize (as may occur in a GIFT cycle). Even when supernumerary oocytes have fertilized in a previous GIFT cycle, we prefer to do a TET cycle.

Finally, in cases scheduled for GIFT in which we obtain fewer than three mature oocytes, the GIFT is cancelled and insemination is delayed and performed in vitro. If two or more embryos are obtained, TET is then carried out. This policy is based on data demonstrating that the pregnancy rate is significantly poorer when immature eggs are transferred for GIFT (8). The tube seems to be a good place for embryo development but not for oocyte maturation.

We feel that by utilizing this policy of patient selection for GIFT versus TET we are able to diagnose a failure of fertilization in many cases of severe male factor and thus not subject the woman to surgery (GIFT) unless embryos are obtained. Furthermore, as micromanipulation techniques improve, TET will be the transfer method of choice in these couples when the woman has functional tubes. We also favor TET as a method of transfer in treating couples in which the man undergoes microscopic epididymal sperm aspiration for congenital absence of the vas deferens (see below).

Transuterine tubal gamete and embryo transfer

Though pregnancy rates with tubal gamete or embryo transfer are superior to those with IVF in most instances, a significant disadvantage of traditional tubal transfer is the necessity for general anesthesia and a surgical procedure (laparoscopy or minilaparotomy). The technique of catheterization of the fallopian tubes transvaginally under ultrasound guidance was proposed to overcome this disadvantage. Jansen and Anderson described a technique for transvaginal tubal catheterization in 1987 (60) and subsequently reported on the use of this technique for intratubal gamete transfer (61) as well as tubal embryo transfer (62). The catheter system consists of a soft Teflon inner catheter introduced through a Teflon outer catheter with a lateral curve at its tip. The outer catheter with a malleable obturator inside is placed transcervically and rotated 90 degrees. Under transvaginal or transabdominal ultrasound guidance, the outer catheter is advanced to the uterine cornua. Catheter placement is confirmed by a combination of ultrasound guidance and tactile sensation. The obturator is then removed and replaced by the inner catheter containing gametes or embryos. This is advanced approximately 4 cm beyond the outer catheter to the ampullary isthmic portion of the tube where the gametes or embryos are delivered.

In 1988 Jansen et al. reported the first pregnancy resulting from transcervical tubal embryo transfer (62). Our group subsequently reported a pregnancy from nonsurgical TET (63). Since Jansen's original report, a number of studies have reported preliminary results with this technique. Lucena et al. reported on seven couples treated with this technique (64). Three of seven couples conceived. Risquez et al. reported five pregnancies in 28 cases of transcervical TET (18% per transfer); however, two of the pregnancies were ectopic (65). Yovich et al. performed transcervical TET in 17 women whose fallopian tubes were inaccessible by the abdominal route but at least one tube was patent (66). Three pregnancies ensued (17% per transfer), and one was ectopic. Scholtes et al. reported a more promising seven clinical pregnancies in 25 transfers (28% per transfer)

(67). Nevertheless a summary of proceedings on transcervical tubal gamete or embryo transfer from the European Society of Human Reproduction and Embryology, Paris, France, March 1990, was not very encouraging, with results appearing somewhat better for TET than for GIFT.

Limitations to this technique include the suboptimal catheter systems so far designed for tubal placement, the theoretical trauma to the endometrium by the catheter, and the possible tubal damage from tubal catheterization. Preliminary studies would suggest that tubal damage is not a major concern. There does, however, appear to be a negative effect on the endometrium, as in cases where tubal catheterization has failed, uterine embryo transfer yields a low pregnancy rate (65). Further refinement of a catheter system may also yield better pregnancy rates. In their report on transcervical TET, Yovich et al. conclude that, though the procedure has potential patient benefits in terms of cost, safety, and minimization of anesthetic procedures, preliminary experience is not encouraging, particularly in cases of known underlying tubal disorder, and that such cases are better treated with conventional IVF (66). Whether pregnancy rates with transcervical gamete or embryo transfer will prove superior to IVF or will approach pregnancy rates obtained with traditional GIFT or TET techniques remains to be seen.

Oocyte donation and tubal transfer

The first successful case of oocyte donation in ART was reported by Lutjen et al. in 1984 (68). IVF and embryo transfer of donated oocytes was performed on a woman with premature ovarian failure (POF). Currently indications for donated oocytes include POF, carriers of a lethal genetic trait, as well as women with a history of a reported poor response in previous ART cycles. Since Lutjen's original report, many investigators have described oocyte donation for IVF cycles, with uniformly good success rates of 25% to 35%. In 1988 we reported the first series of oocyte donation in GIFT cycles, with six of eight patients conceiving (69). Subsequently, other investigators reported similarly excellent results from oocyte donation in GIFT cycles (70). Yovich et al. suggested the use of PROST for oocyte donation cycles (55). They recommended PROST because, in general, tubal transfer gave better results than uterine transfer in their program, and transfer of pronuclear stage embryos allowed for a separation in time between oocyte aspiration and transfer that preserved anonymity of donors (more difficult with GIFT). Success was similarly good.

Currently our protocol for oocyte recipients includes an evaluation cycle in which they receive the following steroid replacement: 1) micronized 17β–estradiol (E_2) orally (Estrace; Mead Johnson, Evansville, Ind.), 2 mg on days 3 through 8, 4 mg on days 9 through 11, and 6 mg on days 12 through 28, in divided daily doses; and 2) progesterone in oil intramuscularly (IM; United Research Laboratories, Philadelphia, Pa.), 100 mg per day, days 16–28. Serum E_2 and progesterone levels are determined by radioimmunoassay on days 8, 11, 15, and 20 of the evaluation cycle, and an endometrial biopsy is performed in the midluteal to late luteal phase. During the cycle of oocyte donation, all recipients follow a similar steroid replacement regimen based on results from the evaluation cycle. Progesterone is begun 2 days before gamete or embryo transfer. If pregnancy results, 8 mg of E_2 and 100 mg of progesterone daily are continued until 60 days from transfer.

In a report from our center, we presented our data comparing pregnancy rates with oocyte donation in cases of IVF, GIFT, and TET (see Table 4.4) (71). Our present results suggest that in cases of oocyte donation there is no significant difference in outcome between IVF and GIFT. However, although the number of cases of TET is small,

the pregnancy rate and implantation rate appear to be slightly higher than that with IVF. We are carrying out a prospective randomized study of IVF versus GIFT and TET for oocyte donation. If GIFT or TET does prove superior, then all patients with a functional fallopian tube should be offered a tubal transfer technique for oocyte donation. The patient will then have to decide whether the increased chance of pregnancy with GIFT or TET compensates for the necessity of a surgical procedure (minilaparotomy or laparoscopy) as opposed to nonsurgical transfer with IVF.

Microscopic epididymal sperm aspiration and tubal embryo transfer

In 1988, our center developed a new treatment protocol involving microscopic epididymal sperm aspiration (MESA) combined with IVF and TET (72). This is principally offered to couples in whom the male partner has congenital absence of the vas deferens (CAV). This condition accounts for 11% to 50% of cases of obstructive azoospermia and has previously been considered untreatable. These patients have been shown to

Table 4.4 Pregnancy rates with oocyte donation

	IVF-ET	GIFT	TET
No. of transfers	51	29	26
Clinical pregnancy	19 (37%)[a]	14 (48%)[a]	15 (57%)[a]
Oocy/embryos tranf.	184	109	102
No. gest. sacs	26	18	24
Implant. rate[b]	14%[c]	16%	23%[c]
Abortion	2 (10%)	4 (28%)	2 (13%)
Ectopic pregn.	0	0	0

[a]Not significant
[b]Implant. rate: number of gestational sacs seen by ultrasound per number of oocytes or embryos transferred
[c]$p < 0.05$

have normal spermatogenesis, theoretically making their sperm capable of fertilizing an egg, yet previous attempts at treatment have been unsuccessful.

The female partners of men with CAV undergo controlled ovarian hyperstimulation in a routine fashion. Following successful ultrasound-guided oocyte retrieval, attention is turned to the male. Scrotal exploration is carried out. The tunica vaginalis is opened, and the epididymis is exposed. With the aid of the operating microscope, a tiny incision is made into the epididymal tunic to expose tubules in the most distal portion of the congenitally blind-ending epididymis. Sperm are aspirated with a number 22 Medicut on a tuberculin syringe directly from the opening in the tubule. Great care is taken not to contaminate the specimen with blood, and careful hemostasis is achieved. The epididymal fluid is immediately diluted with Hepes buffered medium, and a tiny portion is examined for motility and quality of progression. If motility is very poor, another aspiration is made 0.5 cm proximally. Sperm is sought from more and more proximal regions until progressive motility is found. In almost all cases, motile sperm are not obtained until the proximalmost portion of the caput epididymis or vasa efferentia is reached. Two days after insemination, embryos are transferred either to the uterus or to the fallopian tubes.

Results to date are presented in Table 4.5. Among 54 couples with MESA procedure performed, in only two (4%) were no motile sperm recovered, and 61% of the couples had fertilization of oocytes. Eight couples underwent IVF, with only one resulting pregnancy (12%). Twenty-four couples underwent TET, with 12 resulting pregnancies (50%). Overall 24% of couples having MESA performed achieved a pregnancy. It is now our recommendation to perform TET rather than IVF in all such couples if the woman has a patent fallopian tube. Other factors contributing to the success of this technique may include 1) obtaining large numbers of oocytes in order to increase the likelihood of fertilization, and 2) incubation of sperm outside of the milieu of the obstructed epididymis with a Minipercoll preparation. Though experience is preliminary, a combined approach of MESA and TET is very promising for men with CAV.

GIFT in combination with IVF

Only 7 years after its development, GIFT is an established technique for assisted conception in couples in which the woman has at least one patent fallopian tube. IVF, though having a lower success rate, does provide more immediate answers with regard to fertilization capacity. Therefore it was natural that some investigators would propose a combined procedure of GIFT and IVF to provide more information and give a higher chance of pregnancy. In the combined approach, GIFT is carried out in a routine fashion, and 2 to 3 days

Table 4.5 Results of MESA with in vitro fertilization or tubal embryo transfer

No. of cases	Motile sperm	No. of oocytes	No. of mature oocytes	No. of embryos	No. of subjects w/embryos	No. of TET (preg)	No. of IVF-ET (preg)
54	52	835	636	156	33	24 (12)	8 (1)

later, embryos obtained from fertilization of excess oocytes are transferred to the uterus.

Leong et al. reported on a small study comparing GIFT with a combined GIFT and IVF approach (73). They found a lower pregnancy rate with the combined approach (10% vs. 39%). They conclude that GIFT and IVF are neither compatible nor complementary. Theories as to why pregnancy rates are lower with the combined approach are that the uterine embryo transfer may cause trauma to the endometrium, preventing implantation of embryos traveling down the fallopian tubes originating from GIFT; or that if uterine transferred embryos do not survive, toxins may be released that might kill the embryos still in the tube; or that the uterine transferred embryos may initiate implantation (even if they do not ultimately result in a pregnancy), and this may prevent further development and implantation of fallopian tube embryos.

The 1989 IVF-ET Registry for the United States reported an overall 27% clinical pregnancy rate for GIFT and an overall 26% clinical pregnancy rate for combined GIFT and IVF (18).

It is also tempting to speculate that the multiple pregnancy rates that will arise from this combined procedure may be theoretically unacceptable.

With the increasing availability of cryopreservation, it seems as though supernumerary embryos obtained from a GIFT cycle should be cryopreserved for future use rather than transferred to the uterus during the GIFT cycle. Preliminary data would suggest that even in programs in which cryopreservation is not an option, transferring excess embryos to the uterus in a GIFT cycle may be detrimental.

Conclusion

Tubal gamete and embryo transfer are appropriate techniques in couples with at least one normal fallopian

tube. Pregnancy rates and live birth rates are generally reported to be at least 10% higher with GIFT than with IVF (18). These comparisons are, however, difficult to make because of different centers' biases as to which patient populations are treated with GIFT or IVF. A large prospective controlled study between IVF and GIFT in different etiologies of infertility would be helpful.

We feel that IVF, GIFT, and TET should be offered in any center. Appropriate triaging of patients to each technique should maximize pregnancy rates (Fig. 4.1). We recommend that all patients with abnormal or absent fallopian tubes be treated with IVF. Patients with a normal fallopian tube and a severe male factor, significant female antisperm antibodies, or a previous failed GIFT cycle should be treated with TET. All other couples should have an initial GIFT cycle with cryopreservation of supernumerary oocytes.

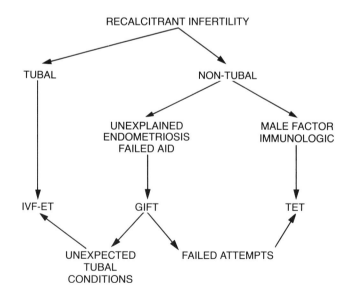

Figure 4.1   Assisted reproductive technology triage.

References

1. Asch RH, Ellsworth LR, Balmaceda JP, Wong PC. Pregnancy after translaparoscopic gamete intra fallopian transfer. Lancet 1984;2:1034–1035.

2. Edwards RG, Steptoe PC. Birth after reimplantation of human embryo. Lancet 1978;2:366.

3. Asch RH. GIFT and associated techniques. In: Johnston I, Balmaceda JP, Asch RH, eds. Gamete Physiology, New York: Serono Symposia Publications from Plenum Press, 1990:287–304.

4. Barad DH, Bartfai G, Barg P, Cohen BL, Feinman M. Gamete intrafallopian tube transfer (GIFT): making laparoscopy more than "diagnostic." Fertil Steril 1988;50(6): 928–930.

5. Pampiglione JS, Bolton VN, Parsons JH, Campbell S. Gamete intra-fallopian transfer combined with diagnostic laparoscopy: a treatment for infertility in a district hospital. Hum Reprod 1989;4(7):786–789.

6. Curole DN, Dickey RP, Taylor SN, Rye PH, Olar TT. Pregnancies in cancelled gamete intrafallopian transfer cycles. Fertil Steril 1989;51(2):363–364.

7. Tzafettas JM, Mukherjee A, Stephanotos A, Papaloucas AC. The purpose of prelaparoscopy transvaginal retrieval of oocytes in a modified GIFT procedure. Hum Reprod 1989;4(7):762–765.

8. Guzick DS, Balmaceda JP, Ord T, Asch RH. The importance of egg and sperm factors in predicting the likelihood of pregnancy from gamete intrafallopian transfer. Fertil Steril 1989;52(5):795–800.

9. Wong PC, Balmaceda JP, Blanco JD, Gibba S, Asch RH. Sperm washing and swim-up technique using antibiotics to remove microbes from human semen. Fertil Steril 1986; 45:97–100.

10. Ord T, Patrizio P, Marello E, Balmaceda JP, Asch RH. Minipercoll: a new method of semen preparation for IVF in severe male factor infertility. Hum Reprod 1990;5(8):987–989.

11. Tucker MJ, Chan YM, Chan SYW, et al. The use of human follicular fluid in gamete intrafallopian transfer. Hum Reprod 1989;4(8):931–936.

12. Fakih H, Vijayakumar R. Improved pregnancy rates and outcome with gamete intrafallopian transfer when follicular fluid is used as a sperm capacitation and gamete transfer medium. Fertil Steril 1990;53(3):515–520.

13. Patrizio P, Asch RH. Intratubal gamete and embryo transfer in male infertility. In: Rajfer J, ed. Common problems in infertility and impotence. Chicago: Year Book Medical Publishers, 1989:137–148.

14. Rodriquez-Rigau LJ, Steinberger E, Weidman ER, et al. Possible role of GIFT for pelvic factor. In: Capitanio GL, Asch RH, De Cecco L, Croce S, eds. GIFT: from basics to clinics. New York: Raven Press, 1989:351–358.

15. Corson SL, Batzer FR, Gocial B, et al. Surgical treatment of endometriosis at the time of gamete intrafallopian transfer. J Reprod Med 1991;36(4):274–278.

16. Yee B, Rosen GF, Cahcon RR, Soubra S, Stone SC. Gamete intrafallopian transfer: the effect of the number of eggs used and the depth of gamete placement on pregnancy initiation. Fertil Steril 1989;52(4):639–644.

17. Pickering SJ, Braude PR, Johnson MH, Cant A, Currie J. Transient cooling to room temperature can cause irreversible disruption of meiotic spindle in the human oocyte. Fertil Steril 1990;54(1):102–108.

18. Medical Research International, Society for Assisted Reproductive Technology, American Fertility Society. In vitro fertilization–embryo transfer in the United States: 1989 results from the IVF-ET registry. Fertil Steril 1991;55(1):14–23.

19. Asch RH. GIFT: indications, results, problems and perspectives. In: Capitanio GL, Asch RH, DeCecco L, Croce S, eds. GIFT: from basics to clinics. New York: Raven Press, 1989:209–228.

20. Craft I, Brisden P. Alternative to IVF: the outcome of 1071 first GIFT procedures. Hum Reprod 1989;4(Suppl): 29–36.

21. Wiedemann R, Noss U, Hepp H. Gamete intrafallopian transfer in male subfertility. Hum Reprod 1989;4 (4):408–411.

22. Cittadini E, Guastella G, Comparetto G, Gattuccio F, Chisnchiano N. IVF/ET and GIFT in andrology. Hum Reprod 1988;3(1):101–104.

23. Cittadini E, Cimino C. Dyspermia and GIFT: results.

In: Capitanio GL, Asch RH, De Cecco L, Croce S, eds. GIFT: from basics to clinics. New York: Raven Press, 1989:391–398.

24. Matson PL, Blackledge DG, Richardson PA, Turner SR, Yovich JM, Yovich JL. The role of gamete intrafallopian transfer in the treatment of oligospermia infertility. Fertil Steril 1987;48(4):608–612.

25. Khan I, Camus C, Staessen C, Wisanto A, Devroey P, Van Steirtghem AC. Success rate in gamete intrafallopian transfer using low and high concentrations of washed spermatozoa. Fertil Steril 1988;50(6):922–927.

26. Rodriguez-Rigau LJ, Steinberger E, Weidmen ER, Smith KD, Ayala C, Gibbons WE. Semen analysis and GIFT. In: Capitanio GL, Asch RH, De Cecco L, Croce S, eds. GIFT: from basics to clinics. New York: Raven Press, 1989:235–244.

27. Al-Shawaf T, Nolan A, Harper J, Serhal P, Craft I. Pregnancy following gamete intra-fallopian transfer (GIFT) with cryopreserved semen from infertile men following therapy to lymphomas or testicular tumor: report of three cases. Hum Reprod 1991;6(3):365–366.

28. Cittadini E, Cimino C. Immunological infertility and GIFT. In: Capitanio GL, Asch RH, De Cecco L, Croce S, eds. GIFT: from basics to clinics. New York: Raven Press, 1989:341–350.

29. Van der Merwe JP, Kruger TR, Windt ML, Hulme VA, Menkveld R. Treatment of male sperm autoimmunity by using the gamete intrafallopian transfer procedure with washed spermatozoa. Fertil Steril 1990;53(4):682–687.

30. Smith DC, Forster MS, Gellert RJ, Ziegler CJ, Daubenmier CA. Gamete or embryo replacement in severely damaged fallopian tubes. Presented at the Thirty-seventh Annual Meeting of the Pacific Coast Fertility Society, Palm Springs, Calif., April 12–16, 1989.

31. Holtz G, Patton GW, Schwartz K, Caines K, Frank S. Gamete intrafallopian transfer in patients at increased risk for ectopic pregnancy. Presented at the Forty-sixth Annual Meeting of the American Fertility Society, Washington, D.C., October 15–18, 1990.

32. Fakih H, Harris G. GIFT in advanced peri-adnexal disease. Presented at the Forty-sixth Annual Meeting of the American Fertility Society, Washington, D.C., October 15–18, 1990.

33. Cefalu E. Cittadini E, Balmaceda JP, et al. Successful gamete intrafallopian transfer following failed artificial insemination by donor: evidence for a defect in gamete transport? Fertil Steril 1988;50(2):279–282.

34. Pilikian S, Watrelot A, Dreyfus JM, Ecochard R, Gennaro JD. Gamete intra-fallopian transfer with cryopreserved donor semen following AID failure. Hum Reprod 1990;5(8):944–946.

35. Fromigli L, Coglitore MT, Roccio C, Belotti G, Stangalini A, Formigli G. One-hundred-and-six gamete intra-fallopian transfer procedures with donor semen. Hum Reprod 1990;5(5):549–552.

36. Kirby CA, Dogfrey B, Warnes GM, Flaherty S, Norman RJ, Matthews CD. In vitro fertilization and gamete intrafallopian transfer following failed donor insemination. Presented at the 7th World Congress on IVF, Paris, France, June 23–July 3, 1991.

37. Romeu A, Muasher SJ, Acosta AA, et al. Results of in vitro fertilization attempts in women 40 years of age and older: the Norfolk experience. Fertil Steril 1987;47(1):130–136.

38. Kerin J, Serafini P, Quinn P, Bernstein S. The effect of maternal age on the pregnancy outcome of IVF and gamete transfer procedures. Presented at the Forty-third Annual Meeting of the American Fertility Society, Reno Nev., September 1987.

39. Penzias AS, Thompson IE, Alper MM, Oskowitz SP, Berger MJ. Successful use of gamete intrafallopian transfer does not reverse the decline in fertility in women over 40 years of age. Obstet Gynecol 1991;77(1):37–39.

40. Asch RH, Ord T, Stone S, Balmaceda JP, Rotsztejn DA. Assisted reproductive techniques in women over 40 years of age: IVF, GIFT, ZIFT, egg donation: is there a best alternative? Presented at the 39th Annual Meeting of the Pacific Coast Fertility Society, Indian Wells, Calif., April 10–14, 1991.

41. Haines CJ, O'Shea RT. Unilateral gamete intra-fallopian transfer: the preferred method? Fertil Steril 1989;51(3):518–519.

42. Haines CJ, O'Shea RT. The effect of unilateral versus bilateral tubal cannulation and the number of oocytes trans-

ferred on the outcome of gamete intrafallopian transfer. Fertil Steril 1991;55(2):423–425.

43. Marconi G, Auge L, Oses R, Quintana R, Raffo F, Young E. Does sexual intercourse improve pregnancy rates in gamete intrafallopian transfer? Fertil Steril 1989;51(2):357–359.

44. Tucker MJ, Wong CJY, Chan YM, Leong MKH, Leung CKM. Postoperative artificial insemination—does it improve GIFT outcome? Hum Reprod 1990;5(2):189–192.

45. Penzias AS, Alper MM, Oskowitz SP, Berger MJ, Thompson IE. Gamete intrafallopian transfer: assessment of the optimal number of oocytes to transfer. Fertil Steril 1991;55(2):311–313.

46. Quigley MM, Sokoloski JE, Withers DM, Richards SI, Reiss JM. Simultaneous in vitro fertilization and gamete intrafallopian transfer (GIFT). Fertil Steril 1987;47(5):797–801.

47. Matson PL, Yovich JM, Bootsma BD, Spittle JW, Yovich JL. The in vitro fertilization of supernumerary oocytes in a gamete intrafallopian transfer program. Fertil Steril 1987;47(5):802–806.

48. McKenna KM, McBain JC, Speirs AL, Jones G, DuPleiss Y, Johnston WIH. The fate of supernumerary oocytes in gamete intrafallopian transfer (GIFT) is not predictive of a poor outcome: the effect of oocyte selection. J In Vitro Fert Embryo Transf 1988;5(5):261–264.

49. Al-Shawaf T, Ah-Moye M, Junk S, Brinsden P, Craft I. Fertilization of supernumerary oocytes following gamete intrafallopian transfer (GIFT): correlation with outcome of GIFT treatment. J In Vitro Fert Embryo Transf 1990;7(2):98–102.

50. Curole DN, Dickey RP, Taylor SN, Olar TT. Correlation of pregnancy after gamete intrafallopian transfer with fertilization and cleavage of sibling oocytes. Fertil Steril 1988;50(5):811–812.

51. Weckstein LN, Balmaceda JP, Ord T, Marello E, Asch RH. Cumulative pregnancy rate from one gamete intrafallopian transfer (GIFT) cycle with cryopreservation of embryos. Presented at the Forty-sixth Annual Meeting of the American Fertility Society, Washington, D.C., October 13–18, 1990.

52. Alam V, Weckstein LN, Balmaceda JP, Ord T, Marello E, Asch RH. Gift and cryopreservation of embryos:

how much can we offer? Presented at the 7th World Congress on IVF, Paris, France, June 23–July 3, 1991.

53. Balmaceda JP, Gastaldi C, Ord T, Borrero C, Asch RH. Tubal embryo transfer in cynomolgus monkeys: effects of hyperstimulation and synchrony. Hum Reprod 1988;3(4):441–443.

54. Devroey P, Braeckmans P, Smith J, et al. Pregnancy after translaparoscopic zygote intrafallopian transfer in a patient with sperm antibodies. Lancet 1986;1:1329–1331.

55. Yovich JL, Blackledge DG, Richardson PA, Matson PL, Turner SR, Draper R. Pregnancies following pronuclear stage tubal transfer. Fertil Steril 1987;48(5):851–857.

56. Balmaceda JP, Gastaldi C, Remohi J, Borrero C, Ord T, Asch RH. Tubal embryo transfer as a treatment for infertility due to male factor. Fertil Steril 1988;50(3):476–479.

57. Yovich JL, Yovich JM, Edirisinghe WR. The relative chance of pregnancy following tubal or uterine transfer procedures. Fertil Steril 1988;49(5):858–864.

58. Devroey P, Camus M, Stuessen C, et al. ZIFT: indications and limitations. In: Capitano GL, Asch RH, DeCecco L, Croce S, eds. GIFT: from basics to clinics. New York: Raven Press, 1989:333–340.

59. Yovich JM, Edirisinghe WR, Cummins JM, Yovich JL. Preliminary results using pentoxifylline in a pronuclear stage tubal transfer (PROST) program for severe male factor infertility. Fertil Steril 1988;50(1):179–181.

60. Jansen RPS, Anderson JC. Catheterization of the fallopian tubes from the vagina. Lancet 1987;2:309–310.

61. Jansen RPS, Anderson JC, Radomic I, Smith J, Sutherland PD. Pregnancies after ultrasound guided fallopian insemination with cryostored donor semen. Fertil Steril 1988;49(5):920–922.

62. Jansen RPS, Anderson JC, Sutherland PD. Nonoperative embryo transfer to the fallopian tube. N Engl J Med 1988;319:288–291.

63. Guidetti R, Balmaceda JP, Ord T, Asch RH. Nonsurgical tubal embryo transfer. Hum Reprod 1990;5(2):221–224.

64. Lucena E, Ruiz JA, Mendoza JC, et al. Vaginal intratubal insemination and vaginal GIFT, endosonographic technique: early experience. Hum Reprod 1989;4(6):658–662.

65. Risquez F, Boyer P, Rolet F, et al. Retrograde tubal transfer of human embryos. Hum Reprod 1990;5(2):185–188.

66. Yovich JL, Draper RR, Turner SR, Cummins JM. Transcervical tubal embryo-stage transfer. J In Vitro Fert Embryo Transf 1990;3(7):137–140.

67. Scholtes MCW, Roozenburg BJ, Alberda AT, Zeilmaker GH. Transcervical intrafallopian transfer of zygotes. Fertil Steril 1990;54(2):283–286.

68. Lutjen P, Trounson A, Leeton J, Findlay J, Wood C, Renou P. The establishment and maintenance of pregnancy using in vitro fertilization and embryo donation in a patient with primary ovarian failure. Nature 1984;307:174–175.

69. Asch RH, Balmaceda JP, Ord T, et al. Oocyte donation and gamete intrafallopian transfer in premature ovarian failure. Fertil Steril 1988;49(2):263–267.

70. Formigli L, Roccio C, Belotti G, Stangalini A, Coglitore MT, Formigli G. Oocyte donation by gamete intrafallopian transfer to amenorrheic and cycling patients given replacement steroids. Hum Reprod 1989;4(7):772–776.

71. Rotszetjn DA, Remohi J, Borrero C, Ord T, Balmaceda JP, Asch RH. Oocyte donation with GIFT, IVF-UT or TET: is there a best alternative? Presented at the Forty-sixth Annual Meeting of the American Fertility Society, Washington, D.C., October 13–18, 1990.

72. Silber SJ, Balmaceda JP, Borrero C, Ord T, Asch RH. Pregnancy with sperm aspiration from the proximal head of the epididymis: a new treatment for congenital absence of the vas deferens. Fertil Steril 1988;50(3):525–528.

73. Leong MKH, Leung CKM, Marriott VM, et al. Comparative study of combined GIFT and IVF-ET with GIFT alone. Hum Reprod 1988;9(7):877–879.

5

Cryopreservation

Patrick Quinn

Introduction

Cryopreservation has become a routine clinical procedure in many clinics utilizing assisted reproductive technologies (ART) to attain pregnancies in subfertile couples; however, several aspects of the procedures used to preserve spermatozoa, oocytes, and embryos require modification and improvement. These changes need to be integrated with prospective clinical and research trials to elucidate what technical factors have the most influence in determining success rates and to minimize confounding factors in the subfertile couple's etiology.

The purposes of this chapter are to review some of the cryobiological principles thought to be important for the preservation of gametes and embryos, to consider the clinical indications and applications for cryopreservation, to comment briefly on the ethical considerations applying to each procedure (including cryobanking), and finally, to summarize current results and areas that show the most potential for advances in the forseeable future.

Historical aspects of cryopreservation

A brief outline of the historical milestones in cryopreservation as it applies to gametes and embryos was given by Quinn (1). With respect to advances that have led to clinical applications of the procedure, the most significant discovery was that of the cryoprotective action of glycerol (2). This was in regard to the cryopreservation of spermatozoa, and its practical application in agriculture, particularly the establishment of banks of frozen bull semen, soon followed. It did not take long for similar methodology to be used for human semen, although few changes to the original methodology occurred until 1963–1964; for a review, see Sherman (3). At this time, the use of liquid nitrogen vapor for freezing and storage in liquid nitrogen was instigated, and few effective changes in the methodology of cryostorage of human semen have occurred since. In the 1970s there was a gradual emergence of national (4) and commercial cryobanks for semen. Concerns regarding the transmission of human immunodeficiency virus (HIV) and other sexually transmitted diseases (STDs) in semen and evidence of such transmission (5) have made it mandatory to use cryopreserved human semen for therapeutic donor insemination (TDI). It is likely that we are now at the stepping-off point for further advances in human sperm cryopreservation, both to increase the efficiency of the process with semen from normal donors and to apply the technique to patients with poor quality semen who desire cryopreservation, such as men with testicular tumors, Hodgkin's disease, and ejaculatory dysfunction.

Successful cryopreservation of mammalian embryos and oocytes lagged several decades behind that achieved with spermatozoa. The logic and techniques used were modeled on those used with semen, but because of the larger cell size of oocytes and embryos, and the relatively low survival rate per cell with spermatozoa, it took some modifications of cooling and thawing rates and cryoprotectant type and concentration before any success was achieved. Then, in 1972, two groups of workers reported successful cryopreservation of eight-cell mouse embryos using dimethylsulfoxide (DMSO) as the cryoprotectant (6,7). In the next 10 to 15 years, the procedures were extended and modified to other species (including humans), embryonic stages, and cryoprotectants. Good reviews of this progress are given in the February 1986 issue of the *Journal of In Vitro Fertilization and Embryo Transfer* and by Whittingham (8).

The first success with the cryopreservation of human embryos was reported in 1983 by Trounson and Mohr (9). They used a methodology with four- and eight-cell embryos similar to that which had worked with cleaving mouse embryos: that is, DMSO as cryoprotectant, slow cooling to a relatively low subzero temperature before transfer to liquid nitrogen (LN), and then a relatively slow warming rate upon thawing. Subsequently, the establishment of successful pregnancies using human blastocysts (10) and zygotes (11) was reported with methodologic changes employed for each specific stage of embryonic development. These results, methodologies, and future prospects will be discussed below.

Routine clinical human oocyte cryopreservation is not yet established as is embryo cryopreservation. The first reported pregnancy using oocyte cryopreservation occurred in 1986 (12), and fewer than 10 pregnancies from cryopreserved oocytes have been reported since then.

In summary, the successful cryopreservation of human gametes and embryos has proceeded in the temporal sequence: sperm, embryos, and oocytes. A few of the major highlights in the evolution of this knowledge are summarized in Table 5.1.

Sperm cryopreservation

As with the cryopreservation of most other cells, the events occurring during cryopreservation of spermatozoa can be divided into three phases: the changes occurring during cooling, storage at final subzero temperature, and the process of thawing and revival of the cells.

Cryophysics

In most cells, including embryos and oocytes, the amount of intracellular water and its conversion to ice crystals upon cooling and subsequent liquefication during warming have to be strictly controlled; however, spermatozoa, because of their relatively compact cellular contents, are not so readily susceptible to the detrimental effects of intracellular ice formation during cooling

(3). For the cryopreservation of spermatozoa, as for other cells, the cells are placed in a biological medium that is supplemented with one or more cryoprotectant agents. The purpose of the cryoprotectant is to regulate the transfer of water across the cell and organelle membranes during freezing and thawing and to minimize the deleterious effects of inappropriate formation of ice crystals. The usual cryoprotectant used for semen is glycerol (5%–10% v/v), and its beneficial effects may be supplemented by the use of a zwitterionic buffer system or egg yolk as an extender or both. The use of DMSO, which has proved suitable for embryos and oocytes, was shown to be less effective than glycerol for the cryopreservation of human semen (3).

The main events occurring during the cooling of spermatozoa in the presence of a cryoprotectant are dehydration and the formation of ice crystals. Dehydration in caused by the influence of hypertonic solution in the extracellular milieu due to the presence of cryoprotectant and on occasion a higher concentration of other solutes, such as sucrose, that do not permeate cell membranes readily. Cell membranes are usually less permeable to these solutes than water, and dehydration by osmosis occurs when the cells are first placed in the cryoprotective medium. Sucrose, which has been used for the cryopreservation of both gametes and embryos, causes an initial dehydration of the cells when they are exposed to it. Ice crystals form in the extracellular solution before they form in the intracellular environment because of the higher initial concentration of solutes intracellularly and hence the lower freezing point. This causes further dehydration during cooling as the concentration of solutes increases extracellularly as more ice forms. The rate at which intracellular ice forms depends then on the initial water content of the cell, the concentration and type of cryoprotectants present, and the rate of cooling. All of these factors have to be optimized so that the amount of intracellular ice formed is compatible with cell survival upon thawing. Excessive dehydration caused by the removal of too much water from the cells and its usual replacement with a permeable cryoprotectant is also detrimental to cell survival, and this has to be optimized also. As described above, with more extracellular ice formation during cooling, the osmotic pressure of the extracellular solution increases, and this can also have a damaging effect on the cells known as the "solution effect." To summarize then, the intention during cryopreservation of spermatozoa and other cells including oocytes and embryos is to dehydrate the cells to an extent compatible with their survival and to use a solution of osmotic pressure such that damaging solution effects do not occur. Upon rewarming, the subsequent rehydration and removal of excess cryoprotective solutes from within the cells has to be optimized so that cryosurvival occurs. Some of the factors influencing the survival of human spermatozoa

Table 5.1 Highlights of gamete and embryo cryopreservation

Contribution	Contributor(s) and date
Discovery of glycerol as a cryoprotectant for spermatozoa	Polge et al., 1949
Cryopreservation of human semen	Sherman, 1953–1954
Use of LN vapor for freezing human semen and storage in LN	Sherman, 1963–1964
Establishment of national and commercial semen cryobanks	Various, 1970s
Cryopreservation of mouse embryos	Whittingham, 1972; Wilmut, 1972
Pregnancies from cryopreserved human embryos	Trounson and Mohr, 1983
Pregnancies from cryopreserved human oocytes	Chen, 1986

after cryopreservation have been summarized by Sherman (3):

1. Temperature shock: Human semen shows little susceptibility compared with some other species, but individuals vary in their response.
2. Cooling rates: Ultrarapid rates ($> 100°C/minute$) are lethal, but slow cooling at rates of 1° to 25°C/minute allow about 70% cryosurvival.
3. Physics of ice crystallization: Intracellular ice formation in spermatozoa is not an important factor, probably because of their relatively dehydrated state to start with; for example, freeze-dried human sperm nuclei can form pronuclei after direct injection into the cytoplasm of hamster oocytes (13). Solution effects during dehydration and the formation of extracellular ice cause the most damage.
4. Cryoprotectant: Glycerol with the use of buffer systems and/or egg-yolk extenders is required.
5. Storage time and temperature: LN at $-196°C$ is the most practical storage facility in large semen cryobanks. There is no loss of cryosurvival after storage in LN, and births have occurred from pregnancies initiated with semen frozen for at least 15 years.
6. Rates of thawing: It appears as if both rapid and slow rates of thawing are compatible with survival. Samples frozen in 2 ml glass ampules then removed from LN and thawed at room temperature (22°C) or in a 37°C water bath survived better than those thawed in a 5°C alcohol bath for 15 minutes (14).
7. Latent cryoinjury: This is apparent after thawing and necessitates the correct timing of insemination in vivo and probably also in vitro.

There is no optimal, universally accepted method for the cryopreservation of human semen that clearly stands alone. It is recommended that clinicians only use a method that in their hands produces normal pregnancy. The many variations that have been used and a concise survey of these factors have been reviewed by Sherman (3).

Clinical indications

The use of frozen semen from male partners or donors has become mandatory because of the risk of HIV transmission (5), as well as difficulties in donor availability for the use of fresh semen and in timing of ovulation in the female (15). The clinical indications for the use of cryopreserved semen have been stated numerous times (3,4,16). They include male infertility, which was the primary cause found in a review of the French national program (4) and comprised both azoospermia (53% of requests) and subfertility (45%) when all other treatment options had failed. Another major reason for the use of cryopreserved donor semen is the presence of genetic risks in the male partner of a couple due to male dominance or recessive inheritable disorders. This accounted for 2% of the approximately 20,000 inseminations conducted in France over the period 1973 to 1988 (4). Some other reasons were also given by Sherman (3) for use of cryopreserved semen:

1. Timed inseminations when the female partner has irregular cycles or special conditions of the female tract.
2. Storage, pooling, and concentration of spermatozoa in oligozoospermic partners to increase the numbers of spermatozoa available for insemination.
3. Use of semen in the temporary absence of the male partner.
4. Preservation of semen before male reproductive tract surgery or chemotherapy or radiotherapy for cancer.
5. Retention of semen from the same donor for subsequent pregnancies.
6. Storage and quarantine of semen during testing of donors for sexually transmitted diseases.

In addition, Trounson et al. (16) found it necessary to establish a semen cryobank because of the number of patients requesting therapeutic donor insemination (TDI) and to meet the demands of donor-husband matching.

As well as screening the male partner of the couple, it is necessary to determine that the female recipient meets certain minimal requirements. In the population studied by Trounson et al. (16), all had at least one patent fallopian tube. This is, of course, necessary for TDI but is not required when in vitro fertilization is performed using cryopreserved spermatozoa. The male partners in the Australian study (16) were also azoospermic or oligozoospermic (spermatozoa $< 20 \times 10^6/$ ml), and the couple had had at least 5 years of sustained infertility. Shapiro (17) also notes that the female recipient should be screened for STDs and should demonstrate ovulation, which should be timed for optimal results. He goes on to state that if the patient subsequently fails to conceive after nine cycles of TDI using cryopreserved semen, she can be evaluated more intensively by way of hysterosalpingography, laparoscopy, and endocrine evaluation as required. Requests for the use of cryopreserved donor semen in the French national program have been exclusively for therapeutic reasons and currently average 3000 per year. Repeat requests for a second or third child total one-third of the annual requests. It is likely that in some clinics in the United States and elsewhere, and it is certainly true of our own program, that cryopreserved donor semen has been used by unmarried single women to achieve a pregnancy.

Donor banks: screening and selection of donors

In France, the recruitment of semen donors is strictly limited to unsolicited volunteers from couples who have had at least one child. About one-third of the donors have been patients who were proceeding to sterilization by a vasectomy. Such strict criteria have not been applied in the majority of other countries.

The selection of donors follows a fairly standard format, which has been described by several authors (3,4,16,17) and can be subdivided into two phases. First, the medical and genetic history of donors and their relatives should be thoroughly investigated, as outlined by Shapiro (17) and given in detail by the American Fertility Society (18). As well as traits due to male dominant and recessive inheritable disorder, a variety of other disorders should be checked for at least three generations (17). Timmons et al. (19) found they could not rely on self-assessment to detect genetic or hereditary problems in donors or recipients even when the person had had formal medical training; ascertainment by counseling and appropriate laboratory testing was also necessary.

Second, a thorough laboratory testing of cryo-survival of spermatozoa to eliminate donors unable to produce a regular supply of sufficient motile spermatozoa of normal morphology capable of producing healthy offspring is necessary. Fairly consistent requirements by most centers undertaking semen cryopreservation involve selecting screened donors whose sample has the following parameters within 1 to 2 hours after ejaculation: volume of at least 1 ml, at least 60% active sperm motility, motile sperm concentration of at least $50 \times 10^6/$ml, and sperm morphology of at least 60% normal oval forms (18). Some variations to these values have been published. For example, sperm concentrations ranging from $50 \times 10^6/$ml to $75 \times 10^6/$ml with at least 50% motility and 70% normal morphology are recommended by particular authors, but the parameters suggested by the American Fertility Society (18), American Association of Tissue Banks (20), and Federation Centre d' Etude et de Conservation du Sperme Humain (CECOS) (4) are all within fairly close agreement. Next, the cryosurvival of frozen-thawed spermatozoa has to reach certain limits. Again, there is a range of values, but as a general rule, at least 50% cryosurvival based on progressive motility is required (3). To attain these requirements, a high number of volunteer donors are rejected (e.g., 38% in the CECOS survey [4]), and because semen quality has lessened during the past 20 years, an even greater proportion of prospective donors face rejection (17).

Ethics for the use of cryopreserved sperm

Mention has already been made of the use of unsolicited volunteer donors in France (4), but the general rule in most other countries is to solicit donors by word-of-mouth, advertisements in college newspapers, and so forth. Ethical considerations of the new reproductive technologies, and specifically the use of donor gametes including spermatozoa, have recently been published by the American Fertility Society (21). The legal and ethical climate for this procedure has evolved somewhat over the years, and certain states in the United States now have laws governing the paternity of a child conceived through TDI. There are still certain reservations about the use of TDI and further technical considerations applying to the use of cryopreserved semen. Most of the biological concerns are unfounded on purely scientific grounds, and it is apparent that self-regulatory peer-group surveillance has and will maintain adequate standards, at least in the United States (3). Returning to specific ethical considerations, many may consider the use of cryopreserved (or fresh) donor semen to produce a child for a single unmarried woman or a lesbian couple unacceptable. However, because of the extreme variations of emotional and societal responses to this issue, the opposing arguments may never be resolved, and we may have to leave it to government decree and the evolution of societal opinion to produce ethical rules at any one time.

Results

Cryopreserved spermatozoa have a decreased functional capacity compared with fresh spermatozoa, for example, in terms of motility, metabolism, and longevity (22), and it has been generally accepted that the fecundability rates in terms of both the pregnancy rate per cycle of TDI and the number of cycles of TDI required to achieve pregnancy are lower with frozen than with fresh donor semen (17). It has also been stated that even in studies that showed no difference between pregnancy rates with the two semen sources, the rates obtained with fresh semen were inordinately low (17). However, it is often not pointed out that there is a wide degree of variability in the etiology of infertility in couples, which could account for differences between centers reporting comparative success rates with fresh and frozen semen. Bordson et al. (23) reported that the fecundability of female patients undergoing TDI with cryopreserved semen was more than doubled when comparing patients with no female factor versus those with a diagnosis of female factor such as endometriosis, pelvic adhesions, tubal disease, or ovulatory dysfunction. When these factors were taken into account, there was no difference between fecundability with fresh semen and that with frozen semen. In several studies reporting a difference, the numbers of motile sperm used for TDI were lower when frozen semen was used than when fresh semen was used (22). Overall, in studies in which some of the etiological variables are more tightly controlled, the data show no difference between the effectiveness of fresh semen and frozen semen provided equivalent numbers of motile spermatozoa are inseminated (4,16,23). Because of the wide variation in reported success rates and a paucity of well-controlled studies that have investigated methodologies that may influence pregnancy rates, it is difficult to assess which factors are relevant. It is generally agreed, however, that the factors that have the most influence are 1) semen quality, 2) cryopreservation methodology, 3) timing of insemination and ovulation, 4) number of oocytes ovulated, and 5) age of recipient. Some of these factors also influence the success rates obtained with fresh semen, and the results available on each topic will be briefly discussed below.

Semen quality: In fertile males probably more than 30 million motile spermatozoa are placed in the cervix at coitus, and the use of at least this number of cryopreserved sperm will probably give the best chance for pregnancy (17). The number of motile spermatozoa that can be recovered from cryopreserved semen is usually less than 30 million and, of course, depends on the initial parameters of the semen before freezing, the extent of dilution with cryoprotectant, and the quantity thawed. Trounson et al. (16) reported that significantly more live spermatozoa were inseminated in patients receiving cryopreserved semen in the months they became pregnant than in those cycles in which pregnancy did not occur. These numbers were 18.3 ± 9.4 million and 14.1 ± 6.5 million ($p < 0.025$), respectively. Also, the longevity of the spermatozoa in the pregnant cycles was greater than in the nonpregnant cycles. A well-designed prospective study was reported by Byrd et al. (24) comparing success rates using cryopreserved washed spermatozoa for intrauterine insemination (IUI) with intracervical insemination (ICI) with thawed semen. The optimum number of motile spermatozoa for achieving pregnancy with IUI was 15 million, whereas with ICI 50 million to 100 million motile sperm were optimal. This indicates the beneficial effects of placing motile spermatozoa closer to the site of fertilization in the fallopian tube. It has also been suggested that too many motile spermatozoa could be used for IUI; Sheldon et al. (25) recommend that not more than 20 million motile spermatozoa be used for IUI in women having multiple follicular development induced with gonadotropin stimulation. They observed a higher incidence of multiple gestations in women undergoing IUI with more than 20 million fresh, washed motile spermatozoa.

Other studies have shown that the motility of donor semen after thawing is one of the contributing factors that has the most influence on success rates, and again, this probably reflects the number of motile spermatozoa reaching the site of fertilization over the ovulation period. The CECOS study (4) reported that the mean success rate per cycle was 7% when the post-thaw motility was 30% to 40% but increased to 17% when the post-thaw motility in the semen was more than 65%. Similar results were reported by Byrd et al. (24). These authors also found that even though some donors had spermatozoa that met the post-thaw survival parameters required (< 50% decrease in motility), the fecundability varied markedly between individual donors. Certain parameters of spermatozoal velocity (linearity, straight-line velocity, and lateral head displacement) were significantly increased in the post-thaw samples of the donors with higher fertility. The phenomenon of variation in donor fecundability was also observed in another study (26) and indicates the need to develop methods to identify this property in donors. Perhaps the French criterion of only using donors from couples who have one or more children (4) and paying closer attention to the sperm velocity parameters measured by Byrd et al. (24) may help ameliorate this problem.

Cryopreservation methodology: As mentioned above, it is difficult to compare the effectiveness of variations in the methodologies used for semen cryopreservation by different laboratories because of the variable success rates. Little has changed in the basic methodology first reported by Sherman in the mid-1960s, and many cryobanks use his basic method involving 5% to 10% glycerol as the cryoprotectant, freezing the samples in LN vapor, and storage in LN (3). The two major areas in which modifications to this basic methodology have been tried are the type of cryoprotectant used and the control of the rate of cooling. Mahadevan and Trounson (27) obtained a higher pregnancy rate using a cryo-preservation medium based on a modified Tyrode's solution containing sucrose, glycine, and glycerol (but no egg yolk) than when an egg yolk–citrate buffer medium was used. Others have reported better cryo-survival of spermatozoa using a zwitterionic buffer system with egg yolk and citrate and glycerol (test-yolk buffer) than when glycerol alone or glycerol–egg yolk–citrate was used (28). Variations in the freezing technique include temperature at addition of glycerol, induction of seeding, and control of the rate of cooling. Critser et al. (29,30) reported better cryosurvival of spermatozoa when glycerol was added to semen at −5°C and the mixture was then held at this temperature for 10 minutes before being seeded and cooled. Serafini and Marrs (31) reported less loss of cryosurvival when semen samples were cooled using a computer-controlled freezing machine that gave a linear rate of cooling at 10°C per minute than when the samples were cooled in LN vapor. Ragni et al. (32) have confirmed that the computer-controlled freezing method is superior to the LN vapor method for the cryopreservation of semen from men with testicular tumors or Hodgkin's disease.

Timing of insemination and ovulation: Healthy spermatozoa need to be in the upper fallopian tube within 24 hours of ovulation. The importance of insemination to cover the most likely time of ovulation has been emphasized in several studies; see review by Kerin and Quinn (33). Since cryopreserved spermatozoa maintain their motility for a shorter period than fresh spermatozoa, more precise timing of insemination and/or several inseminations over the several days when ovulation is expected are necessary.

The importance of accurate timing of IUI in relation to ovulation in patients undertaking insemination with fresh spermatozoa is illustrated in the data reported by Kerin and Quinn (33). When a single IUI was performed the day after the peak levels of serum luteinizing hormone (LH) were reached, the conception rates were more than twice as high as when a single IUI was given on the day that the peak serum LH levels occurred. IUI on the day after the peak serum LH values would be closer to the expected time of ovulation. Similar observations have been reported with IUI using cryopreserved semen (24). Using single inseminations, Byrd et al. (24) found that maximum conception rates occurred when IUI was performed 10 to 20 hours after the urinary LH peak, whereas with ICI the best time was 0 to 10 hours. These authors also found that the number of inseminations using IUI with cryopreserved semen was important; they observed a conception rate of 11.6% per cycle with two inseminations, one given on the day of the LH peak and the second on the following morning, but the pregnancy rate fell significantly to 7.0% when only one insemination was given. There was no significant difference between pregnancy rates with single and double inseminations with ICI, the values being 4.3% and 3.7%, respectively. In contrast to these observations, significantly higher pregnancy rates were reported with ICI with two inseminations, one given the day of and the other the day after the urinary LH peak (34). Despite the paucity of well-controlled studies of TDI using cryopreserved semen, the limited data available do show that IUI gives superior pregnancy rates than ICI when the inseminations are correctly timed in relation to the expected time of ovulation. Better pregnancy rates with IUI than with ICI have also been reported with fresh semen (35). It is likely that the methodology used to wash cryopreserved semen for IUI would be important to obtain the maximum number of motile spermatozoa for placement close to the site of fertilization. In this regard, we have found that washing cryopreserved semen by a discontinuous Percoll gradient method results in the collection of more motile spermatozoa with a better capacity to penetrate zona-free hamster oocytes than when corresponding aliquots from the same thawed sample were prepared by a centrifugation and swim-up method (Table 5.2). Using the Percoll gradient method for collecting washed spermatozoa from cryopreserved donor semen, we have obtained 17 clinical pregnancies in a series of 59 patients (29%) undergoing from one to six IUI cycles.

Number of oocytes: No reports have been published on the effect of the number of oocytes ovulated in relation to pregnancy rates when TDI has been carried out with cryopreserved semen. However, it has been hypothe-

sized that the increased ovulatory rate obtained by the use of human menopausal gonadotropin (hMG) stimulation in IUI cycles using washed spermatozoa from freshly collected semen was partly responsible for the enhanced cycle fecundity, which was comparable to that obtained by in vitro fertilization–embryo transfer (IVF-ET) or gamete intrafallopian transfer (GIFT) (36). The increased number of ovulated oocytes would also contribute to the high multiple pregnancy rate (29%) reported in this study and in other studies using hMG stimulation in IUI cycles (25). It would be likely, therefore, that superovulation in conjunction with IUI with washed spermatozoa obtained from cryopreserved semen could enhance pregnancy rates.

Age of recipient: A direct relationship between the age of the female recipients undergoing TDI with cryopreserved donor semen and successful pregnancy rates has been reported by the French national program involving more than 2000 women whose husbands were azoospermic (37). The cumulative success rates and mean conception rates per cycle of insemination with cryopreserved donor semen were similar in women aged up to 30 years. However, in women aged 31 years and older, the success rate significantly declined, and the decline was even greater for women over 35. Similarly, in a smaller group of 154 patients, Byrd et al. (24) reported a decline in pregnancy rates with increased age of the treated women. Therefore, the age of the female recipient has to be taken into account when comparing different treatments using cryopreserved semen both within and between different centers.

Table 5.2 Comparison of two methods for the recovery of washed spermatozoa from cryopreserved semen

Sample	Mean ± SE
Thawed semen before wash	
Concentration ($\times 10^6$/ml)	66±12
Motility (%)	25±5
Centrifugation and swim-up	
Motile concentration ($\times 10^6$/ml)	6.3±1.7
Motility (%)	38±6
SPA[a] (%)	15±3
Fertility index[b]	0.18±0.06
Percoll gradient centrifugation	
Motile concentration ($\times 10^6$/ml)	13.3±2.9[c]
Motility (%)	38±5
SPA[a] (%)	33±4[c]
Fertility index[b]	0.47±0.10[c]

[a]SPA, zona-free hamster oocyte sperm penetration assay
[b]Fertility index: number of penetrating spermatozoa in total number of oocytes inseminated
[c]Values significantly ($p < 0.001$) higher than corresponding figures for centrifugation and swim-up method (sign test)

Oocyte cryopreservation

Successful oocyte cryopreservation has remained elusive in all groups of mammals in which this procedure has been attempted, unlike the situation for embryo cryopreservation. The much larger size of oocytes and embryos compared with most other cells in the body has necessitated a different approach for the addition of cryoprotectants and the rate of cooling of the cells. Basic differences in the developmental state of the nuclear material and cytoplasm have made oocytes much more refractory than embryos to successful cryopreservation.

Cryophysics

The general principles concerning the dehydration of cells during cooling, the formation of ice crystals within cells and the surrounding extracellular medium, and the use of cryoprotectants with variable degrees of cellular permeability to bring about the optimal rate of dehydration of cells during cooling have already been outlined in the section of sperm cryopreservation. One of the major differences between the cryopreservation of spermatozoa and that of oocytes and embryos is the much larger size of oocytes and embryos. The size of the cell is a major determinant of the rate at which water can leave the cell during dehydration induced by cooling and extracellular ice formation, and is dependent on the ratio of volume to surface area of the cell. Because this ratio is very high in the oocyte and the large spherical cells of embryos, cooling rates 10 to 100 times lower than those used to cryopreserve spermatozoa, red blood cells, or cell lines have been required. This principle was first applied in the successful cryopreservation of mouse embryos (6,7). The other component of cryopreservation that has to be taken into account with oocytes and embryos is the formation of intracellular ice crystals. The amount of ice crystal formation can be regulated by at least two factors: first, the dehydration of the cells by relatively impermeable solutes such as sucrose before extracellular ice formation is induced at seeding, and second, the subzero temperature at which the cooling program is terminated before the cells are transferred to LN. If the amount of intracellular ice is relatively high, as occurs when slow cooling is terminated between −30° and −40°C, the cells survive better if thawing is carried out rapidly (500°C/minute or faster). It is thought that this allows for the rapid thawing of the intracellular ice crystals. On the other hand, if slow cooling is terminated at −50° to −80°C, the cells have had more time to dehydrate further, they contain fewer ice crystals, and upon thawing, the best survival rates are obtained when they are warmed somewhat slower at 4° to 25°C per minute to allow for adequate rehydration.

A third option for the cryopreservation of oocytes and embryos is the process of vitrification. Vitrification refers to the solidification of a liquid into a glass state by extreme elevation of viscosity during cooling and does not involve the process of crystallization. Vitrification of cryopreservative solutions will occur when the concentration of cryopreservatives is sufficiently high and the cooling rate is sufficiently rapid (∼ 2500°C/minute), as occurs when the sample is placed directly into LN (38). It is thought that embryos may also vitrify intracellularly when slow cooling is terminated between −25° and −45°C and they are then transferred to LN (39). This is probably because the concentration of intracellular solutes has been sufficiently increased by dehydration during slow cooling but ice crystal formation has not yet occured. It has been found that the best method for thawing oocytes and embryos cryopreserved by vitrification is to warm them rapidly at 500°C or more per minute to allow the water molecules in the vitrified glass state to be converted directly to the liquid state and to avoid the formation of ice crystals that would occur if the warming rate were slower.

Another method of cryopreservation utilizing the quick and inexpensive benefits of vitrification is the process termed ultrarapid cooling (40). In this procedure oocytes or embryos are exposed for a brief time (2–3 minutes) to a cryoprotective medium containing 3.5 to

4.5M DMSO and 0.25 to 0.3M sucrose and then transferred to LN; the cells are thawed by rapid warming. Vitrification probably occurs using these concentrations of DMSO and sucrose (41).

Clinical indications

The cryopreservation of oocytes for clinical reasons can be divided into two main areas. First, as with semen cryopreservation for men at risk of losing reproductive function because of radiotherapy or chemotherapy for cancer, or for other various conditions of pelvic disease or surgery, oocyte cryopreservation would allow women to store their gametes for similar reasons. Most ART clinics receive requests for oocyte cryopreservation for these reasons each year, and if a successful method were available, the numbers of women seeking such an option would undoubtedly increase. The second benefit of oocyte cryopreservation occurs in couples in which the wife undergoes ovarian hyperstimulation for oocyte retrieval with the intention of having the resulting oocytes and/or embryos transferred back to her. Since it is medically unacceptable to transfer more than three or four oocytes or embryos in a single cycle because of the increased risk of multiple gestations, the majority of couples request cryopreservation of the embryos resulting from the in vitro insemination of the excess oocytes for their future use. However, some couples may wish to donate some of their excess oocytes to another infertile couple to be inseminated by spermatozoa of the husband of the recipient infertile couple. Oocyte cryopreservation would allow the donor couple the option of a final decision on the fate of their oocytes when the number of mature oocytes retrieved is known. Under these circumstances, as well as in the case in which oocytes are retrieved from a specific oocyte donor, oocyte cryopreservation would also overcome problems of synchronization between the cycles of the donor and recipient women.

Donor banks: screening and survival

The screening and selection of oocyte donors should follow the same requirements for a thorough medical and genetic history of the donor and her relatives as does the selection of semen donors. In addition, results obtained with freshly donated oocytes indicate that the age and previous parity of the donor influence the success of the outcome obtained (42). It would be difficult to apply the biological criteria used for the selection of semen donors based on gamete survival after cryopreservation for oocyte donors. Nevertheless, it is most likely that there would be variation between individuals in oocyte cryosurvival just as there is for embryo and semen cryosurvival. Perhaps survival outcome on subsequent thawing of the oocytes collected in the first cycle of the retrieval from an oocyte donor could be used to select donors more likely to produce oocytes capable of surviving cryopreservation.

Ethics

The ethical considerations regarding oocyte cryopreservation will remain hypothetical until a practical method of successful cryopreservation is perfected. However, considering the legal cases that have arisen concerning the disposition of frozen embryos when the gamete providers are in disagreement upon divorce or one or both partners die before the frozen embryo has been thawed and utilized, some guidelines would seem appropriate. Professional societies in most countries where ART is an established clinical procedure have provided such guidelines, as have government-appointed committees, but on the whole the recommendations and laws have centered mainly on the consideration of cryopreserved embryos.

On purely scientific grounds, one might assume that the ethical considerations applying to the use of cryopreserved semen would apply equally to cryopreserved oocytes. However, disparity in the number of viable gametes available in men compared with those in women, the medical intervention required to retrieve the oocytes, and the emotional aspects attached to gestation would require somewhat different and more flexible considerations for oocytes cryopreserved for use by the female provider or for donation to other infertile couples. The Orwellian prospect of donor factories and gestational surrogates raises diverse opinions concerning the rights of the individual and society in these matters. Thus, the intentions of the donors regarding the disposition of their gametes and any rights or relationship with subsequent offspring need to be clearly set out in an appropriate informed-consent document. A more thorough coverage of the legal and ethical considerations involving gametes and embryos is given elsewhere in this volume.

Results

The first report of a successful pregnancy in humans originating from cryopreserved oocytes was that of Chen in 1986 (12), and two other groups reported pregnancies in the following year (43,44). Since that time, however, no further successes have been reported. In all three of the above reports, DMSO was used as the cryoprotectant, and the oocytes were slowly cooled to $-40°C$ or to $-70°$ to $-80°C$ before transfer to LN; this is the basic methodology used by Whittingham (45), who was the first to report the successful cryopreservation of mammalian (mouse) oocytes and the birth of live young derived from the oocytes. Even in the mouse, the results of Whittingham and subsequent reports by others (46,47) show that the oocyte is much more intractable to cryopreservation than the embryo, and a similar situation occurs with human oocytes. Because of the demand for an effective method to cryopreserve human oocytes, intensive studies have been undertaken with both mouse and human oocytes to elucidate the problems and how they can be overcome.

It is now evident that slow cooling and exposure of oocytes to cryoprotectants even before freezing induce changes that affect the fertilizing potential of the oocyte, disrupt the meiotic spindle, and cause subsequent chromosome anomalies (46,48–51). Several studies have shown that oocytes incubated at $4°C$ or exposed to DMSO or propanediol undergo a premature zona reaction, which probably originates from a precocious release of the cortical granules (48,52), events that normally follow fusion of the fertilizing spermatozoan with the oolemma and prevent polyspermy. Indeed, the reduced fertilization rate of mouse oocytes exposed to $4°C$ or cryopreserved can be circumvented if the zona pellucida is removed prior to insemination (48) or if the barrier of the zona is breached by drilling (53). Similarly, the penetration of cryopreserved zona-free hamster oocytes by human spermatozoa is equivalent to that of freshly collected oocytes (54). The presence of serum during exposure of mouse oocytes to DMSO and during cryopreservation can alleviate the deleterious effects of these procedures on the zona pellucida by reducing the conversion of the zona pellucida glycoprotein ZP2, one of the sperm-binding proteins, to its modified form ZP2f, which is unable to bind sperm (50). The presence or absence of serum in the solutions used for the cryopreservation and handling of oocytes prior to and after freeze-thawing may explain some of the variations in the success rates of cryopreservation of mouse oocytes that have been reported (46,47,55). Cooling oocytes has also been shown to disrupt their microtubule system, the human oocyte being more susceptible to this than mouse oocytes (49). Subsequent chromosome anomalies have been reported after fertilization of frozen-thawed mouse oocytes (47,51).

Since slow cooling of oocytes appears to aggravate problems with fertilization and nuclear normality, more rapid cooling by vitrification may be one way to ameliorate the situation. Successful survival and development in vitro of mouse oocytes that have been vitrified or cryopreserved by ultrarapid cooling have been reported (56,57). There have been conflicting reports, however, of the normality of conceptuses derived from vitrified mouse oocytes (51,56). This may be due to the extended exposure time (5–10 minutes at room temperature) of the oocytes to the vitrification solutions before plunging in LN used by Kola et al. (51) rather than the shorter exposure time (5–10 seconds) used by Nakagata (56). Evidence that rapid cooling of human oocytes is more effective than slow cooling is illustrated in Table 5.3.

Survival, fertilization, and cleavage of embryos arising from vitrified human oocytes has also been reported (60). It has also been found that a high proportion (80%) of freshly collected human oocytes was capable of surviving vitrification when frozen by an ultrarapid procedure utilizing 3.5M DMSO and 0.5M sucrose (61). The ability of these oocytes to be fertilized was not assessed, however. Finally, attempts have been made to freeze immature oocytes. It has been found that mouse oocytes at the germinal vesicle stage, although capable of surviving freeze-thawing, do not produce viable embryos unless they are first matured in vitro, so that extrusion of the first polar body occurs prior to cryopreservation (55). However, when primary follicles isolated from immature mice were frozen, thawed, placed in collagen gels, matured by a combined in vitro culture, and inserted under the kidney capsule of recipients, some of the enclosed oocytes matured, were fertilized in vitro, and developed into viable offspring upon transfer to recipients (62).

In summary, the cryopreservation of human oocytes is still very experimental, although there has been limited success by some workers. Undoubtedly, further progress in this area will occur, and oocyte storage banks will be established. The method most likely to be successful with oocytes will probably be one involving vitrification by ultrarapid cooling.

Embryo cryopreservation

Cryophysics

This aspect of embryo cryopreservation has been covered adequately in the previous sections on sperm and oocytes. To reiterate, embryos require slow cooling to allow for adequate dehydration, and the warming rates are related to the amount of intracellular water remaining when the cells are finally placed in LN. More data are emerging that the vitrification procedure using higher concentrations of one or more permeable cryo-preservatives together with a relatively impermeable cryoprotectant such as sucrose will become the most practical method for routine human embryo cryo-preservation in clinical ART programs. In this method, the embryos will be placed in a cryoprotectant medium that will allow for sufficient dehydration and then placed directly in LN. A rapid thawing regimen will be

Table 5.3 Survival and fertilization of human oocytes cryopreserved by two methods involving the use of propanediol and sucrose and different cooling rates

Oocytes	No. of oocytes	
	Method 1[a]	Method 2[b]
Frozen	16	36
Surviving	8 (50%)	1 (3%)
Fertilized	3[c]	0

[a]Renard et al. (58): cryoprotectant medium 2.2M propranediol/0.5M sucrose; transferred from room temperature to −30°C and held for 30 minutes before plunging in LN.

[b]Lassalle et al. (59): cryoprotectant medium 1.5M propranediol/0.2M sucrose; seeded at −7°C, cooled at 0.3°C per minute to −30° before plunging in LN.

[c]One of the fertilized oocytes had three pronuclei.

used to allow for rapid transition of intracellular water from the glass to liquid state without any intervening formation of ice crystals, which have been shown to be lethal to the cells. The cryoprotectants will finally be removed by dilution of the embryos by passage through a series of media containing decreasing concentrations of sucrose.

Clinical indications

The indications for human embryo cryopreservation have been stated on several occasions previously (1). The clinical (and ethical) considerations of the Ethics Committee of the American Fertility Society on the cryopreservation of human (pre-) embryos have recently been published (21). Following the successful use of embryo biopsy for genetic screening prior to embryo replacement (63), cryopreservation of biopsied embryos will become an increasingly important procedure as methods to diagnose more genetic diseases in the small amounts of cellular material available from cleaving embryos or blastocysts become available.

Donor banks

The use of cryopreserved embryos for donation to other unrelated infertile couples or for transfer to a gestational surrogate recipient is becoming a practical option in some ART programs. Our own experience with such procedures is shown in Table 5.4. The success rate in this small group of patients is more than acceptable. Note the two pregnancies obtained when embryos were shipped from countries overseas, indicating the international aspects of embryo donation. In another pregnant patient receiving donated embryos, the two embryos transferred were from two different donors.

Standards for screening and selection of the donors (and gestational surrogate recipients) should be the same as those used for gamete donors in terms of genetic and medical histories.

Ethics

Again the ethics of embryo cryopreservation have been considered in some detail previously (21,64), and once again the caveat that an appropriate informed-consent document be agreed upon to protect all parties involved cannot be overemphasized.

It has been pointed out that the use of the term "pre-embryo" to describe the conceptus from the time of fertilization to the appearance of the primitive streak has been based more on reasons of public policy concerning the moral status of the conceptus than on scientific grounds (65,66). Indeed, the editor of *Nature* described it as a "cosmetic trick" (66). The terms

Table 5.4 Results of transferring cryopreserved embryos to genetically different recipients, 1989–1991

Stage of embryos	No. of patients	No. of embryos		Pregnancies per ET
		Thawed	Survived	
Surrogates				
D1	22	67	48 (72%)	6/22[a] (27%)
D2	2	5	5	0/2
D6	2	2	2	1/2
D1 + D2	1	3 + 2	2 + 2	0/1
Donation				
D1	1	2	2	1/1[b]
D2	1	2	2	1/1
Overall	29	83	63 (76%)	9/29 (31%)—8 delivered or ongoing

[a]Two patients had embryos shipped from overseas. One of these patients had three cycles of transfer of embryos from the same genetic mother; she was not pregnant in the first, had a spontaneous abortion in the second, and is currently pregnant after the third attempt.
[b]The two embryos were from two different donors.

"preimplantation embryo," morula, and blastocyst, together with zygote, two-cell, four-cell, eight-cell embryo, and so on, have been used for many years, have a precise definition, and seem adequate for use in most scientific and medical journals.

Results

National statistics for the United States and Australia have been reported (67,68) and show that for clinics performing 50 or more transfers on an annual basis, the clinical pregnancy rate is 14% with an ongoing pregnancy rate of 70% of the clinical pregnancies. These numbers are similar but significantly lower than those reported for transfer of fresh embryos in IVF (67,68).

Our own results using cryopreservation of embryos for the 4 years 1987 through 1990 are shown in Table 5.5. The success rates are very similar to the national results given in the two reports mentioned above. Our experience with transfer of cryopreserved embryos to surrogate gestational carriers and recipients of donated embryos has already been mentioned (see Table 5.4).

Table 5.5 Results of cryopreservation at the Institute for Reproductive Research, Los Angeles, California, 1987–1990

Day of freezing	No. of patients	Embryo survival	Pregnancies per ET	Ongoing pregnancies
1	345	668/897 (74%)	43/314 (14%)	29 (67%)
2	116	196/243 (81%)	8/104 (8%)	4 (50%)
5–6	64	76/106 (72%)	7/50 (14%)	5 (71%)
Total	525	940/1246 (75%)	58/468 (12%)	38 (66%)

Table 5.6 Comparison of using BSA versus patient's serum as the protein supplement in cryoprotectant medium

Protein	No. of patients	Embryo survival	Pregnancies per ET	Ongoing pregnancies
BSA[a]	18	41/48 (85%)	4/16 (25%)	4
POS[b]	36	74/100 (74%)	4/31 (13%)	3

[a]BSA, bovine serum albumin, 5 mg/ml
[b]POS, patient's own serum, 20% (v/v)

Mention should be made of some of the modifications we have made to simplify the procedure. These include the use of bovine serum albumin (BSA) versus human serum as the protein source in the cryopreservative medium, seeding at $-5°C$ rather than $-7°C$, and dilution of the cryoprotectant from the embryos by their passage through medium containing sucrose only. The results are shown in Tables 5.6, 5.7, and 5.8. The use of BSA as the protein supplement is necessary in some cases when a blood sample has not been obtained from the patient and serum from another person has not been used. Nevertheless, despite the lack of difference in results when BSA or human serum was used, we still prefer to use 20% human serum as the protein supplement. This is because of the possible beneficial cryoprotectant properties of serum and the

Table 5.7 Seeding at $-5°C$

Day of freezing	No. of patients	Embryo survival	Pregnancies per ET	Ongoing pregnancies
1	10	21/29 (72%)	1/9	1/1
2	4	9/11 (82%)	1/4	1/1
6	2	2/5 (40%)	0/1	—
Total	16	32/45 (71%)	2/14 (14%)	2/2

known protective effects of serum on oocytes during cryopreservation. Seeding at −5°C rather than −7°C is based on the assumption that it is better to induce ice-crystal formation closer to the freezing point of the cryo-protectant solution to minimize temperature changes due to the release of the latent heat of crystallization. The only drawback to this procedure is that it has to be done relatively quickly with little exposure of the sample to ambient room temperature, which could raise its temperature above the freezing point. However, one can check that ice-crystal formation has indeed occurred and avoid supercooling by monitoring the sample before the temperature has dropped very far. Of more practical use is the dilution of the thawed sample by the simplified protocol outlined in Table 5.8. Instead of decreasing the propanediol concentration from 1.0 to 0.5M in the presence of 0.2M sucrose before transfer of the thawed embryos to wash media as was proposed originally (59), we placed the contents of the thawed straw directly into 0.2M sucrose solutions with no propanediol for 5 minutes, then 0.1M sucrose for 5 minutes, and then washed twice to retrieve the embryo. This slightly shortens the time the embryos spend in

dilution media and reduces the number of different types of media required. Since this modified procedure produces the same embryo survival and pregnancy rate in our laboratory as does the original protocol, we now routinely use it.

A final comment is required with respect to the use of vitrification/ultrarapid freezing for the cryo-preservation of human embryos. Because this method has proved successful with mouse embryos (40,69,70), it is to be expected that it should be tried and prove useful with human embryos. Several groups have obtained pregnancies using this procedure (71–73), and it is my opinion that the method will become routine and the one of choice for human embryo cryopreservation in the near future. Because of the simplicity of its nature and its low cost, this procedure should make cryopreservation of cleaving human embryos available to all ART programs no matter what their budget.

Acknowledgments: I thank Denny Cook for typing the manuscript and Kay Quinn for statistical advice.

Table 5.8 Use of a modified dilution protocol for the recovery of thawed human embryos

Day of freezing	No. of patients	Embryo survival	Pregnancies per ET	Ongoing pregnancies
1	113	247/337 (78%)	16/102 (16%)[a]	10
2	22	40/48 (83%)	2/20 (10%)[a]	2

The thawed straw contents were emptied into 0.2M sucrose and incubated 5 minutes, then transferred to 0.1M sucrose for 5 minutes, then washed twice in sucrose-free medium (5 minutes each).
[a]Not significantly different from results using protocol of Lassalle et al. (59); data not shown.

References

1. Quinn P. Success of oocyte and embryo freezing and its effects on outcome with in vitro fertilization. Semin Reprod Endocrinol 1990;8:272–280.

2. Polge C, Smith AU, Parkes AS. Revival of spermato-zoa after vitrification and dehydration at low temperatures. Nature 1949;164:666.

3. Sherman JK. Cryopreservation of human semen. In: Keel BA, Webster BW, eds. Handbook of the laboratory diagnosis and treatment of infertility. Boca Raton, Fla.: CRC Press, 1990:229–259.

4. Federation CECOS, LeLannou D, Lansac J. Artificial procreation with frozen donor semen: experience of the French Federation CECOS. Hum Reprod 1989;4:757–761.

5. Stewart GJ, Tyler JPP, Cunningham AL, et al. Transmission of human T-cell lymphotropic virus type III

(HTLV-III) by artificial insemination by donor. Lancet 1985; 2:581–585.

6. Whittingham DG, Leibo SP, Mazur P. Survival of mouse embryos frozen to −269°C. Science 1972;178:411–414.

7. Wilmut I. Effect of cooling rate, warming rate, cryoprotective agent and stage of development on survival of mouse embryos during cooling and warming. Life Sci 1972;11:1071–1079.

8. Whittingham DG. Principles of embryo preservation. In: Ashwood-Smith MJ, Farrant J, eds. Low temperature preservation in medicine and biology. Tunbridge Wells: Pitman Medical, 1980.

9. Trounson AO, Mohr L. Human pregnancy following cryopreservation, thawing and transfer of an eight-cell embryo. Nature 1983;305:707–709.

10. Cohen J, Simons RF, Edwards RG, Fehilly CB, Fishel SB. Pregnancies following the frozen storage of expanding human blastocysts. J In Vitro Fert Embryo Transf 1985;2:59–64.

11. Testart J, Lassalle B, Belaisch-Allart J, et al. High pregnancy rate after early human embryo freezing. Fertil Steril 1986;46:268–272.

12. Chen C. Pregnancy after human oocyte cryopreservation. Lancet 1986;1:884–886.

13. Uehara T, Yamagimachi R. Microsurgical injection of spermatozoa into hamster eggs with subsequent transformation of sperm nuclei into male pronuclei. Biol Reprod 1976;15:467–470.

14. Cohen J, Felten P, Zeilmaker GH. In vitro fertilizing capacity of fresh and cryopreserved human spermatozoa: a comparative study of freezing and thawing procedures. Fertil Steril 1981;36:356–362.

15. Marrs RP, Brown J, Quinn P. Gamete and embryo cryopreservation. ·Advantages, techniques and results. In: Soules MR, ed. Controversies in reproductive endocrinology and infertility. New York: Elsevier, 1989:321–331.

16. Trounson AO, Mahadevan M, Wood J, Leeton JF. Studies on the deep-freezing and artificial insemination of human semen. In: Richardson D, Joyce D, Symonds M, eds. Frozen human semen. London: Royal College of Obstetrics and Gynaecology, 1979:173–183.

17. Shapiro SS. Therapeutic donor insemination. Establishing protocols for effective practice. In: Soules MR, ed. Controversies in reproductive endocrinology and infertility. New York: Elsevier, 1989:205–228.

18. American Fertility Society. New guidelines for the use of semen donor insemination: 1990. Fertil Steril 1990; 53(Suppl 1):1s–13s.

19. Timmons MC, Rao KW, Sloan CS, Kirkman HN, Talbert LM. Genetic screening of donors for artificial insemination. Fertil Steril 1981;35:451–456.

20. American Association of Tissue Banks. Standards of tissue banking. Arlington, Va., 1989.

21. American Fertility Society. Ethical considerations of the new reproductive technologies. Fertil Steril 1990;53(Suppl 2):1s–109s.

22. Richter MA, Haning RV, Shapiro SS. Artificial donor insemination: fresh versus frozen sperm; the patient as her own control. Fertil Steril 1984;41:277–280.

23. Bordson BL, Ricci E, Dickey RP, Dunaway H, Taylor SN, Curole DN. Comparison of fecundability with fresh and frozen semen in therapeutic donor insemination. Fertil Steril 1986;46:466–469.

24. Byrd W, Bradshaw K, Carr B, Edman C, Odom J, Ackerman G. A prospective randomized study of pregnancy rates following intrauterine and intracervical insemination using frozen donor sperm. Fertil Steril 1990;53:521–527.

25. Sheldon R, Kemmann E, Bohrer M, Pasquale S. Multiple gestation is associated with the use of high sperm numbers in the intrauterine insemination specimen in women undergoing gonadotropin stimulation. Fertil Steril 1988;49:607–610.

26. Thorneycroft IH, Bustillo M, Marik J. Donor fertility in an artificial insemination program. Fertil Steril 1984;41:144–145.

27. Mahadevan M, Trounson AO. Effect of cryoprotective media and dilution methods on the preservation of human spermatozoa. Andrologia 1983;15:355–366.

28. Prins GS, Weidel L. A comparative study of buffer systems as cryoprotectants for human spermatozoa. Fertil Steril 1986;46:147–149.

29. Critser JK, Huse-Benda AR, Aaker DV, Arneson

BW, Ball GD. Cryopreservation of human spermatozoa. I. Effects of holding procedure and seeding on motility, fertilizability and acrosome reaction. Fertil Steril 1987;47:656–663.

30. Critser JK, Arneson BW, Aaker DV, Huse-Benda AR, Ball GD. Cryopreservation of human spermatozoa. II. Postthaw chronology of motility and of zona-free hamster ova penetration. Fertil Steril 1987;47:980–984.

31. Serafini P, Marrs RP. Computerized staged-freezing technique improves sperm survival and preserves penetration of zona-free hamster ova. Fertil Steril 1986;45:854–858.

32. Ragni G, Caccamo AM, Dalla Serra A, Guercilena S. Computerized slow-staged freezing of semen from men with testicular tumors or Hodgkin's disease preserves sperm better than standard vapor freezing. Fertil Steril 1990;53:1072–1075.

33. Kerin J, Quinn P. Washed intrauterine insemination in the treatment of oligospermic infertility. Semin Reprod Endocrinol 1987;5:23–33.

34. Centola GM, Mattox JH, Raubertas RF. Pregnancy rates after double versus single insemination with frozen donor semen. Fertil Steril 1990;54:1089–1092.

35. Cruz RI, Kemmann E, Brandeis VT, et al. A prospective study of intrauterine insemination of processed sperm from men with oligoasthenospermia in superovulated women. Fertil Steril 1986;46:673–677.

36. Dodson WC, Whitesides DB, Hughes CL, Easley HA, Haney AF. Superovulation with intrauterine insemination in the treatment of infertility: a possible alternative to gamete intrafallopian transfer and in vitro fertilization. Fertil Steril 1987;48:441–445.

37. Federation CECOS, Schwartz D, Mayaux MJ. Female fecundity as a function of age. Results of artificial insemination in 2193 nulliparous women with azoospermic husbands. N Engl J Med 1982;306:404–406.

38. Fahy GM, MacFarlane DR, Angell CA, Meryman HT. Vitrification as an approach to cryopreservation. Cryobiology 1984;21:106–121.

39. Rall WF, Polge C. Effect of warming rate on mouse embryos frozen and thawed in glycerol. J Reprod Fertil 1984;70:285–292.

40. Trounson A, Peura A, Kirby C. Ultrarapid freezing: a new low cost and effective method of embryo cryopreservation. Fertil Steril 1987;48:845–850.

41. Shaw JM, Kola I, MacFarlane DR, Trounson AO. An association between chromosomal abnormalities in rapidly frozen 2-cell mouse embryos and the ice-forming properties of the cryoprotective solution. J Reprod Fertil 1991;91:9–18.

42. Sauer MV, Paulson RJ, Macaso TM, Francis-Hernandez M, Lobo RA. Establishment of a nonanonymous donor oocyte program: preliminary experience at the University of Southern California. Fertil Steril 1989;52:433–436.

43. Al-Hasani S, Deidrich K, van der Ven H, Reinecke A, Hartje M, Krebs D. Cryopreservation of human oocytes. Hum Reprod 1987;2:695–700.

44. Van Uem JF, Seibzehnrubl ER, Schuh B, Koch R, Trotnow S, Lang N. Birth after cryopreservation of unfertilized oocytes. Lancet 1987;1:752–753.

45. Whittingham DG. Fertilization in vitro and development to term of unfertilized mouse oocytes previously stored at −196°C. J Reprod Fertil 1977;49:89–94.

46. Trounson A, Kirby C. Problems in the cryopreservation of unfertilized eggs by slow cooling in dimethyl sulfoxide. Fertil Steril 1989;52:778–786.

47. Carroll J, Warnes GM, Matthews CD. Increase in digyny explains polyploidy after in-vitro fertilization of frozen-thawed mouse oocytes. J Reprod Fertil 1989;85:489–494.

48. Johnson MH, Pickering SJ, George MA. The influence of cooling on the properties of the zona pellucida of the mouse oocyte. Hum Reprod 1988;3:383–387.

49. Pickering SJ, Braude PR, Johnson MH, Cant A, Currie J. Transient cooling to room temperature can cause irreversible disruption of the meiotic spindle in the human oocyte. Fertil Steril 1990;54:102–108.

50. Vincent C, Turner K, Pickering SJ, Johnson MH. Zona pellucida modifications in the mouse in the absence of oocyte activation. Mol Reprod Dev 1991;28:394–404.

51. Kola I, Kirby C, Shaw J, Davey A, Trounson A. Vitrification of mouse oocytes results in aneuploid zygotes and malformed fetuses. Teratology 1988;38:467–474.

52. Schalkoff ME, Oskowitz SP, Powers RD. Ultrastructural observations of human and mouse oocytes treated with cryopreservatives. Biol Reprod 1989;40:379–393.

53. Carroll J, Depypere H, Matthews CD. Freeze-thaw-induced changes of the zona pellucida explains decreased rates of fertilization in frozen-thawed mouse oocytes. J Reprod Fertil 1990;90:547–553.

54. Quinn P, Barros C, Whittingham DG. Preservation of hamster oocytes to assay the fertilizing capacity of human spermatozoa. J Reprod Fertil 1982;66:161–168.

55. Schroeder AC, Champlin AK, Mobraaten LE, Eppig JJ. Developmental capacity of mouse oocytes cryopreserved before and after maturation in vitro. J Reprod Fertil 1990;89:43–50.

56. Nakagata N. High survival rate of unfertilized mouse oocytes after vitrification. J Reprod Fertil 1989;87:479–483.

57. Surrey ES, Quinn PJ. Successful ultrarapid freezing of unfertilized oocytes. J In Vitro Fert Embryo Transf 1990;7:262–266.

58. Renard J-P, Nguyen B-X, Garnier V. Two-step freezing of two-cell rabbit embryos after partial dehydration at room temperature. J Reprod Fertil 1984;71:573–580.

59. Lassalle B, Testart J, Renard J-P. Human embryo features that influence the success of cryopreservation with the use of 1,2 propanediol. Fertil Steril 1985;44:645–651.

60. Trounson A. Preservation of human eggs and embryos. Fertil Steril 1986;46:1–12.

61. Pensis M, Loumaye E, Psalti I. Screening of conditions for rapid freezing of human oocytes: preliminary study toward their cryopreservation. Fertil Steril 1989;52:787–794.

62. Carroll J, Whittingham DG, Wood MJ, Telfer E, Gosden RG. Extra-ovarian production of mature viable mouse oocytes from frozen primary follicles. J Reprod Fertil 1990;90:321–327.

63. Handyside AH, Kontogianni EH, Hardy K, Winston RML. Pregnancies from biopsied human preimplantation embryos sexed by Y-specific DNA amplification. Nature 1990;344:378–380.

64. Board of Trustees, American Medical Association. Frozen pre-embryos. JAMA 1990;263:2484–2487.

65. Biggers JD. Arbitrary partitions of prenatal life. Hum Reprod 1990;5:1–6.

66. Kelly J. Pre-embryos. Lancet 1990;1:116.

67. Medical Research International, Society for Assisted Reproductive Technology, American Fertility Society. In vitro fertilization–embro transfer (IVF-ET) in the United States: 1989 results from the IVF-ET registry. Fertil Steril 1991;55:14–23.

68. National Perinatal Statistics Unit, Fertility Society of Australia. IVF and GIFT pregnancies: Australia and New Zealand. Sydney: National Perinatal Statistics Unit, 1990.

69. Wilson L, Quinn P. Development of mouse embryos cryopreserved by an ultra-rapid method of freezing. Hum Reprod 1989;4:86–90.

70. Kasai M, Komi JH, Takakamo A, Tsudera H, Sakurai T, Machida T. A simple method for mouse embryo cryopreservation in a low toxicity vitrification solution, without appreciable loss of viability. J Reprod Fertil 1990;89:91–97.

71. Trounson AO. Cryopreservation. Br Med Bull 1990;46:695–708.

72. Gordts S, Roziers P, Campo R, Noto V. Survival and pregnancy outcome after ultrarapid freezing of human embryos. Fertil Steril 1990;53:469–472.

73. Barg PE, Barad DH, Feichtinger W. Ultrarapid freezing (URF) of mouse and human preembryos: a modified approach. J In Vitro Fert Embryo Transf 1990;7:355–357.

6

Laboratory Function for the Assisted Reproductive Technologies

David R. Meldrum

T h e ability to sustain gametes and embryos outside the body with minimum effects on their metabolic and functional integrity is probably the most important variable in the success of the assisted reproductive technologies (ART) and in the remarkable variation of success rates among programs. The oocyte is a highly complex, very large cell, that must maintain full metabolic function allowing it to resume meiosis, to undergo normal fertilization, and to develop to the four-to-eight-cell stage before the embryonic genome finally becomes activated (1). At the time of aspiration, the oocyte is usually at metaphase II, with its chromosomes distributed on an extremely delicate microtubular spindle. Formation and fusion of the male and female pronuclei are complex processes requiring an intricate series of events. Cytoplasmic maturation must be adequate to provide for sufficient metabolic machinery to form a multicelled embryo. Suboptimal conditions may result in abnormalities of fertilization or cleavage or simply in failure of ongoing development and implantation.

Basic laboratory setup and equipment

Construction and physical setup

Ideally, all laboratory functions should be carried out in the same general area to achieve optimal efficiency of personnel. If necessary, gametes and embryos can be transported in appropriately buffered media at 37°C, probably without detriment. The wet area for preparation of culture materials, the sperm preparation area, and the area for handling animal embryos should be separate from the human embryo culture laboratory. Flooring, walls, and ceilings should be designed for optimal sterility. Air for the embryo laboratory should be high-energy particle absorption (HEPA) filtered with positive outflow, and the air intake should be at an area free from odors. New construction can lead to dust and odors that could profoundly influence the culture system. Adequate time should be left before active use of the area. Critical items of equipment should be on emergency power supply.

Equipment

Main incubators: The embryo culture laboratory will require an adequate number of tissue culture incubators to limit door openings to a minimum. Fewer are needed if they incorporate a system for rapid recovery of carbon dioxide (CO_2) level or if an accessory mobile incubator is used for oocyte and embryo manipulations in a controlled environment (2). It is best to use brands of incubators that other successful programs have used, to avoid unrecognized embryotoxicity. New incubators can have a strong plastic odor and should be tested with a bioassay for toxicity before use. Trimix incubators allowing control of oxygen (O_2) as well as CO_2 levels require a nitrogen tank to adjust O_2 concentration and introduce further electronic and mechanical points that could fail. Some teams use an inner sealed vessel (e.g., desiccator) that has a gas flow-through from a tank or is gassed and then sealed. Advantages are that the CO_2 level is protected from incubator failure and that 5% O_2 can be used. Disadvantages are the cost of the mixed gas, potential for failure due to gas running out, and potential for embryotoxicity and temperature fluctuations.

Microscopes: A good quality dissecting microscope is needed for oocyte identification and grading and for evaluation of pronuclei and embryo morphology. If it is used inside a 37°C environment, a stage must be used that will not become excessively hot. If used in ambient conditions, a stage warmer will help it to maintain body temperature. An inverted phase-contrast or interference-contrast microscope is needed if oocytes are evaluated for the first polar body. It is also needed to confirm polypronuclear oocytes, since vacuoles can have the appearance of a nucleus. Such "pseudopronuclei" can be associated with normal evolution of pregnancy (3).

Meters for pH and osmolarity: A highly accurate pH meter should be readily available to check media periodically after equilibration and to monitor handling procedures to ensure that excessive pH drifts are being avoided. A thin electrode allows testing of small aliquots in a culture tube with enough stability under ambient conditions to obtain an accurate reading. Media are adjusted to 278 to 284 mosmol/kg, which requires a highly accurate osmometer.

Laminar flow hoods: Preparation and aliquoting of media must be carried out in a sterile environment within a laminar flow hood. Adequate flow and sterility should be verified on a regular schedule, and the working surface should be sterilized periodically with alcohol. Ultraviolet lights are commonly used for further control of surface bacteria.

Portable incubator/isolette: To avoid pH and temperature shifts of media, a pediatric isolette or similar device can be modified to house a dissecting microscope and working area. A CO_2 controller can be mounted within it (2). Humidification can be provided by ultrapure water. Temperatures should be monitored in each area where materials are set or examined. Carbon dioxide levels should be checked regularly by the same external device used for the main incubators. Each time the program stops between series, all surfaces within the isolette should be cleaned and then wiped with alcohol to prevent contamination. Such chambers are commercially available but can be economically fashioned using simple components and a used isolette.

Water baths: Any sera used for cell culture must be heat-inactivated (56°C for 30 minutes) to remove complement. Documentation of times and temperatures is particularly important for any donor sera, since this inactivates the human immunodeficiency virus (HIV) (4).

Analytical balance: Materials for weighing media should be dedicated for only that function and should be located in the embryo laboratory. Provided weighing of media solutes is highly accurate, reproducible osmolarity and pH should be consistently achieved. If any unusual value is obtained, the medium should be discarded and a new batch prepared.

Culture medium

Type

The most common medium used has been Ham's F10. To make it more closely approximate tubal fluid, the Ham's F10 has been modified (5), or the appropriate solutes have been mixed without Ham's F10 and described as "human tubal fluid" (HTF) (6). Both human and animal results have suggested that at least 5mM potassium is necessary for optimal embryo development (6). In fact, the potassium concentration of the fallopian tube is 20 to 30mM. The modified Ham's F10 introduced by Lopata has 8mM potassium after adjusting osmolarity (5). It has been suggested that Ham's F10 would be improved if hypoxanthine was deleted from the recipe since it is a meiosis inhibitor (7). Several other media are used. There is no evidence that one is superior to the others.

Preparation

Water: There have been numerous indications that water purity is of utmost importance (8). Most commonly either in-house milli-Q (Millipore Corp., Bedford, Mass.) reverse osmosis deionized water or commercial water of high-performance liquid chromotography (HPLC) grade or tissue-culture grade has been used. Endotoxin can contaminate water purification systems through even minor bacterial growth. This should be tested with a simple kit. Routine mouse embryo assays are not sensitive enough to detect endotoxin, which has been related to reduced fertilization of human eggs and increased fragmentation of embryos (9). Endotoxin may be of particular concern when openings are made in the zona to aid fertilization, since zona-free mouse embryos manifest increased sensitivity to endotoxin (10).

Solutes: Added solutes provide a major source for embryotoxicity. It is best to use the same exact components as those used by a highly successful program. Chemical purity does not equate to lack of embryotoxicity. Reagents of tissue-culture grade are often used, but that label does not guarantee good results with embryos.

Antibiotics: Penicillin and streptomycin are usually added to media and may be particularly important with transvaginal retrieval. Streptomycin preparations are prone to embryotoxicity. We have tested several in order to find one completely free of adverse effects on mouse embryos. It is best to keep it in powder form until the medium is mixed.

Preparation materials: Preparation materials can add minor amounts of toxicity and should be tested. Reusable materials should be kept to a minimum and prepared through a full tissue-culture wash including multiple washes and soaks of ultrapure water. Osmolarity is adjusted to 278 to 284 mosmol/kg. After overnight equilibration, pH should be between 7.35 and 7.45.

Toxicity testing: Media and any materials contacting the culture system should be tested with a bioassay that evaluates any adverse effects on reproductive cells in culture (11,12). In approximate decreasing order of sensitivity, these are hamster sperm motility (8), mouse one-cell embryo (13) or zona-free two-cell embryo (10), two-cell mouse embryo (11), and human sperm (14). Human sperm, although least sensitive, can be used as an ongoing quality control step. For each normal male, overnight motility should decrease by no more than 5% to 10% over control if an appropriate protein source is used during processing. Although hamster sperm are highly sensitive to decreases of water quality (8), we have found that not all embryotoxicity is detected by that assay. Also, we have found that our particular two-cell assay (B6C3F1, 8- to 10-week-old female × B6C3F1 male; no protein added) is more sensitive when compared with the one-cell model. This could be because of methodology or strain. We collect the tubes in an area remote from the culture laboratory so as to not have to bring the animals into the laboratory. This or other procedural factors could make it more sensitive. Each batch of medium should be tested for ideal quality control, but at the minimum whenever there is any change of one of the components. Medium is generally not used for more than 4 weeks before a new batch is prepared. Our media are prepared and tested weekly.

Protein supplements: Albumin and serum have protective effects on sperm during washing and centrifugation (15) and aid capacitation. Both purified albumin (16) and some individual sera (17) can contain material that is toxic to reproductive cells. It is not clear whether albumin, patient's serum, or fetal cord serum have any positive effect on egg or embryo culture, although one study showed a significantly higher rate of pregnancy with fetal cord serum than with patient's preovulatory ("maternal") serum (5). Serum could act either by adding embryotrophic growth factors or by absorbing

toxic substances in the media. Ideally, each individual serum specimen is assessed in a mouse embryo assay for toxicity, and only nontoxic sera are then used (18). Some programs have used a designated donor to make this process more efficient. There may be an advantage to immediate separation of the serum, since platelets are a source of embryotoxicity (19). Donor sera should be tested for HIV and hepatitis B and C and should be heat-inactivated to inactivate complement and HIV. Sera should not be pooled, which could increase the number of patients exposed to any infectious agent in a particular serum specimen. The usual concentration of serum has been 7% to 15% in the insemination medium and 15% in the medium used after fertilization is identified ("growth medium").

Coculture using "helper" cells: A number of studies on animal embryos have demonstrated improved results when embryos are cultured over a monolayer of various cell types, with improved morphologic appearance of the embryos as well as improved rates of pregnancy following transfer. The first clinical application of this modality was by Wiemer et al. (20) using fetal bovine uterine fibroblasts. Following verification of fertilization, human zygotes were placed in culture with or without an underlying cell monolayer. The incidence of fragmentation was significantly reduced, and the pregnancy rate increased from 17% to 35%. Bongso et al. have shown similar reductions of embryo fragmentation using cocultures of human fallopian tube epithelial cells (21). Menozo et al. have shown beneficial effects with monkey kidney (Vero) cells (22). Thus the beneficial effects on embryo growth do not appear to be specific to cell type or to the reproductive tract. Effects have been attributed either to positive embryotrophic factors or to simple removal of toxic contaminants from the media. This is an important distinction, since in the latter instance, improvement of the culture conditions could make use of cocultures unnecessary. A distinct disadvantage of these systems is the difficult and time-consuming task of maintaining these cell lines. Their growth rate will influence effects on media pH, and any impaired viability could obviate beneficial effects. Even groups experienced in the use of these cell lines have substantial times when they are not growing satisfactorily. A further drawback of coculture is that the accompanying blastomere swelling (20) is incompatible with zona micromanipulation techniques, causing loss of individual cells through the opening in the zona.

Culture materials: Anything contacting the media ("contact materials") either should be tested for embryotoxicity or should be processed through a tissue-culture wash that incorporates multiple rinses and soaks in ultrapure water. Sterilization should be by dry heat, which does not deposit any potentially embryotoxic residue, as can occur with autoclaving or ethylene oxide. Even materials sold for tissue cultures have variable and occasionally marked embryotoxicity, sometimes varying from batch to batch or even within sleeves packaging several dishes or tubes. Therefore as a further precaution, we rinse each tube or dish with culture medium before use. When filter-sterilizing media, we routinely flush disc filters and discard the first 30 to 40 cc with large filter units (23). In general we avoid nondisposable materials in case the quality of the wash might vary. To avoid use of a volumetric flask, we have calculated the amount of water that must be pipetted into the solutes to achieve the desired total volume. Aspiration needles should not be reused owing to toxicity, and aspiration of urine should be avoided owing to marked embryotoxicity (12). We routinely place a new CO_2 tank on the mouse embryo incubator before moving it to the human laboratory. Tanks should be dedicated for use only with the particular gas being delivered.

Culture environment

Temperature

The oocyte appears to be particularly sensitive to reduced temperature. A reduction to room temperature has been shown to cause disorganization of the chromosome spindle, resulting in chromosome maldistributions (24). Even minor temperature decreases have been associated with decreased fertilization and pregnancy outcome (25). To minimize changes, we rinse the collecting system with warm media, aspirate the folliclar fluid into a tube within a heating block, and place the tube immediately into the pediatric isolette. The main incubator is then opened only once for each procedure. Since the chamber temperature drops with each door opening, and this is not reflected in the readout, a significant and prolonged drop of chamber temperature can go unrecognized. The use of the isolette is a major advantage in keeping the incubator environment as stable as possible. Use of a gas flow-through system must allow for adequate warming since the cold tank gas together with heat absorption accompanying humidification of the gas can substantially lower temperature in the culture chamber. Although fertilized eggs and embryos are probably much less sensitive to temperature shifts, we utilize the pediatric isolette for all manipulations for whatever benefit that might accrue. Temperatures should be monitored in all areas where oocytes and embryos are placed, by laboratory thermometers, which are in turn checked by a highly accurate reference thermometer on a regular basis.

Carbon dioxide

Bicarbonate-buffered media used in in vitro fertilization (IVF) require approximately a 5% CO_2 environment to maintain a physiologic pH. This is provided in the incubator or mobile isolette by a CO_2 sensor that adjusts the CO_2 level in the presence of humidity to the desired level. If CO_2 is utilized as a flow-through system from a tank of dry gases, the resulting actual level of CO_2 when humidity is added in the culture chamber will be lower. This can be adjusted by requesting a mixture slightly in excess of 5%. With the modified Ham's F10 recipe that we use (5), approximately 5.5% CO_2 is required to achieve a pH of 7.4 with humidity and about 5.8% CO_2 as a dry gas.

The level of CO_2 must be monitored, before any breech of the culture environment, by means of an independent device. Although other methods are available, the Fyrite (Bacharach Inc. Pittsburg, Pa. is the most widely used. It must be properly maintained to avoid inaccuracy. An additional check on CO_2 level is the pH of the media after overnight equilibration. Given accurately weighed solutes, media pH should be highly reproducible from week to week. Otherwise the accuracy of the CO_2 level should be suspect.

Oxygen

Mouse embryos develop slightly but significantly better in 5% O_2 compared with room air (21% O_2). It is not clear whether there is any advantage for human embryos, and most IVF programs do not utilize 5% O_2. Use of the lower O_2 level requires either a trimix incubator or a mixed gas (5% CO_2, 5% O_2, and 90% nitrogen). In the former case, the nitrogen tank adds one further source of embryotoxicity, and the O_2 sensor and solenoid valve add further points for mechanical failure. The trimix gas in turn has the disadvantage of possible embryotoxic contaminants added during preparation or from the tank itself, as well as the temperature effects mentioned above. At one point in the past, we considered converting to such a system, but our mouse embryo assay did not perform as well as in West Los Angeles air.

Humidity

Large pans of ultrapure water may be placed in the bottom of the incubator to provide humidity. The water should be changed frequently, and the pan should be periodically sterilized to avoid growth of organisms. If a gas flow-through system is used, the gas may be warmed and humidified by bubbling it through a flask of ultrapure water.

Ambient air

Air within the laboratory should be free of particles and odors, which could be embryotoxic. The air intake should be located to bring in high-quality air. High-energy particle absorption (HEPA) filters should be used to provide air quality similar to that of an operating room. Use of pesticides or volatile cleansing materials should be avoided. It is our routine to do detailed cleaning two to three times per year between series. With a sticky mat outside the door, foot covers, filtered air, and hand scrubbing, there is no need for more frequent cleaning except for periodic alcohol cleaning of working surfaces.

Embryo handling and transfer

Protection against temperature and pH shifts

Loss of both heat and CO_2 under ambient conditions is a function of the surface-to-volume ratio of the culture medium and time. With 1.0 ml of medium in a Falcon organ culture dish (3037; Falcon Plastics, Cockeysville, Md.), pH will be outside the physiologic range within 1 to 2 minutes, whereas the same volume in a 5 ml tube will be more stable (2). Dishes should not be under ambient conditions for more than 1 minute. To minimize pH shifts, use of 2 to 3 ml of media, use of a CO_2-controlled mobile isolette (2), and transfer to buffers having physiologic pH at ambient CO_2 levels have all been utilized. Another effective means to slow loss of heat and CO_2 is to use an overlay of equilibrated washed paraffin or mineral oil (26). With the latter technique, particular attention must be paid to avoid introduction of embryotoxicity from the oil (27). Time out of the incubator should be limited to 1 minute with 1 ml in a dish and to a few minutes under oil, but is not constrained in proper buffers or in a CO_2-controlled isolette. Heat loss can be moderated by warming trays and warmed microscope stages. A warming enclosure is available for the Nikon inverted microscope, to which we have also added a CO_2 controller. If individual dishes are used, multiple openings of the main incubator are required. The temperatures and CO_2 shifts of the culture chamber can be marked and will add together with the shifts that have already occurred in the sample being examined. For example, two door openings of the incubator can reduce the CO_2 level to 1% or less, and recovery will occur over 15 to 30 minutes. Temperature can drop several degrees. These changes *are not* reflected in the digital displays. The CO_2 will simply cycle faster, and by the time there is a marked drop in the digital readout, the chamber CO_2 level is less than 1%. Because of these various factors, we have felt that the ideal system is the use of a temperature and CO_2-controlled isolette, with a minimum number of breaches of the main incubator environment. We have continued to use 5 ml tubes because of their stability. They are more difficult to transfer in and out of, but are easier to transfer to and from the incubator by carrying them within a 100 ml beaker.

Protection against equipment failure

All critical equipment items should be on emergency back-up power. Surge protectors should be used to avoid interference with internal circuitry. Alarms should be utilized on incubators and low-level alarms on embryo freezers. These can be connected to the hospital switchboard if they are not audible to persons in the area at all times. An alternative is an automatic system (Sensiphone; Phonetics Inc., Media, Pa.), which will monitor various functions and dial a series of numbers on a dedicated telephone line. The latter is most practical for programs in office settings and is the method that we currently use. Liquid nitrogen tanks should also be checked mechanically for level. This method is alone sufficient except for rare failure of the tank insulation, which leaves only several hours until loss of the contents. Because of the impact of such a catastrophic event, we have also used the low-level alarm. Gas tanks should be set up with a back-up with an automatic low-level switch or a simpler tandem arrangement with the second stage of the back-up tank set at a lower level than that of the primary tank. All line connections should be secure.

Manipulation

For transfers from tube to dish or dish to dish, we have used borosilicate glass Pasteur pipettes that have been soaked and rinsed in ultrapure water and dry-heat sterilized. They are placed in the pediatric isolette and warmed prior to use. If disposable pipetting devices are used, they must be tested for toxicity.

Oocyte identification, grading, and preincubation

If an isolette chamber is not used, heating blocks, heating trays, and stage warmers should be used, and rapid handling is essential. Use of buffers to keep pH stable under ambient conditions makes speed less important. We have found that aspirates can be poured into a Petri dish. Most oocytes are identified under the naked eye by their clear surrounding mucus-like cumulus. The dish can then be partially emptied and tipped to layer out and examine and grade the oocyte under the dissecting microscope. A mature oocyte has a dispersed cumulus and radiating, dispersed corona, whereas an immature oocyte lacks cumulus and has a tight corona. Oocytes may also be graded as intermediate. Some laboratories utilize an inverted microscope to look for the first polar body or a germinal vesicle. It is not clear whether the information gained is worth the potential disturbances of osmolarity and pH that occur with extended observation of the oocyte in a thin layer of surrounding fluid. Oocytes are then washed to remove blood (28) and meiosis inhibitors that may be present in follicular fluid. They are then placed in culture in a tube or dish for a period of time before adding sperm. Several years ago, Trounson and coworkers demonstrated a marked increase of fertilization and pregnancy with preincubation of oocytes for 5 to 7 hours before addition of sperm (29). Some workers have suggested that this period could be varied according to morphology of the cumulus and corona, but it has been shown that there is little correlation between these findings and the actual morphology of the oocyte (30). Some have suggested that preincubation could be varied according to the presence of the first polar body. However, this does not ensure adequate cytoplasmic maturation, which may be important to provide the metabolic machinery to form a capable embryo. A longer than usual interval can be allowed for those oocytes not yet at metaphase II. However, it is inconvenient to inseminate oocytes during the evening or night and to perform fertilization checks at multiple times. Furthermore, the benefit derived from resulting embryos may be small, since their less mature status may reflect a poor follicle environment. For all these reasons, we routinely pre-incubate oocytes with cumulus for 6 to 8 hours. For oocytes without cumulus or with a germinal vesicle, it has been conventional to preincubate for 24 to 36 hours pending morphologic maturation, but these embryos appear to seldom result in implantation. Exposure to gonadotropins (31), mature granulosa cells, or mature follicular fuild (32) may aid maturation and fertilization, but whether these can increase implantation is not clear. We seldom make the effort to screen microscopically for oocytes lacking cumulus but would incubate these for 24 to 36 hours in 50% mature follicular fluid.

Sperm collection and preparation

Abstinence of 2 to 4 days will avoid aberrations of sperm function due to unusual abstinence periods. Short absti-nence may be beneficial with antisperm antibodies. The collection vessel should be verified to be nontoxic by checking overnight sperm motility, or, as we have done, a wide-mouthed Teflon jar can be used and processed through the tissue-culture wash following a period of boiling in detergent. Collection should take place in a private, relaxed setting, with adequate materials to provide sexual arousal. After cleansing the hands and penis, the specimen is ejaculated directly into the sterile container. After 30 minutes, processing is carried out. In the case of sperm antibodies, the fertilization rate is significantly increased by ejaculation directly into 50% serum followed by immediate centrifugation (33).

The objectives of sperm processing are to remove seminal plasma, to retrieve adequate sperm of high motility and penetrating capacity, and to obtain a specimen with minimal possibility of bacterial contami-nation. A two-step wash and swim-up has been the most common method used. An appropriate source of protein will help to preserve sperm motility with washing (15). A highly motile sperm preparation is obtained with minimal bacterial contamination (34,35), but a relatively low yield of the motile sperm population is achieved. Percoll (Pharmacia Laboratories, Pis-cataway, N.J.) achieves a highly motile specimen, high yield, and a clean specimen and is therefore well suited to specimens with reduced count or motility (36) or suspected infection (37). It generally improves the sperm penetration assay (36), but we have seen individual cases in which this method has a clear adverse effect on sperm function in penetrating hamster eggs. A number of other methods, such as Nicodenz (38), swim-up into hyaluronic acid (39), and glass wool column (40), have been reported. None appears to have specific advantages although the yield is particularly high with glass wool.

Sperm penetrating capacity tends to improve with Percoll or with exposure to follicular fluid or test-yolk buffer. Fertilization has been reported to improve with all three methods (36,41,42), but responses can be quite individual. We currently evaluate sperm function with these three methods and swim-up so that the best method can be selected for each individual male.

Sperm density used for oocyte insemination for the normal male has been most commonly in the range of 50,000 to 100,000 motile sperm per milliliter. With male factor, improved fertilization is obtained with 500,000/ml (43). With high antisperm antibody binding, addition of a million or more motile sperm will generally provide an adequate number of antibody-free sperm (44).

If an adequate number of sperm is difficult to achieve, several maneuvers may be helpful. Frozen specimens may be stored if post-thaw survival is adequate. An additional collection can be done with storage for 1 to 2 days in test-yolk buffer at 4°C (45). An additional collection 30 to 60 minutes after the initial specimen is very worthwhile, particularly with male factor (46). Finally, insemination volume can be reduced under oil, or multiple oocytes can be inseminated in a single tube or dish.

For some men, the sperm may have difficulty traversing the cumulus and corona. Hyperactivation is required for this to occur readily. In one study of men with normal semen analysis who had failed to fertilize in a prior cycle, fertilization significantly improved by removing the cumulus and corona with hyaluronidase (47).

Reinsemination following failure of pronuclear formation is of relatively little benefit except with donor sperm (48) or with a fresh collection of husband's sperm (49). Use of frozen donor or husband's sperm (50) for the primary insemination is highly effective provided the semen has normal characteristics and post-thaw motility. With frozen sperm it is probably best not to have a long interval between preparation and insemination, since penetrating ability drops off rapidly.

Fertilization check

Dissection of the cumulus and coronal cells can be done by aspirating the oocyte back and forth through a drawn pipette or by sweeping these cells aside by means of 26 gauge needles. The latter technique requires more manual dexterity. Polypronuclei should be confirmed under the inverted microscope so that oocytes with vacuoles ("pseudopronuclei") are not discarded (3). If pronuclear formation is not checked, polypronuclear embryos may be inadvertently chosen for transfer. Although these embryos generally have irregular morphology, some may have superior appearance.

Embryo transfer

Timing

Transfer is most commonly carried out at 2 days of culture and is the surest approach because of the vast experience with that timing. Concern is that with earlier transfer, the uterine cavity may not be supportive of embryos, whereas with later transfer, embryo viability may be compromised by suboptimal culture conditions. Transfer of sperm and eggs several hours after retrieval has been associated with low results. Similar results have been achieved with day 1 and day 2 transfers (51), although a much larger experience would be necessary to ensure reasonably equivalent outcome. It has been suggested that a day 1 transfer should be considered whenever suboptimal culture conditions have been detected (51). Results with day 3 transfers have been conflicting, with one uncontrolled study reporting miscarriage to be higher (52) and one randomized study finding a lower rate of fetal loss (53). As culture conditions continue to improve, later times of transfer may prove to be worth reexamining.

Technique

Many different transfer catheters are available. Most incorporate a flexible, soft Teflon catheter within a more rigid guide. The guide is used to point the inner catheter in the approximate direction of the cervical canal. The inner catheter then "walks" its way along the canal. Other catheters have a more rigid memory. A curve is matched to the configuration of the canal. These catheters are passed more by feel. Reuse of catheters may introduce toxicity and is best avoided. Most programs load the embryos in 50 μl of medium or less, since the uterine cavity in some women may not accommodate larger amounts. Air should be considered as part of total volume, particularly with use of the lithotomy position, since air could rise toward the upper fundus and displace the embryos downward (18). A continuous fluid column may aid in accuracy of fluid delivery, by avoiding compressible air (54). Uncontrolled studies have suggested improved rates of implantation by using a high concentration of serum, possibly by promoting embryo retention through increased viscosity of the transferred fluid. However, the pH of this high serum concentration is quite alkaline (2). Therefore, we have preferred to maximize embryo retention by transferring in approximately 20 μl of growth medium (18). We use a highly accurate air-tight microliter syringe to maximize accuracy of the ejected volume.

Transfer should be atraumatic. Any slight bleeding could displace the embryos from the uterine cavity and reduce the chance of success (55). We have found it very valuable to do a rehearsal of the transfer, with careful mapping of the direction and curve of the canal at a time removed from the treatment cycle. The value of this has been recently shown (56). Some have used ultrasound guidance (57), but this has not been shown to improve results.

To avoid contamination of the uterine cavity, which could impair implantation, we wash the cervix with cotton swabs soaked with culture medium and give a single 100 mg capsule of doxycycline on the morning of transfer. Most teams use the dorsal lithotomy position. The knee-chest position allows the uterine fundus to be dependent during transfer but is more physically and psychologically difficult for the patient. The uterus tends to fall forward, and more frequently cervical traction is required to position the cervix for transfer. Attempts should be made to swab away mucus that could be carried up on or within the catheter tip and result in trapping or adherence of embryos. The catheter is gently passed to 0.5 cm from the top of the uterine cavity. After ejecting the fluid, the catheter is withdrawn slightly. One minute is given to allow dispersion of the fluid. On removal, the catheter is turned 90 degrees to sweep off any adhering material and to cover the track to prevent fluid from following the catheter out.

Following transfer, the catheter should be examined and flushed to detect any residual embryos. Most often they are found in the tip of the catheter, but occasionally they can adhere to mucus at the catheter tip. With micromanipulation, rarely a retained embryo is noted with a partially or completely empty zona, indicating compression has occurred, for example, due to lumen narrowing from a mucus plug (J. Cohen, personal communication). Smooth transfer technique may be particularly important with openings in the zona. If the catheter does not pass very readily, adjustments should be made to improve passage. We have found that traction on the cervix using a 4-0 suture on a small cutting needle (e.g., PS 2; Ethicon Inc., Somerville, N.J.) aids passage of the catheter with minimal or no cramping or pain. Following transfer a variable period of bed rest is ordered, usually head-down and with the uterine fundus most dependent. Our routine has been 3 hours.

Quality control

Reagents

Solutes, antibiotics, proteins, water, and other components of the culture medium must be of the highest quality. Sources and lot numbers and expiration dates must be recorded. They must be stored and mixed in such a way that no contamination can occur, preferably within the "clean room" reserved for human embryo culture. A further level of assurance is achieved by using only components used by other highly successful IVF programs.

Materials

All materials that contact the culture, directly or indirectly, must be subjected to a tissue-culture wash or to toxicity testing using a bioassay. The culture medium should also be tested regularly. Since minor embryotoxicity can be present on any material, rinsing with culture medium is a good precaution. Particular attention should be paid to collection and preparation of serum additives. For example, the red top vacutainer is highly embryotoxic (58). Ideally each individual serum should be tested with a bioassay.

Equipment

All equipment must be regularly serviced and calibrated against external standards. For example, incubator CO_2 level can be verified directly using a Fyrite and indirectly by monitoring pH following equilibration.

Personnel

Persons handling human gametes and embryos must have an adequate period of training and must work under direct supervision until an adequate level of competency can be verified. Each person should be required to do a minimum number of cases per year. With cryopreservation, competency should ideally be tested for each individual by demonstrating adequate survival and development of mouse embryos. Likewise, animal models should be used to gain adequate expertise in micromanipulation prior to handling human material.

Recording

All findings, manipulations, and results pertaining to clinical material should be recorded on standardized sheets and should be part of the patient's record. Information on freezing methods and locations of embryos must be kept in two separate sites.

All data on reagents (sources, lot numbers, expiration dates), function checks (pH, Fyrite checks, incubator and refrigerator temperatures), media parameters (date of preparation, pH, osmolarity, toxicity testing), personnel requirements, work schedules, and actions should be recorded and available for inspection.

Procedure manuals

Every detail of every procedure used should be outlined in a procedure manual. Evidence of initial and periodic review by the laboratory and medical directors ensures that all procedures are well defined, without any arbitrary variations introduced at the bench. Only through standardized protocols is it possible to associate poor or good results with specific techniques. If any substantial change is made, and other procedures are kept consistent, only then can one suspect that any suboptimal technique has inadvertently been introduced. Individual exceptions should be described and the reasons given. Procedures should be defined for responding to any out-of-range values or unusual occurrences.

Safety precautions for laboratory personnel

Nontoxic, powderless gloves should be worn whenever handling any biologic specimen. Laboratory cover-gowns and eye protection should be worn if any possibility of splashing is present. Personnel should be aware of precautions necessary to avoid exposure to aerosols during centrifugation. Vaccination for hepatitis B should be offered and encouraged. Both male and female partners under treatment should be tested periodically (e.g., every 6 months) for HIV and hepatitis B. Safety goggles and appropriate gloves should be worn when handling liquid nitrogen. Bare legs can also be unsafe in the event of a liquid nitrogen spill. Liquid nitrogen should not be handled in a limited closed space without a low O_2 level alarm.

References

1. Tesarik J, Kopecny V, Plachot M, Mandelbaum J. Activation of nucleolar and extranucleolar RNA synthesis and changes in the ribosomal content of human embryos developing in vitro. J Reprod Fertil 1986;78:463–470.

2. Chetkowski RJ, Nass TE, Matt DW, et al. Optimization of hydrogen-ion concentration during aspiration of oocytes and culture and transfer of embryos. J In Vitro Fert Embryo Transf 1985;2:207–212.

3. Van Blerkom J, Bell H, Henry G. The occurrence, recognition and developmental fate of pseudo-multipronuclear eggs after in vitro fertilization of human oocytes. Hum Reprod 1987;2:217–224.

4. Spire B, Barre-Sinoussi F, Dormont D, Montagnier L, Chermann JC. Inactivation of lymphadenopathy-associated virus by heat, gamma rays, and ultraviolet light. Lancet 1985;1:188–189.

5. Leung PCS, Gronow MJ, Kellow GN, et al. Serum supplement in human in vitro fertilization and embryo development. Fertil Steril 1984;41:36–39.

6. Quinn P, Kerin JF, Warnes GM. Improved pregnancy rate in human in vitro fertilization with the use of a medium based on the composition of human tubal fluid. Fertil Steril 1985;44:493–498.

7. Warikoo, PK, Bavister BD. Hypoxanthine and cyclic adenosine 5-monophosphate maintain meiotic arrest of rhesus monkey oocytes in vitro. Fertil Steril 1989;51:886–889.

8. Bavister BD, Andrews JC. A rapid sperm motility bioassay procedure for quality-control testing of water and culture media. J In Vitro Fert Embryo Transf 1988;5:67–75.

9. Fishel S, Jackson P, Webster J, Faratian B. Endotoxins in culture medium for human in vitro fertilization. Fertil Steril 1988;49:108–111.

10. Montoro L, Subias E, Young P, Baccaro M, Swanson J, Sueldo C. Detection of endotoxin in human in vitro fertilization by the zona-free mouse embryo assay. Fertil Steril 1990;54:109–112.

11. Ackerman SB, Stokes GL, Swanson RJ, Taylor SP, Fenwick L. Toxicity testing for human in vitro fertilization programs. J In Vitro Fert Embryo Transf 1985;2:132–137.

12. McDowell JS, Swanson RJ, Maloney M, Veeck L. Mouse embryo quality control for toxicity determination in the Norfolk in vitro fertilization program. J In Vitro Fert Embryo Transf 1988;5:144–148.

13. Davidson A, Vermesh M, Lobo RA, Paulson RJ. Mouse embryo culture as quality control for human in vitro fertilization: the one-cell versus the two-cell model. Fertil Steril 1988;49:516–521.

14. Critchlow JD, Matson PL, Newman MC, Horne G, Troup SA, Lieberman BA. Quality control in an in vitro fertilization laboratory: use of human sperm survival studies. Hum Reprod 1989;4:545–549.

15. De Ziegler D, Cedars MI, Hamilton F, Moreno T, Meldrum DR. Factors influencing maintenance of sperm motility during in vitro processing. Fertil Steril 1987;48:816–820.

16. Caro CM, Trounson A. The effect of protein on preimplantation mouse embryo development in vitro. J In Vitro Fert Embryo Transf 1984;1:183–187.

17. Shirley B, Wortham JWE, Peoples D, White S, Cordon-Mahony M. Inhibition of embryo development by some maternal sera. J In Vitro Fert Embryo Transf 1987; 4:93–97.

18. Meldrum DR, Chetkowski R, Steingold KA, de Ziegler D, Cedars MI, Hamilton M. Evolution of a highly successful in vitro fertilization–embryo transfer program. Fertil Steril 1987;48:86–93.

19. Jinno M, Iida E, Iizuki R. A detrimental effect of platelets on mouse embryo development. J In Vitro Fert Embryo Transf 1987;4:324–330.

20. Wiemer KE, Cohen J, Amborski GF, et al. In-vitro development and implantation of human embryos following culture on fetal bovine uterine fibroblast cells. Hum Reprod 1989;4:595–600.

21. Bongso A, Soon-Chye NG, Sathananthan H, Lian NP, Rauff M, Ratnam S. Improved quality of human embryos when co-cultured with human ampullary cells. Hum Reprod 1989;4:706–713.

22. Menozo YJR, Guerin JF, Czyba JC. Co-culture of human embryos with Vero cells. Biol Reprod 1990;42:301–306.

23. Harrison KL, Sherrin A, Hawthorne TA, Breen TM, West GA, Wilson LM. Embryotoxicity of micropore filters used in liquid sterilization. J In Vitro Fert Embryo Transf 1990;7:347.

24. Pickering SJ, Braude PR, Johnson MH, Cant A, Currie J. Transient cooling to room temperature can cause irreversible disruption of the meiotic spindle in the human oocyte. Fertil Steril 1990;54:102–108.

25. Abramczuk JW, Lopata A. Incubator performance in the clinical in vitro fertilization program: importance of temperature conditions for the fertilization and cleavage of human oocytes. Fertil Steril 1986;46:132–134.

26. Quinn P, Warnes GM, Kerin JF, Kirby C. Culture factors in relation to the success of human in vitro fertilization and embryo transfer. Fertil Steril 1984;41:202–209.

27. Fleming FP, Pratt HMP, Braude PR. The use of mouse preimplantation embryos for quality control of culture reagents in human in vitro fertilization programs: a cautionary note. Fertil Steril 1987;47:858–860.

28. Daya S, Kohut J, Gunby J, Younglai E. Influence of blood clots in the cumulus complex on oocyte fertilization and cleavage. Hum Reprod 1990;5:744–746.

29. Trounson AO, Mohr LR, Wood C, Leeton JF. Effect of delayed insemination on in vitro fertilization, culture and transfer of human embryos. J Reprod Fertil 1982;64:285–294.

30. Laufer N, Tarlatzis BC, De Cherney AH, et al. Asynchrony between human cumulus–corona cell complex and oocyte maturation after human menopausal gonadotropin treatment for in vitro fertilization. Fertil Steril 1984;42:366–372.

31. Prins GS, Wagner C, Weidel L, Gianfortoni J, Marut EL, Scommegna A. Gonadotropins augment maturation and fertilization of human immature oocytes in vitro. Fertil Steril 1987;47:1035–1037.

32. Cha KY, Koo JJ, Choi DH, Han SY, Yoon TK. Pregnancy after in vitro fertilization of human follicular oocytes collected from non-stimulated cycles, their culture in vitro and their transfer in a donor oocyte program. Fertil Steril 1991;55:109–113.

33. Elder KT, Wich KH, Edwards RG. Seminal plasma anti-sperm antibodies and IVF: the effect of semen sample collection into 50% serum. Hum Reprod 1990;5:179–184.

34. Forman R, Guillet-Rosso F, Fari A, Volante M, Frydman R. Testart J. Importance of semen preparation in avoidance of reduced in vitro fertilization results attributable to bacteria. Fertil Steril 1987;47:527–530.

35. Wong PC, Balmaceda JP, Blanco JD, Gibbs RS, Asch RH. Sperm washing and swim-up techniques using antibiotics removes microbes from human semen. Fertil Steril 1986; 45:97–100.

36. Berger T, Marrs RP, Moyer DL. Comparison of techniques for selection of motile spermatozoa. Fertil Steril 1985;43:268–273.

37. Sun LS, Gastaldi C, Peterson EM, de la Maza LM, Stone SC. Comparison of techniques for the selection of bacteria-free sperm preparations. Fertil Steril 1987;48:659–663.

38. Gellert-Mortimer ST, Clarke GN, Baker HWG, Hyne RV, Johnston WIH. Evaluation of Nycodenz and Percoll density gradients for the selection of motile human spermatozoa. Fertil Steril 1988;49:335–341.

39. Huszar G, Willetts M, Corrales M. Hyaluronic acid (Sperm Select) improves retention of sperm motility and

velocity in normospermic and oligospermic specimens. Fertil Steril 1990;54:1127–1134.

40. Van der Ven HH, Jeyendran RS, Al-Hasani S, et al. Glass wool column filtration of human semen: relation to swim-up procedure and outcome of IVF. Hum Reprod 1988;3:85–88.

41. Ghetler Y, Ben-Nun J, Kaneti H, Jaffe R, Gruber A, Fejgin M. Effect of sperm preincubation with follicular fluid on the fertilization rate in human in vitro fertilization. Fertil Steril 1990;54:944–946.

42. Katayama KP, Stehlik E, Roesler M, Jeyendran RS, Holmgren WJ, Zaneveld LJD. Treatment of human spermatozoa with an egg yolk medium can enhance the outcome of in vitro fertilization. Fertil Steril 1989;52:1077–1079.

43. Diamond MP, Rogers BJ, Vaughn WK, Wentz AC. Effect of the number of inseminating sperm and the follicular stimulation protocol on in vitro fertilization of human oocytes in male factor and non-male factor couples. Fertil Steril 1985;44:499–503.

44. Hamilton F, Gutlay-Yeo AL, Meldrum DR. Normal fertilization in men with high antibody sperm binding by the addition of sufficient unbound sperm in vitro. J In Vitro Fert Embryo Transf 1989;6:342–344.

45. Cohen J, Fehilly CB, Walters DE. Prolonged storage of human spermatozoa at room temperature or in a refrigerator. Fertil Steril 1985;44:254–262.

46. Tur-Kaspa I, Dudkiewicz A, Confino E, Gleicher N. Pooled sequential ejaculates: a way to increase the total number of motile sperm from oligozoospermic men. Fertil Steril 1990;54:906–909.

47. Lavy G, Boyers SP, De Cherney AH. Hyaluronidase removal of the cumulus oophorus increases in vitro fertilization. J In Vitro Fert Embryo Transf 1988;5:257–260.

48. Trounson A, Webb J. Fertilization of human oocytes following reinsemination in vitro. Fertil Steril 1984;41:816–819.

49. Ashkenazi J, Feldberg D, Dicker D, Shelef M, Goldman GA, Goldman JA. Reinsemination in human IVF with fresh versus initial semen: a comparative study. Eur J Obstet Gynecol Reprod Biol 1990;34:97–101.

50. Morshedi M, Oehninger S, Veeck LL, Ertunc H, Bocca S, Acosta AA. Cryopreserved/thawed semen for in vitro fertilization: results from fertile donors and infertile patients. Fertil Steril 1990;54:1093–1099.

51. Quinn P, Stone BA, Marrs RP. Suboptimal laboratory conditions can affect pregnancy outcome after embryo transfer on day 1 or 2 after insemination in vitro. Fertil Steril 1990;53:168–170.

52. Van Os HC, Alberda AT, Janssen-Caspers HAB, Laerentveld RA, Scholtes MCW, Zeilmaker GH. The influence of the interval between in vitro fertilization and embryo transfer and some other variables on treatment outcome. Fertil Steril 1989;51:360–362.

53. Edwards RG, Fishel SB, Cohen J, et al. Factors influencing the success of in vitro fertilization for alleviating human infertility. J In Vitro Fert Embryo Transf 1984;1:3–23.

54. Poindexter AN, Thompson DJ, Gibbons WE, et al. Residual embryos in failed embryo transfer. Fertil Steril 1986;46:262–267.

55. Englert Y, Puissant F, Camus M, Van Hoeck H, Le Roy F. Clinical study on embryo transfer after human in vitro fertilization. J In Vitro Fert Embryo Transf 1986;3:243–246.

56. Mansour R, Aboulghar M, Serour G. Dummy embryo transfer: a technique that minimizes the problems of embryo transfer and improves the pregnancy rate in human in vitro fertilization. Fertil Steril 1990;54:678–681.

57. Strickler RC, Christianson C, Crane JP, Curato A, Knight AB, Yang V. Ultrasound guidance for human embryo transfer. Fertil Steril 1985;43:54–61.

58. Haimovici F, Hill JA, Anderson DJ. Variables affecting toxicity of human sera in mouse embryo cultures. J In Vitro Fert Embryo Transf 1988;5:202–206.

7

Gamete and Embryo Micromanipulation

Jacques Cohen
Jamie Grifo
Henry E. Malter
Beth E. Talansky

Introduction

These are exhilarating times for in vitro fertilization (IVF) specialists. The days of routine laboratory IVF, simple isolation of sperm and oocytes for fertilization followed by selection of embryos for cryopreservation or replacement, appear to be over. Micromanipulation procedures applied to gametes and embryos are providing a range of novel techniques that may alter the IVF laboratory dramatically, expanding its applications to men with severely impaired testicular function and bridging the gaps between reproductive physiology, experimental embryology, and molecular genetics. Although some applications are particularly related to important issues involved in the human field, for instance, microsurgical fertilization and preimplantation genetics, other micromanipulation techniques, routine in animal husbandry, like artificial twinning and blastocyst reconstitution, have not yet become popular among IVF practitioners. This chapter will provide an introduction to some micromanipulation methods being applied on an experimental basis in some IVF centers.

More than 75 pregnancies worldwide have been obtained following the application of microsurgical fertilization techniques in couples in whom the male partners had severely abnormal semen and who would have had little or no chance producing offspring with conventional IVF. A large section of this chapter is therefore dedicated to mechanisms involved in the fertilization process and modes of bypassing the zona pellucida (ZP), since this forms a major barrier inhibiting gamete fusion in instances of male factor infertility. A second section is allocated to the exciting potential of single-cell genetics for assessment of embryos at risk for genetic disease, a field generally described as preimplantation genetic diagnosis. Finally, some attention is paid to as yet hypothetical procedures, like polyspermy correction, assisted hatching, and germ cell line therapy through gene insertion.

Fertilization and assisted fertilization

Successful mammalian fertilization results from the fine coordination of two very complex reproductive systems. The molecular, biochemical, and physical processes that occur independently in the male and female systems are subject to disruption and dysfunction at many levels. In addition, the concurrence of events necessary for normal fertilization is particularly sensitive to interruption. In the discussion that follows, we will present a necessarily limited description of normal fertilization, describe defects in sperm-egg interaction, and introduce some of the ways in which micromanipulation has been used experimentally to overcome these defects. While this discussion of fertilization is not designed to be a comprehensive review of all aspects of sperm-egg interaction, it will provide an explanation of basic elements that are involved in the development of micromanipulative technology for assisting the fertilization process in vitro.

Sperm-egg interaction

Upon leaving the testis, mammalian spermatozoa undergo a process of maturation in the epididymis that is necessary for the initial achievement of fertilizing capability. Epididymal sperm maturation is a multifactorial process that involves the acquisition of motility, the alteration of nuclear, membrane, and tail components, and the integration of new cell surface macromolecules (1,2). After ejaculation, mature epididymal sperm must undergo further capacitation, either in the female reproductive tract or in vitro, prior to fertilization. The process of capacitation is poorly understood, but it probably involves the removal or alteration of substances on the plasma membrane (1,3). One important consequence of capacitation is that the sperm of some species, including the human, become hyperactivated. Hyperactivation results in a distinctive, vigorous form of motility that has been correlated with the ability of the sperm to cross the ZP and to effect fertilization (4).

Once the spermatozoa have acquired the capability to fertilize, they must penetrate the egg investments—the cumulus oophorous and the ZP. The cumulus consists of specialized follicular cells and an extracellular matrix that is largely composed of mucopolysaccharide. In most mammals, the cumulus mass is retained close to the ovulated oocyte(s). The ZP is a thick, acellular layer composed of several sulfated glycoproteins. Both of these structures present a barrier to sperm penetration, and sperm motility alone is not enough to overcome these obstacles. Enzymatic activity is also necessary for efficient fertilization. A number of hydrolytic enzymes are contained within the acrosome, a cap-like lysosomal structure that covers the anterior portion of the sperm nucleus (5). The best characterized of the acrosomal enzymes are acrosin and hyaluronidase (6). These and other enzymes are released during the acrosome reaction (AR); during this exocytotic event, the outer acrosomal membrane fuses with the overlying plasma membrane, and the contents of the acrosome escape through the fenestrations that result. Although the AR is naturally induced by contact with the ZP, and possibly by the cumulus, it also occurs spontaneously in vitro (7–10).

To penetrate the cumulus cell mass, sperm must be capacitated and have intact acrosomes (11,12). Once the cumulus is penetrated, some sperm undergo the AR and release hyaluronidase. The cumulus matrix, which consists mainly of hyaluronic acid, is consequently dispersed. The passage of all sperm through the cumulus may therefore be facilitated by the AR of a portion of the sperm population (13).

The process of fertilization is initiated when the sperm attach to the ZP; firmer sperm binding results when sperm receptors present on the zona encounter a complementary egg-binding protein on the surface of the sperm head. This receptor-mediated binding is species specific and plays a significant role in restricting interspecies fertilization. In the mouse, the specific ZP sperm receptor has been termed ZP3 and is one of three glycoproteins that compose the ZP (14). Only sperm with intact acrosomes are capable of binding to the ZP. Exposure to ZP3 induces the AR; the release of acrosin aids in the passage of sperm across the ZP (15,16). In the mouse, the sperm passes through the zona at a rate of 1 μm per minute (17).

Once it has traversed the ZP and enters the perivitelline space, the sperm fuses with the vitelline membrane. Only acrosome-reacted sperm are capable of completely fusing with the plasma membrane (18). Microvilli on the surface of the oocyte envelope the sperm during fertilization, and the sperm is then drawn into the oocyte by microvillar action (19). Sperm motility is therefore not required for penetration into the oocyte; in fact, motility usually ceases upon first contact with the vitellus.

The principal block to polyspermy in mammals is at the level of the ZP. During oocyte development, lysosome-like organelles called cortical granules develop from the Golgi complex and gradually move to the periphery of the cytoplasm (20). Upon fertilization, the contents of the cortical granules are released into the perivitelline space. The release of various hydrolytic enzymes during the cortical reaction causes structural changes in the ZP. The ZP3 molecule is altered so that further sperm binding is prevented, and structural changes occur in ZP2, one of the other zona glycoproteins, that cause the zona to become hardened (21). These changes in the structural molecules of the ZP comprise the zona reaction and constitute the slow block to polyspermy. A rapid block may also be operative in some mammals. A transient membrane depolarization

occurs when the sperm first contacts the vitellus. It has been postulated that in some lower animals this change in membrane potential effects a block to further sperm penetration. It is possible that the same mechanism is operative in the mammalian system, although it remains to be convincingly demonstrated (22).

Micromanipulation

The development of gamete micromanipulation technology has enabled the reproductive biologist to circumvent any inefficient steps in the fertilization process that might prevent sperm-egg fusion from reaching completion. The protocols utilized in most mammalian IVF procedures are conducive to incorporation of microsurgical fertilization. Conditions and materials to which oocytes are exposed may be artificially modified in order to facilitate the physiologic and biochemical prerequisites to fertilization.

To date, three major categories of assisted fertilization by gamete micromanipulation have been explored in several mammalian systems. The first involves the creation of an artificial gap in the ZP. Subsequently, the micromanipulated oocyte is inseminated according to standard IVF protocols. These procedures have been broadly termed "zona drilling." A second category of micromanipulation techniques directed at facilitating sperm-egg interaction is the subzonal insertion (SZI) of sperm. More invasive than zona drilling, SZI completely bypasses the ZP and involves direct placement of sperm into the perivitelline space. Finally, the third and most invasive form of microsurgical fertilization is the microinjection of sperm into the cytoplasm of the oocyte. This method entails the traversal of all outer barriers of the oocyte: the cumulus-corona complex, the ZP, and the vitelline membrane.

Zona drilling (zona micromanipulation): In the original zona drilling procedure, developed in the mouse model, the oocyte was secured by suction on a holding pipette and a microneedle loaded with acid Tyrode's solution was brought into contact with a restricted region of the ZP (23). A minute volume of solution was gently released from the microneedle until the point at which the zona was breached. In some cases, when the procedure was done more aggressively, the opening in the zona became obvious as the underlying oocyte protruded from the site of manipulation. Routine insemination followed the procedure. In the mouse model the creation of an artifical gap in the zona was associated with increased rates of fertilization at both normal and reduced sperm concentrations. Initial pronuclear formation was observed about 45 minutes earlier in manipulated groups than in controls. In addition, zona drilling resulted in rates of supernumerary sperm penetration that did not differ from those in zona-intact controls. Mouse zygotes that resulted from assisted fertilization by zona drilling, when transferred to the oviducts of pseudopregnant foster female mice, gave rise to normal live young. These results were very encouraging. The zona drilling procedure exposed sperm to a region of direct access to the oocyte but also allowed the majority of the ZP to retain the physiologic function of helping to block polyspermic fertilization.

To develop zona drilling as a potential tool for clinical IVF, further animal studies were undertaken. Since replacement of pronuclear stage zona-drilled embryos did not allow for direct observation of embryonic development, cleavage to the blastocyst stage was observed in vitro following micromanipulation (24). The result of these investigations demonstrated that frequently, after the creation of a relatively large hole in the ZP, the embryo tended to protrude through the gap as development progressed. This sometimes resulted in embryonic development both inside and outside the zona, or in the loss of intact blastomeres. When a portion of the blastocyst protruded

through the small gap in the zona, the resulting constriction frequently caused the formation of twin blastocysts (24,25). Also, hatching routinely occurred one day early in micromanipulated embryos (25).

Removal of a portion of the ZP is effective in exposing sperm directly to the oocyte. That the sperm are actually utilizing the artificially created gap to gain access to the egg has been demonstrated by several techniques. It is known that, in the mouse, premature induction of the AR prevents fertilization of zona-intact oocytes (26). With this in mind, Gordon and Talansky (1986) induced the AR in populations of mouse sperm with dibutycyclic guanosine monophosphate (dB cGMP), and demonstrated that these acrosomeless sperm were able to penetrate zona-drilled oocytes, but not zona-intact oocytes (23). Conover and Gwatkin (1988) exposed oocytes to an antibody to ZP3 and showed that these oocytes could not be penetrated without micromanipulation by zona drilling (27). We have since shown that a method of zona drilling greatly increases the rate of fertilization in a strain of random-bred mice that is normally refractory to sperm penetration in vitro (28). These results all indicate that sperm are indeed traversing the opening in the ZP following micromanipulation.

Since the results of the initial animal studies were encouraging, micromanipulation-assisted fertilization was applied to clinical IVF (29). Although fertilization was frequently achieved, embryonic cleavage was frequently abnormal, and no pregnancies resulted after uterine replacement. The human ZP differed from the mouse zona in its response to acid Tyrode's solution. While the outer layer of the human zona was easily dissolved by the acidic solution, the inner, more resistant layer required longer exposure in order to be completely breached. Alternative enzymatic methods for opening the human ZP were attempted; however, due to species differences in the sensitivity to artificial agents for zona dissolution, the treatments ideal for other mammalian models, such as the mouse, were not effective for use with human oocytes (30).

In order to apply assisted fertilization by zona drilling as a viable clinical tool, alternative methods for opening the ZP were sought. Among the procedures that were attempted in animal and human models were zona cutting and cracking (31,32). Cohen et al. (1988), however, developed a mechanical procedure for introducing a gap in the mammalian ZP that resulted in the first human pregnancy from microsurgical fertilization (33). This method, termed partial zona dissection (PZD), involves the use of a sucrose solution to shrink the oocyte so that a glass microneedle can be introduced into the perivitelline space without damaging the oocyte. The microneedle is threaded through one side of the ZP at the 1 o'clock position and out through the side of the zona at the 11 o'clock position. The oocyte is released from the holding pipette, which is then used to massage the portion of the ZP that is incorporated between the points at which it is pierced by the microneedle. After repeated massage by the holding pipette, the oocyte drops off, and the result is a clear slit in the zona where the microneedle was threaded. Following this procedure, the oocyte is removed from the sucrose solution, reexposed to medium of normal osmolarity, and inseminated.

The clinical use of PZD has been highly successful. To date, more than 30 live births have resulted from this method of microsurgical fertilization, and many pregnancies are ongoing. These clinical data will be discussed in detail below.

What types of fertilization disorders may be alleviated by zona micromanipulation procedures such as zona drilling or PZD? Initially, zona drilling was devised as a method for assisting fertilization in cases in which sperm were available only in reduced numbers. In instances of oligospermia, insemination of zona-intact oocytes frequently results in low rates of fertilization (34). Animal models have exemplified the usefulness of micromanipulation. After zona drilling was performed, insemination with sperm counts as low as 10 sperm per egg was associated with fertilization rates that were significantly higher than those of zona-intact controls. Similar results were obtained in mouse studies involving other forms of zona breaching (32).

As discussed above, the motility that is acquired and enhanced during sperm development is important for penetration through outer egg investments. It has been shown, however, that motility may not be necessary for traversal through the plasma membrane. In 1982, Cohen et al. noted that human spermatozoa which lacked progressive motility were able to penetrate zona-free hamster oocytes (35). Subsequently, Aitken et al. (1983) indicated that sperm from a patient with Kartagener's syndrome, an immotile-cilia syndrome, were able to penetrate zona-free hamster oocytes (36). These were interesting observations in spite of the fact that hamster egg penetration by human sperm is not representative of physiologic gamete interaction. Thus, sperm with nonprogressive, abnormal, or limited motility may be relatively inefficient in traversing only the outermost barriers of the oocyte. Several investigators have applied the use of zona drilling to "rescue" the fertility of mice that carry, for instance, some genetic defect that renders them incapable of fertilizing a zona-intact oocyte. For example, zona drilling was used to overcome the infertility in male mice that were heterozygous for the t haplotype ($T/t^{w5/w71}$) (37). Spermatozoa from such mice which transmit the t haplotype have severely reduced motility and a consequent inability to penetrate intact zonae pellucidae. Other animal models have demonstrated the application of zona manipulation for sperm in which abnormal morphology was linked to an inability to penetrate intact zonae pellucidae. Gordon et al. (1990) generated a transgenic mouse pedigree in which male homozygotes were sterile (38). Ultrastructural studies showed severe flagellar defects in the sperm of the affected males, and it was felt that this condition led to motility disorders which rendered the sperm incapable of penetrating outer egg investments. These sperm were incapable of penetrating an intact ZP and could only fertilize eggs after zona drilling was performed. Although there is no direct human analogy to this model, it demonstrates that motility defects resulting in infertility can be overcome with zona drilling. Other types of morphologic anomalies such as severe teratozoospermia have been clinically treated by application of zona manipulation (38,39).

In addition to the aforementioned sperm factors, micromanipulation may be useful when the ZP is impenetrable even by "normal" sperm. Those glycoproteins composing the ZP which serve primarily as sperm receptors, if masked in some way, will cause the zona to be refractile to sperm binding and penetration. In the human, antibodies to sperm can be present in the follicle and may result in infertility due to prevention of fertilization (40). Furthermore, properties of the ZP are altered with time in culture and exposure to serum (41,42). The zona hardening that results from in vitro culture can inhibit sperm penetration. In both of these instances, it may be possible to bypass the zona barrier with microsurgical fertilization.

Subzonal insertion (SZI) of sperm:

A second method of assisted fertilization utilizing micromanipulation is SZI. In this procedure, the ZP is not merely opened but is functionally and physically bypassed. Sperm are aspirated into a hollow microneedle and are deposited into the perivitelline space of the oocyte. Like zona drilling methods, SZI has been attempted in both animal and human models. However, because it involves placement of preselected sperm directly into the perivitelline space, SZI poses a greater challenge to the oolemma than the previously discussed forms of micromanipulation. It is necessary to account for both the quality and quantity of spermatozoa involved in SZI. As we have discussed, only sperm that have undergone capacitation and the AR will be capable of fusing with the eggs' plasmalemma. Since the ZP is no longer involved in the selection process, it may be necessary to use artificial induction of the AR to ensure that the "selected" sperm will be capable of fertilization. Thus, in terms of sperm "handling," SZI is difficult. Spermatozoa of certain mammalian species are fragile and prone to mechanically caused damage. Therefore, in addition to physiologic preparation, in order to maximize the efficiency of sperm delivery during SZI several animal models have been investigated.

Much progress has been made in refining the use of perivitelline sperm insertion in the mouse model. In 1986, Barg et al. attempted to introduce immobilized, yet acrosome-reacted sperm into the perivitelline space of oocytes (43). Results indicated that sperm rendered immotile by several methods (e.g., cold exposure, treatment with calcium ionophore, mechanical immobilization) after subzonal insertion were unable to fuse with the oocyte and form pronuclei. These results raised the possibility that the methods used to immobilize or acrosome-react the sperm might have disrupted the integrity of the sperm membrane so as to render it incapable of fertilization. In fact, it was subsequently shown that even acrosome-reacted sperm require a functional ion pump (Na^+K^+ ATPase) in order to fuse with the vitelline membrane of the oocyte (26). It is possible that the contact between sperm and microneedle as described by Barg et al. (1986) disrupted a membrane function which was associated with motility and the ability of the sperm to undergo normal fusion with the egg (43). Other groups who attempted SZI using motile sperm that were not artificially induced to undergo the AR showed that such sperm could penetrate the oocytes, albeit at a low rate (44). Yamada et al. (1988) used a protocol in which mouse spermatozoa were exposed to a cyclic nucleotide treatment that induced the AR without affecting motility before SZI was performed (26,45). This treatment led to higher rates of fertilization than were previously attained in the mouse model. Finally, full embryonic development was achieved in a mouse SZI study by Mann, who placed mouse sperm capacitated under "normal" conditions in a viscous solution of methylcellulose (46). This treatment served to slow the motility and facilitate capture of the spermatozoa into the microneedle. It is likely that exposure to the methylcellulose protected vulnerable mouse sperm from the mechanical and physiologic damage caused by aspiration into the microneedle that was reported in previous studies (43). Mann (1988) was the first to report live births after performance of SZI (46). Others have tried to combine the use of methylcellulose with various methods of AR induction in order to improve the results of SZI by generating more uniform populations of acrosome-reacted sperm (47).

Finally, SZI has been modified further for use in other mammalian species. For example, in the rabbit efficient microinjection of sperm into the perivitelline space has been facilitated by exposing the oocyte to hyperosmotic solutions such as those used in the PZD procedure (48). Here, fertilization occurred in the absence of acrosome-reacting agents. Thus, in order to develop the most suitable animal model for clinical SZI, it is important to bear in mind that conditions ideal for gamete fusion differ among the mammalian species that have been discussed. The requirements for single versus multiple sperm insertion within an individual species like the mouse may differ. Furthermore, the ideal methods for AR induction may also vary among species such as the mouse and the rabbit.

The need to identify treatments specifically applica-ble to the induction of capacitation and the AR in human spermatozoa was investigated in a heterospecific model. Since hamster oocytes are receptive to human sperm penetration, they provide another system by which to test several sperm preparation protocols (49). The induction of the AR prior to SZI significantly increased the rate of human sperm penetration of hamster oocytes (50). Sperm that were artificially acrosome-reacted with calcium ionophore penetrated oocytes at a higher rate than untreated sperm. This finding contrasts with the observations of the mouse homospecific model by Barg et al. (43). A higher rate of penetration was observed when sperm were acrosome-reacted by freeze-thaw. The optimal number of inserted sperm was five in both cases; lower penetration rates resulted when fewer sperm were inserted, and multiple sperm penetration increased significantly when more than five sperm were inserted.

Some of the developmental work on SZI has come to fruition in the clinical laboratory. Successful application of a method for synchronizing capacitation in which sperm are incubated in medium in which strontium chloride is substituted for calcium has been reported (51,52). This method enabled the investigators, for the first time, to obtain fertilization after a single, motile spermatozoon was placed under the human ZP. Subsequently, others reported a pregnancy after transfer of multiple (7–10) sperm under the ZP (53). Special methods of sperm preparation were not used in this study. Fertilization in human oocytes injected with immotile sperm from a male with Kartagener's syndrome has also been reported (54). This result is yet another contrast with the inability to obtain fertilization with immotile mouse sperm and emphasizes the distinction between different mammalian systems in the application of SZI (43). Recently, we have applied SZI to severe cases of male factor infertility (55). The data obtained from these clinical trials have clarified several biological principles and raised several interesting questions pertaining to mammalian fertilization. For example, although both PZD and SZI may be effective treatments for cases of extreme teratozoospermia, it has become clear that those embryos derived from SZI implant at a significantly higher rate than those resulting from the PZD procedure. A possible explanation for this phenomenon as well as further results are offered in the clinical discussion of micromanipulation.

Direct sperm microinjection: The third alternative for using micromanipulation to facilitate sperm-egg interaction involves the direct microinjection of sperm into the cytoplasm of the egg. This invasive technique involves circumvention of all oocyte barriers, including the plasma membrane. Microinjection of sperm or sperm nuclei into the ooplasm has been attempted in both mammalian heterospecific (56) and homospecific (43,57,58) models. Though these initial attempts occasionally resulted in formation of male pronuclei, death of the oocyte was frequent. The success of microinjection is dependent on several factors. The ability of the oocyte to undergo activation and pronuclear formation is partially affected by the sperm treatment utilized to induce capacitation, the acrosome reaction, as well as by nonspecific cytoplasmic factors (59,60). In addition, in order to demonstrate the viability of the procedure, animal models should be chosen in which it is possible to obtain at least some cleavage development. Successful embryonic cleavage to blastocysts has been attained after sperm microinjection in cattle (61,62) with the use of various capacitating and acrosome-reacting agents such as calcium ionophore. In the rabbit microinjection has led to pronuclear formation, embryonic cleavage, and the birth of normal live offspring (60,63,64). Thus, it has been confirmed that a microinjection procedure in which all

natural barriers to sperm-egg interaction are bypassed may be a viable method with which to achieve fertilization.

What is the reality of applying such technology to clinical IVF? There is undoubtedly a subset of gamete defects that might be refractory to SZI. Severe morphologic defects (65), including complete absence of an acrosome, may render sperm incapable of undergoing the interactions necessary for fusion and may require application of microinjection. This hypothesis has been tested by Lazendorf and coworkers (1988), who demonstrated that sperm with defects specific to the acrosome and related structures were able to decondense in the cytoplasm of hamster oocytes (65). In addition, similar studies have been carried out using spare human oocytes and sperm. These investigators demonstrated that, to a limited extent, human oocytes were capable of surviving microinjection and were able to support formation of male and female pronuclei (66). Although these data are somewhat encouraging, assisted fertilization by direct sperm microinjection remains a tedious and difficult procedure. It will be necessary to demonstrate sperm microinjection as a viable and repeatable method for achieving fertilization, which poses minimal danger to the oocyte, before it can be considered a microsurgical method with which to assist human fertilization.

Biological aspects of zona pellucida micromanipulation

The evolution of gamete micromanipulation not only has introduced an important and novel approach to treating fertilization disorders, but also has provided new insight into the biology of fertilization in different mammalian systems. Results of several studies have clarified the role served by the ZP in the oocytes' block to polyspermy. While limited levels of polyspermy have been reported in the mouse model with the use of zona drilling and partial zona dissection (23), these rates increase when such techniques are applied to the human oocyte (29,67). It is known that in the mouse, there is a slow and partial block to polyspermy at the level of the plasma membrane (68). On the other hand, the polyspermy control in the human oocyte seems to be more dependent on the function of the ZP (29,67). Whether or not the human vitelline membrane maintains slow and transient function has not yet been determined. However, results of clinical trials of SZI which show that polyspermy increases with increased numbers of sperm placed in the perivitelline space emphasize the minor role played by the plasma membrane in polyspermy prevention (39).

During the initial phases of clinical PZD, it was noted that the degree of polyspermic fertilization was reduced as the interval between exposure to sucrose and insemination was increased (67). It was postulated that the sucrose was somehow affecting the sperm receptivity of the plasma membrane. This effect became increasingly apparent with time. The hypothesis was tested further in a trial of PZD performed on day-old re-inseminated oocytes (69). By varying the periods of exposure to sucrose following micromanipulation, it was demonstrated that polyspermy rates were significantly altered by changing the interval during which oocytes were exposed to sucrose. The investigators suggested that the changes in the cell membrane resembling activation were triggered by sucrose. Whether such changes involve any of the biological processes associated with physiologic "activation" (10) such as calcium oscillations and metabolic alterations remains unclear. Whatever the mechanism, however, the receptivity and fusogenic characteristics of the oocyte plasma membrane are subject to effects of the micromanipulation protocol (most likely related to sucrose exposure). Such technical details appear to have profound consequences for subsequent sperm–egg interaction.

Zona manipulation has also helped to elucidate the biological role of the mammalian egg surface during fertilization. In a recent investigation, PZD was used in conjunction with IVF to study the function of the heterogenous surface structure of the mouse and hamster oocyte (28). Specifically, the function of the microvillus-free area of the vitellus associated with the first polar body was examined by performing PZD both in proximity and opposite to this area of the egg surface. Inseminations of such oocytes revealed clear differences in sperm-egg interactions that were dependent on the site of zona manipulation. The experimental design supported the fact that sperm made contact and interacted with the oocyte at the site of micromanipulation. Furthermore, manipulation of the ZP at a region opposite the first polar body, and therefore away from the microvillus-free area, consistently resulted in higher rates of fertilization than when PZD was performed near the polar body. This indicates that in some mammalian species, zona manipulation, for assisting fertilization, should be done at a region away from the polar body. Whether these results are applicable to human IVF is not clear. However, clinical data in which the site of PZD in relation to the polar body has been carefully recorded suggests that the human oocyte may not have a functional microvillus-free area. In fact, the results seem to indicate that in the human oocyte, zona dissection near the polar body favors supernumerary sperm entry. It may be that in the absence of a (functional) microvillus-free region, the enlarged PVS created by the polar body acts as a "sink" in which sperm may accumulate.

Clinical microsurgical fertilization

Human IVF can be considered a treatment for limited gamete interaction since sperm and eggs are placed in close proximity under carefully optimized conditions (34). However, the presence of sperm abnormalities, and possibly oocyte abnormalities as well, often results in a complete failure of fertilization even by the most carefully optimized application of the standard technique. In addition, a number of infertile men with very few live spermatozoa in their semen are refused access to IVF centers. Various micromanipulation strategies, discussed in the previous section, have been suggested for the promotion of sperm-egg fusion in these couples. Of these methods, only PZD and SZI have been applied successfully in the human (53,70).

Partial zona dissection

Partial zona dissection has produced pregnancies in more than 10 different IVF centers. We have applied it to 174 couples with male factor infertility at Reproductive

Biology Associates in Atlanta, Georgia, and the Center for Reproductive Medicine and Infertility of the New York Hospital–Cornell Medical Center (Table 7.1). Basically, three groups of patients were admitted for these studies. The first group, which comprises approximately half of the total number of patients, had severely abnormal semen analyses (71,55) and failed to fertilize all oocytes in a previous IVF cycle. Some of these patients failed to fertilize when IVF was repeated several times. The second group had not been accepted for regular IVF by any other programs, including our own. These patients' semen analyses were considered highly abnormal, and only a maximum of 50,000 motile spermatozoa could be retrieved from their semen, even if the last sperm pellet was resuspended in a small

Table 7.1 Results of PZD trials with ZP-intact controls (117 cycles in male factor couples) performed at Reproductive Biology Associates between March 1988 and September 1990 and 57 similar cycles performed at the Center for Reproductive Medicine and Infertility (New York Hospital–Cornell Medical Center) between October 1989 and September 1990

Parameter	Cohen et al., 1990	Tucker et al., 1990	Cohen et al., 1991[a]	Total
Fertilization of ZP-intact (ZI) eggs	42/129 (33%)	33/254 (13%)	NA	NA
Fertilization (PZD eggs)	75/138 (54%)	73/281 (26%)	97/267 (36%)	245/686 (36%)
Replacements/cycles	37/47 (79%)	30/70 (43%)	38/57 (67%)	105/174 (60%)
ZI embryos replaced	24	20	17	61
PZD embryos replaced	55	40	78	173
Fetuses/embryos replaced	15/79 (19%)	17/60 (28%)	16/95 (17%)	48/234 (21%)
Clinical pregnancy	10	16	12	38
Ongoing/delivered	8	13	9	30
Preg. from PZD embryos only	2	4	4	10
Preg. PZD/ZI mixed	8	12	6	26
Clin. preg./cycle	10/47 (21%)	16/70 (23%)	12/57 (21%)	38/174 (22%)
Clin. preg./transfer	10/37 (27%)	16/30 (53%)	12/38	38/105 (36%)

[a]ZI control oocytes only occasionally used

volume of 20 to 50 μl. Such patients were advised to have microsurgical fertilization rather thana standard IVF cycle. The third group (approximately 30% of those selected for PZD) had not attempted IVF previously (some were not acceptable to other IVF programs), and all had male factor infertility of intermediate severity. Since the chances of fertilization would be somewhat reduced among these patients, micromanipulation was performed on some of their oocytes, while other oocytes were left intact. A fourth group of patients with abnormal semen analyses were not considered suitable for PZD since many motile spermatozoa were recovered from their semen and they had never had IVF before.

Combined results of the first three groups of couples are summarized in Table 7.1. Fertilization rates were always significantly higher in PZD oocytes than in zona-intact oocytes (67,71). However, one should not compare fertilization rates of both groups of oocytes in men who were selected according to different criteria. For example, the fertilization of oocytes subjected to PZD by spermatozoa from men who were not able to fertilize oocytes in a previous regular IVF cycle is significantly higher than that of ZP-intact control oocytes. However, it is approximately the same as that of regular IVF in couples who were selected for PZD but who never had IVF before. Some of the patients received only embryos that had undergone PZD whereas others received ZP-intact controls and PZD embryos. A small number of patients had only ZP-intact control embryos replaced, and two of them became pregnant. Overall though, at least 10 pregnancies were produced following replacement of only micromanipulated embryos, and in several other patients twin pregnancies were obtained following replacement of one control embryo combined with one or more PZD embryos. Of all embryos 21% implanted successfully, and 22% of the patients had a clinical pregancy (Table 7.1). We have postulated recently that the high incidence of implantation could be explained by the presence of the artificial gap in the ZP, facilitating the blastocysts to shed the ZP during hatching (72,73). This assumption has led to several investigations attempting to introduce a micromanipulation method, which we have named "assisted hatching," possibly suitable for all IVF embryos and applied shortly before transfer (see below).

Subzonal sperm insertion and frequency of gamete fusion

The concept that most spermatozoa in the ejaculate are unable to fertilize—even those from fertile men—and represent chiasmatic errors occurring during spermatogenesis is not well founded. The question related to the fertilizing ability of individual human spermatozoa is not only intriguing scientifically, it is also important to know how many spermatozoa from fertile and infertile men can fuse with the oolemma if one wants to use SZI as an alternative to regular IVF. Much of our knowledge of the mechanisms involved in human fertilization is derived from observations made during therapeutic IVF. The number of spermatozoa incubated with oocytes varies depending on the techniques used and the expected fertilizing ability of motile spermatozoa from each individual. With possibly few exceptions, hundreds or even thousands of motile spermatozoa will interact during several hours with the ZP. In spite of this, the rate of monospermic fertilization of mature oocytes exceeds 70%, with only 5% incidence of polyspermy. The methodology followed in different laboratories, and hence the use of varying sperm concentrations for the insemination of oocytes, does not appear to affect the incidence of fertilization and polyspermy. IVF laboratories inseminate oocytes with sperm concentrations ranging from 0.5×10^5/ml to 5×10^5/ml. Nevertheless, fertilization rates differ only marginally.

The fact that reduced numbers of spermatozoa used for insemination lead to fertilization rates similar to those resulting from insemination with higher numbers of sperm suggests—assuming competition between spermatozoa is not altered by varying concentrations—that a substantial number of human spermatozoa are capable of traversing the ZP and fertilizing the oocyte. Recently we performed an SZI study in couples with male factor infertility by inserting between one and 20 motile spermatozoa in the perivitelline space of fresh mature oocytes (39). Sixteen percent of individual spermatozoa were able to fuse with the oolemma and form a pronucleus. It is therefore not surprising that fertilization following SZI increased when more spermatozoa were inserted. However, the incidence of polyspermy also increased, especially when more than two live sperm cells were introduced into the perivitelline space. Insertion of more than eight spermatozoa resulted in 100% polyspermy, indicating that sperm cells derived from infertile men are capable of multiple fusion with the oolemma.

More than half of motile spermatozoa from men with normal semen analyses are able to fuse with the oolemma when inserted directly into the perivitelline space of morphologically normal mature one-day-old oocytes. This conclusion was obtained from the use of SZI techniques in oocytes that failed to fertilize following insemination in a group of couples with various types of infertility (Table 7.2). Instead of regular reinsemination, SZI was performed. Sperm-egg fusions were counted by addition of all pronuclei of all zygotes, and the final number was diminished by the number of zygotes in order to correct for the inclusion of female pronuclei (one per zygote). Fifty-five fusions (23%) were counted following the insertion of 240 sperm cells. The rate of sperm fusion was higher (39%) when only those patients whose sperm function was considered normal were assessed. The degree of normality was based on the semen analyses and initial fertilization rates following insemination.

In order to calculate the potential of normally motile spermatozoa to fuse with the oolemma, one has to consider the fertilizing potential of each individual oocyte. It is likely that certain oocytes cannot be fertilized even if they have an extruded polar body. Some of the oocytes reinseminated by SZI had refractile bodies (74), and others had dark vacuolized cytoplasm. The fusing potential of motile human spermatozoa from men with normal semen analyses should therefore be based on potentially fertilizable eggs. Of 68 subzonally inserted spermatozoa, 41 (59%) of those from such men fused with the oolemma in 13 morphologically normal eggs (Table 7.2). From these results it can be concluded that the human oolemma has little protective mechanism against multiple sperm fusion, since the vast majority of aged oocytes subjected to SZI became polyspermic. The latter finding is in agreement with previous observations assessing the fertilizing capacity of men with abnormal semen following zona drilling (29,67). Others have suggested that the human oolemma, and not the ZP, is the main barrier to polyspermy (59,60). Such conclusions, though drawn

Table 7.2 Sperm-egg fusion following subzonal insertion

Type of infertility	SZI performed at	No. of fusing sperm/no. of inserted sperm
Male factor	Insemination	70/438 (16%)
Male factor	Reinsemination	6/108 (6%)
Tubal/idiopathic (all oocytes)	Reinsemination	49/132 (37%)
Tubal/idiopathic (morphologically normal oocytes)	Reinsemination	41/69 (59%)

from the application of SZI, were based on sperm populations with a known reduction in fertilizing ability. It is also feasible that swelling sperm heads were present in some of the oocytes studied but were unclear due to the nature of zygote assessment. The mechanism of polyspermy can only be evaluated using normal fertile spermatozoa, and the current observations leave little doubt as to the efficiency of the human zona reaction and the relatively poor ability of the oolemma to prevent multiple sperm fusion.

Subzonal sperm insertion for treatment of infertile men

Subzonal sperm insertion in oocytes from couples in whom the men were considered infertile has led to pregnancies at four different centers (53,55,70). To evaluate the potential applications of PZD and SZI, we have recently assessed both techniques simultaneously by comparing them in sibling oocytes in couples with male factor infertility in whom regular IVF had failed previously or in whom normal fertilization was likely to be reduced owing to severe semen abnormalities. In addition, the embryonic morphology and implantation potential of PZD and SZI embryos from couples with extreme forms of teratozoospermia was compared using retrospective analyses of videotapes of microsurgically fertilized embryos shortly before replacement. The morphology of these micromanipulated embryos was compared to those of ZP-intact embryos cultured under identical conditions and replaced concurrently. Previously, it was demonstrated that the percentage of spermatozoa with normal shape assessed with strict criteria was the only semen criterion correlated with the implanting capacity of PZD embryos (39,75).

Of the 47 couples included in this study, 24 (51%) had a previous IVF failure and 36 (77%) had severe male factor (groups A and B; Table 7.3). Fertilization rates among groups of oocytes in patients who had SZI,

PZD, and zona-intact control oocytes inseminated were not different. Rates of polyspermy for all SZI and PZD eggs were 20% and 26%, respectively. The rate of fertilization in SZI eggs (37/125, 30%) was significantly higher ($p < 0.01$) than in PZD eggs (11/86, 13%) in cases where ZP-intact control eggs could not be included due to extremely low sperm numbers (see rows three and four in Table 7.2). This indicates that the PZD technique requires higher motile sperm concentrations than SZI. Surprisingly, fertilization appeared higher in SZI eggs from patients with a previous failure of fertilization (48/129, 37%) than in patients who never had an IVF attempt before (17/125, 14%). This possibly demonstrates that the latter group of patients were selected using very low cutoff criteria.

Despite the severity of their sperm profiles, 70% of the patients had an embryo replacement, and nine of them became clinically pregnant (19%). Five of these pregnancies were established in patients in whom only SZI embryos were available. One of these was a twin pregnancy. One quadruplet pregnancy was established in a patient who had two SZI, one PZD, and one ZP-intact embryo replaced. One patient became pregnant after replacement of control embryos only, and two other pregnancies were established in patients who had both PZD and SZI embryos replaced. The range of the number of possible implantations attributed to microsurgical embryos only is indicated for each group in Table 7.3.

Subzonally inserted embryos from men with extreme teratozoospermia are able to implant at a significantly higher rate than PZD embryos from a comparable group of men (Table 7.4). Because of the possibility of mixed embryo transfers (SZI and/or PZD and/or ZP-intact control), the range of minimum and maximum implantation rates must be compared for each group; both analyses were significant. If it is assumed that a minimum number of embryos from microsurgical fertilization implanted, then none of the 18 PZD embryos from couples with extreme teratozoospermia implanted. Under these conditions, SZI appears significantly more successful; at least 6/15 (40%) of the embryos implanted. The same significance was found when the assumption was made that the maximum number of embryos implanted was derived from microsurgical fertilization. Again SZI appeared more effective than PZD in this particular group of patients. Using the same mode of comparison, PZD appeared more successful than SZI in men with moderate teratozoospermia; however, the trend was not significant due to the small sample size (Table 7.4).

The total number of abnormal embryo characteristics in PZD embryos was not different from that in SZI embryos (an average of 2.4 and 2.9, respectively).

Table 7.3 Results of 47 cycles (male factor couples) in which SZI was performed and PZD occasionally

Allocation of oocytes	Previous failure of fertilization (patient group)[a]	Incidence of fertilization per oocyte[b] [cycles with fertilization]			Percentage of polysp. zygotes (PZD)[SZI]	Proportion of cycles with transfer	Incidence of implantation	
		ZP-intact control	PZD	SZI			Per embryo (min.–max. from PZD) [min.–max. from SZI]	Per patient (min.–max. from PZD) [min.–max. from SZI]
All SZI	Yes (A)	—	—	8/26 [4/4]	[13]	4/4	3/7 [3–3]	2/4 [2–2]
All SZI	No (B)	—	—	2/37 [2/5]	[0]	2/5	1/2 [1–1]	1/5 [1–1]
SZI/PZD	Yes (A)	—	10/55 (18%)[c] [8/15 (53%)]	30/75 (40%)[c] [12/15 (80%)]	(50) [17]	12/15	2/29 (0–1) [1–2]	2/15 (0–1) [1–2]
SZI/PZD	No (B)	—	1/31 (3%) [1/7 (14%)]	7/50 (14%) [3/7 (43%)]	(0) [43]	2/7	0/4	0/7
SZI/PZD/ ZP-intact	Yes (A)	6/24 (25%) [2/5 (40%)]	4/20 (20%) [1/5 (20%)]	10.28 (36%) [4/5 (80%)]	(0) [0]	5/5	1/11 [1–1]	1/5 [1–1]
SZI/PZD ZP-intact	No (C)	16/47 (34%) [7/11 (64%)]	16/42 (38%) [7/11 (64%)]	8/38 (21%) [6/11 (55%)]	(19) [38]	8/11	6/27 (1–2) [2–3]	3/11 (1–2) [1–2]
All cycles				65/254 (26%) [31/47 (66%)]	(26) [20]	33/47 (70%)	13/80 (16%) (1–3) [8–10]	9/47 (19%)[d] (1–3) [6–8]

[a]A, previous failure of regular IVF; B, not acceptable for regular IVF due to low sperm numbers; C, acceptable for IVF, but reduced fertilization anticipated
[b]Based on cleaved embryos only
[c]p<0.02 (chi-square analysis)
[d]One singleton pregnancy from ZP-intact embryos

However, the distribution of abnormal embryos in both groups was different when it was correlated with teratozoospermia. For example, PZD embryos from extreme teratozoospermic patients were more frequently abnormal (defined as having at least two abnormalities) than embryos from moderate teratozoospermic patients (94% vs. 56%, respectively). On the other hand, most abnormal SZI embryos (87%) were associated with cases of moderate teratozoospermia (Fig. 7.1).

A plausible explanation for the observation that embryos derived from routine IVF as well as PZD rarely implant when the spermatozoa are obtained from extreme teratozoospermic men, while SZI embryos appear unaffected, is that it may be a result of the insemination procedure. PZD and ZP-intact embryos are usually inseminated with large numbers of spermatozoa, many of which are immotile due to the complexity of the semen profiles. These ostensibly inert spermatozoa may interfere with normal development of ZP-intact or PZD embryos by releasing toxic elements, such as free radical oxygen species (76). The intact ZP may normally function as a partial filter, protecting the

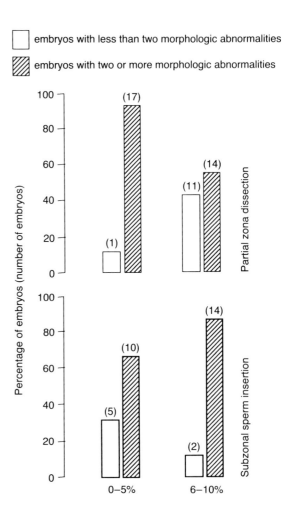

Fig. 7.1   Effect of sperm morphology on embryonic morphology following PZD or SZI. Sperm morphology was assessed with strict criteria, whereas embryonic morphology was based on retrospective analyses of videotapes, scoring 11 parameters for each embryo.

Table 7.4   Effect of teratozoospermia on the implanting capacity of PZD and SZI embryos

Mode of micromanipulation	Minimum and maximum no. of embryos implanting (%)	
	Normal sperm 0%–5%	Normal sperm 6%–10%
Partial zona dissection	0/18–3/18[a] (0%–20%)	5/25–7/25 (20%–28%)
Subzonal sperm insertion	6/15–7/15[a,b] (40%–47%)	1/16–1/16[b] (7%–7%)

[a]Comparisons of minimal and maximal proportions; both $p<0.05$
[b]Comparisons of minimal and maximal proportions; $p<0.05$ and $p<0.02$, respectively

oocyte and zygote from environmental damage. This protection may become ineffective by partial or complete removal of the ZP. Embryos from SZI are likely to be less affected by the environment as they are not exposed to heterogenous sperm populations and other seminally derived components, but are only presented with a few spermatozoa during micromanipulation.

It is more difficult, however, to provide an explanation for the frequent abnormality and lack of viability of SZI embryos from couples in which the men had moderate teratozoospermia. Polyspermy occurs more frequently when more normal specimens are used during PZD. Similarly, some of the SZI embryos in the current study may have been polyspermic, and this may have been overlooked by the observers.

In conclusion, techniques such as PZD and SZI are advantageous in cases of extreme male factor infertility. They can be used either simultaneously on sibling oocytes or, if indicated, individually. On the basis of the preliminary findings presented above, SZI should be applied to extreme forms of male factor infertility, whereas PZD may be more beneficial in cases of moderately abnormal semen profiles.

Enucleation for the correction of polyspermy

The block to supernumerary sperm penetration in the human oocyte seems to reside principally at the level of the ZP. When the ZP is compromised through microsurgical fertilization procedures, an increase in the incidence of polyspermic fertilization occurs (60,77,78). The rate of polyspermy following PZD in our program has consistently been approximately 25%. Also, in rare cases, IVF cycles have been observed in which a high degree of polyspermy occurs in the absence of ZP micromanipulation. The ability to control polyspermy or to correct the genetically abnormal embryos that result from it would be of obvious value to clinical IVF.

There is a large body of research regarding genetic manipulation in rodents and large animals based on techniques for the vital, intact removal of mammalian pronuclei (79,80). It would seem that these techniques could be modified and used to simply remove the extra sperm pronucleus, thereby returning the zygote to a normal genetic complement. Preliminary experiments toward this goal have been reported by several groups (77,78,81).

The survival rate in our enucleation work is 84%, and most of the surviving embryos exhibit further development. A real assessment of embryonic development was compromised by the desire to perform ultrastructural and genetic analysis. The embryos of those patients who consented to provide blood for genetic analysis were cryopreserved at the two- to four-cell stage for subsequent polymerase chain reaction screening of genetic makeup. Most of the embryos of those patients who did not consent were fixed for ultrastructural analysis; either 3 hours after enucleation or at syngamy. Some embryos were occasionally left and observed for development. Cleavage was definitely observed in 62% of the enucleated embryos. However, accounting for those that appeared healthy but were fixed prematurely, this rate could increase to 79%. Both the ultrastructural and genetic analyses are in progress, and no data are yet available.

The real issue in using enucleation to correct polyspermy is the correct identification of the supernumerary male pronuclei. This identification is simple in rodent zygotes, in which nuclear size and the presence of sperm tail remnants, as well as position in relation to the second polar body, are all valid criteria. In human zygotes, size appears to be a random variable, and sperm tail remnants can almost never be identified by vital microscopic observation (78,82). Pronuclei that are farthest from the second polar body are being selected for removal, and genetic analysis will, one hopes, vindicate this as being a valid criterion for identification. Ultrastructural analysis could show that the procedure is not resulting in hidden damage to the cytoskeleton or other components of the ooplasm. Despite the physical success of the enucleation procedure, until it is certain that this procedure produces normal, diploid embryos with both a maternal and paternal component, clinical application would be highly ill-advised.

The embryonic zona pellucida, micromanipulation, and hatching

The molecular structure of the mammalian embryonic ZP as it undergoes hatching is largely unknown, but it appears that the ZP matrix alters with time. Evidence suggests that hatching may occur via any of the following three mechanisms: uterine enzymes digest the zona from the outside; embryonic proteases digest the zona from the inside; and the zona is thinned through increased proliferation and pressure from the expanding blastocyst. Evidence for these three routes exists in the mouse, whereas embryonic proteases appear to be absent in several other species (83). Expansion and thinning of the ZP appear to be essential for hatching and are observed in most mammalian species. In the rabbit, hatching occurs only when the number of cells is minimal, and ZP rupture appears to be associated with proliferation and physical expansion. Rhesus monkey blastocysts also require a minimal diameter in order for hatching to occur (84).

Human embryos are usually transferred at the cleaved embryo stage, owing to increased embryonic demise with prolonged culture. Only one in four fully expanded blastocysts derived from in vitro fertilized ovarian human oocytes will hatch (85,86). This provides evidence that human blastocysts are capable of hatching in the absence of uterine lysins, but also demonstrates that zonae are often resilient to dissolution. The incidence of blastocyst formation and hatching can be increased by culturing human embryos on monolayers of reproductive tract cells (86,87). This finding supports the argument that many in vitro fertilized embryos are deficient in the amount of zona lysins needed to initiate and complete hatching.

Although introducing an incision in the zona pellucida is a simple procedure, it may have important consequences for further embryonic development. For instance, microorganisms, viruses, and cytotoxins present in the insemination suspension could invade and infect the embryo via the artificially produced gap in the zona (see section on microsurgical fertilization). Immune cell invasion through gaps in the zona may cause embryonic death prior to the formation of tight junctions (88). Blastomeres may be lost through large holes, possibly causing embryonic death or vesiculation (24). Although it is difficult to monitor such events following embryo replacement, a trial that addressed some of these problems has been conducted in PZD patients (89). Every other patient received corticosteroids and antibiotics for 4 days in order to counteract the potential effects of immune cell invasion. The rationale for corticosteroid administration was to reduce the number of intrauterine immune cells. Seven of the eight pregnancies obtained following PZD occurred in the experimental group, and although this represented a relatively small group of patients, immunosuppression is now routinely applied to patients whose oocytes or embryos are micromanipulated.

Disruption of the zona by micromanipulation may not only lead to loss of embryonic tissue but also have profound consequences on the hatching process, a prerequisite for implantation. Both the timing and morphology of the hatching process in vitro of mouse and human PZD embryos are altered (78). The ZP does not thin as it does normally during blastocyst expansion, and hatching occurs earlier and at a higher frequency. Though the sample sizes in the original studies were relatively small (67), human PZD embryos implanted better than zona-intact embryos. This notion is sustained in studies presented here (Table 7.1).

Assisted hatching

Assisted hatching of cleaved embryos was applied to 99 patients using PZD as the technique to open the ZP (72,73). Embryos allocated for replacement were micromanipulated in alternate patients. This resulted in an experimental group (patients whose embryos were micromanipulated) and a control group (patients whose embryos had intact ZP). The ZP of a total of 144 fresh two- to eight-cell embryos were thus micromanipulated. All embryos appeared intact following micromanipulation, and none of the blastomeres were damaged. Positive β-human chorionic gonadotropin was confirmed in 17 (34%) of the 51 control patients who received zona-intact embryos and in 24 (50%) of the 48 assisted hatching patients. The incidence of clinical pregnancy increased from 26% in the control group to 46% per embryo replacement in the experimental group, a significant improvement ($p < 0.05$; chi-square test). Moreover, embryonic implantation increased from 13% to 22% ($p < 0.05$). Half of the pregnancies in the experimental group were either twin or triplet pregnancies. On the basis of these experiments, it has been postulated that approximately one-quarter of all IVF embryos have the ability to implant, that a substantial number of IVF embryos are unable to breach the zona at the time of hatching, and that many can be rescued by opening their ZP several days earlier. It is as yet unclear whether assisted hatching using PZD should be applied as part of the standard IVF procedure. Only 7% of human embryos treated with assisted hatching implanted when we applied PZD in 20 couples at the IVF program at Cornell in 1989. This series of investigations was not performed as part of a prospective randomized trial. However, the implantation rate of zona-intact embryos in this program normally exceeds 10%, indicating that PZD holes in the ZP may also have an adverse effect on implantation. This may be due to many differences between culture methods and replacement procedures between the two IVF programs at the time.

Though the hatching process may be inhibited following IVF (or perhaps even following natural fertilization), it may not always be advantageous to perform assisted hatching on an embryo using the PZD technique 2 days after egg collection. Zona hardening alters the resilience of the ZP to the PZD technique; the incisions are easier to make and may be smaller than those made prior to fertilization. The absence of zona thinning and expansion during expulsion of the blastocyst through the narrow artificial opening may cause constriction of the trophoblast and the inner cell mass. Indeed, trophoblast tissue may be lost when the blastocyst squeezes through the narrow gap. At least one of the twins obtained following assisted hatching was monozygotic and miscarried in the second trimester of gestation. Another disadvantage of the PZD procedure for assisted hatching during the early cleaved embryo stage may be the loss of blastomeres or even the whole embryo during the replacement procedure (C. B. Fehilly, unpublished observations). Mucus and tissue are frequently collected in the transfer catheter at the time of cervical insertion. Although ZP-intact embryos usually squeeze past such obstacles unharmed, embryos with holes in their ZP are damaged easily and may be lost upon release into the uterine cavity. Results may improve by enlarging the artificial hole and patching it with a self-digesting biological gel to improve its strength during embryo replacement and reduce intra-uterine immune invasion. Alternatively, embryos may be micromanipulated with acidic medium to increase the the size of the opening after the formation of constructional junctions between the blastomeres. This may avoid the hazards imposed on the embryos during replacement and would facilitate trophoblast expulsion during hatching. Recently it was demonstrated that desmosomes and gap junctions occur during the third cleavage division in the human (90). Indeed, biopsy techniques applied to eight-cell embryos with the use of acidic medium apparently facilitate hatching (91).

Preimplantation genetic diagnosis

Prenatal genetic analysis is currently limited to the postimplantation period. Couples at risk of transmitting genetic disorders undergo prenatal testing during the first trimester of gestation by chorionic villus sampling, or during the second trimester by amniocentesis. Pregnancies found to be genetically abnormal are terminated. Although such procedures are routine, some maternal risk may be involved. Comparatively, in vitro fertilization (IVF) combined with preimplantation genetic analysis is a less invasive option. The morbidity and mortality associated with IVF is less than for termination.

Transvaginal ultrasound-guided oocyte aspiration recovery has replaced laparoscopy, simplifying the IVF procedure. The expansion of moleculer genetics in parallel with that of the assisted reproductive technologies has resulted in a greater understanding of genetic disease. The polymerase chain reaction, for example, which allows for the amplification of DNA sequences up to a millionfold, has dramatically increased the sensitivity and speed with which genetic analysis can be accomplished. It is now theoretically possible to analyze a single cell removed from an early embryo and provide specific genetic diagnosis prior to embryo replacement (Table 7.5). A vast amount of literature on animal embryo manipulation demonstrates the safety and feasibility of these techniques. Furthermore, the proce-

dures have been successfully applied to human embryo biopsy in the experimental setting. Further advances in the sensitivity of genetic analysis will likely increase their applicability. The use of these procedures in the clinical setting is imminent. This section will review the literature that has led to developments which have made embryo biopsy possible.

Embryo manipulation vis à vis embryo biopsy

To successfully sample a preimplantation embryo, a cell or number of cells must be removed without altering growth or development. In addition, the procedure must be efficient enough so that a high percentage of sampled embryos will produce viable offspring. Finally, sampled material must be genetically and biochemically representative of the whole embryo and must be easy to analyze.

Embryo manipulation in laboratory animals has shown that early embryos are to some degree resistant to microsurgery. A method for culture of micro-manipulated sheep embryos and its use to produce monozygotic twins was described by Willadsen (88). Blastomeres from two- and four-cell sheep embryos

Table 7.5 Diseases amenable to preimplantation genetic diagnosis

X-linked diseases
Lesch-Nyhan syndrome
Duchenne muscular dystrophy
X-linked mental retardation
Adrenoleukodystrophy

Single gene defects
Sickle-cell anemia
Thalassemia
Cystic fibrosis
Tay-Sachs disease

were separated and inserted into empty zonae obtained from porcine oocytes. The single blastomere and zona was then transferred to an agar solution and allowed to congeal in a thin pipette. A second agar cylinder containing the first agar chip and several zonae was solidified and transferred to the ligated oviduct of a recipient. Although a small proportion of embryos are damaged by the micromanipulation technique, the procedure is now a routine mode for twinning in bovine and ovine models. It demonstrates that a single blastomere from a two-cell embryo can produce full, liveborn offspring. Production of identical twins by bisection of blastocysts in the bovine model has also been described (92). In this study, 8-day embryos were recovered by nonsurgical methods from superovulated crossbred heifers. Expanded blastocysts with identifiable inner cell mass and trophoblast were released from the zona pellucida and bisected. Each half blastocyst was placed into an empty zona pellucida and cultured for an additional 2 hours. These embryos were then transferred. This study demonstrates that, despite some cellular differentiation which occurs by the blastocyst stage, it is possible to produce identical cattle twins by bisection of the blastocysts. A similar study was performed by Nagashima et al. (93). In this study, monozygotic mouse twins were produced from microsurgically bisected morulae. After pretreatment for ZP softening and decompaction, approximately 80% of the morulae were bisected without visible cell damage. They were then cultured and classified as normal blastocysts, abnormal blastocysts, or trophectodermal vesicles. Approximately 60% of embryos manipulated by this method produced normal appearing blastocysts. From 30 normal blastocysts, eight twin fetuses were obtained. This study again demonstrated the ability of the early embryo to withstand traumatic injury and still produce viable offspring. In a similar study performed in horses, Allen and Pashen described production of mono-

zygotic horse twins by embryo micromanipulation (94). In this study, evacuated pig zona pellucidae were used to make 27 micromanipulated half-embryos and 17 quarter-embryos from 19 two- to eight-cell embryos recovered surgically from pony mares. Subsequent transfer of 13 half-embryos and 17 quarter-embryos resulted in 10 established pregnancies, including two monozygotic pairs. From a breeder's standpoint, these methods have clear commercial significance. Information gained from these experiments is potentially useful when one considers the possibility of sampling the early human embryo to obtain genetic diagnosis prior to implantation.

Biopsy techniques and analysis of embryonic health

The first successful diagnosis carried out in the pre-implantation period was performed by Gardner and Edwards in 1968 (95). Rabbit blastocysts were sexed karyotypically by removing a segment of trophectoderm cells. They confirmed the diagnosis of the newborn rabbits resulting from the transfer of these blastocysts to host mothers. These techniques have been improved and are now performed routinely to sex cattle blastocysts for use in commercial embryo transfer. While trophectoderm biopsy is an alternative for pre-implantation diagnosis, this method will probably have limited success in humans. Currently, IVF technology and culture methods do not allow for routine recovery of human blastocysts. Approximately 30% to 40% of human embryos cultured in vitro will proceed to the blastocyst stage, and only a fraction of these will expand and hatch. While blastocysts can be recovered from the uterus by transcervical flushing, this is an inefficient procedure (96,97). The advantage of trophectoderm biopsy is that more cells are available for analyses and that it circumvents the IVF procedure. Additional material makes complex genetic analysis more feasible.

Embryo biopsy at earlier stages of development will yield only one to three cells.

Currently, most biopsy techniques are applied at the four- to eight-cell stage. The focus on pre-implantation diagnosis has centered at this stage, since four- to- eight-cell embryos are routinely obtained from IVF programs. Some investigators, however, are focusing on polar body biopsy as an indirect method for preimplantation genetic diagnosis (98). This method is limited to the situation in which the mother is a carrier and the genetic status of the oocyte can be determined indirectly by accessing the first polar body.

There are a number of animal models for preim-plantation genetic diagnosis. Monk et al. described a pre-implantation diagnosis of deficiency of hypoxanthine phosphoribosyl transferase (HPRT) in a mouse system for Lesch-Nyhan syndrome (99). In this study, they mated heterozygous carrier females with normal males. Offspring from this mating should contain 50% normal males, 50% affected males, 50% normal females, and 50% carrier females. Embryos were obtained and sam-pled at the eight-cell stage. Using a microenzyme assay, the investigators were able to analyze HPRT activity and adenine phosphoribosyltransferase in single blastomeres, and thus categorize the embryo as "affected" or "nor-mal." Their analysis was done rapidly enough to allow embryos to be transferred during the same cycle. Sub-sequent analysis of the resulting offspring showed that the selective procedure had been successful (100). This work was extended by performing trophectoderm bi-opsy in mouse embryos at the blastocyst stage. Embryos were removed from the uterus, diagnosed, and returned within 2 days without the need for cryopreservation. In a similar fashion, affected male embryos as well as carrier female embryos were identified in offspring (100). These studies utilized the microenzyme assay as a mechanism for diagnosing the presence or absence of a gene product: in this case, an enzyme activity.

Trophectoderm biopsy was also performed in marmoset monkeys (101). Using micromanipulation techniques, a tear was made in the zona pellucida opposite the inner cell mass of 8-day blastocysts. This tear facilitated the controlled herniation of trophec-todermal cells as the blastocysts expanded. The her-niated trophectoderm was cut off by free hand and the biopsied blastocysts were transferred to recipients. Normal offspring were born. However, there was a clear requirement for luteal phase support in the form of human chorionic gonadotropin. Biopsies of 30 to 50 cells of the 10-day-old blastocysts were cultured in vitro, and trophoblast vesicles with an excess of 1000 cells were obtained. However, biopsies from 9-day-old blastocysts contained fewer than 20 cells and formed a monolayer of binucleated and multinucleated cells with limited cell replication. Pregnancies were obtained by this method. A pregnancy was also obtained from a biopsied blastocyst that had been frozen. This technique could potentially be applied to humans.

Mouse model systems were utilized to develop four- to eight-cell embryo biopsy techniques. Wilton and Trounson reported a successful single cell removal with cryopreservation of preimplantation mouse em-bryos (102). They described a method of removing a single blastomere from a four-cell mouse embryo that did not compromise continued development in vitro or in vivo. When transferred to pseudopregnant mice, 60% of biopsied embryos and 64% of control embryos implanted and 53% of biopsied and control embryos developed into fetuses. Embryos biopsied in this fashion could be successfully cryopreserved by ul-trarapid freezing, even though there was a puncture site in the ZP. The incidence of implantation and that of fetal development of biopsied frozen-thawed embryos were identical to those of controls (103). Wilton and Trounson also described the ability to culture a single blastomere removed from early stage embryos. More than 90% of biopsied and control embryos reached the blastocyst stage after 48 hours of culture. Implantation rates of biopsied embryos were greater than 53%. Blastomeres were also cultured in vitro with extracellular matrix components to enhance proliferation. Components such as fibronectin, laminin, nidogen, or a complex thereof have been utilized. After 6 days in culture, between 10 and 20 cells were obtained using extracellular matrix components. These techniques would allow embryo biopsy coupled with cryopreservation to obtain a complex of preimplantation diagnoses using a single blastomere. Many copies of the genetic material could be obtained for analysis by various techniques including karyotyping, in situ hybridization, and DNA amplification.

Finally, Handyside and coworkers have successfully biopsied human four-cell embryos and sexed them using a Y-chromosome-specific primer pair (103). They were able to remove a single cell and determine embryonic gender with no apparent consequences. Biopsied embryos developed to the blastocyst stage at the same rate as control embryos. The single cell recovered from the biopsy procedure was analyzed by DNA amplification techniques that amplify Y-chromosome-specific sequences. The efficiency of this procedure was confirmed by analyzing the cultured biopsied by both polymerase chain reaction and in situ hybridization, and in all cases of normal embryos the analyses agreed. They extended this work by using these techniques clinically to identify female embryos for transfer in couples at risk of transmitting sex-linked disorders. In these couples 50% of the male embryos would be affected by the disorder. By transferring only the female embryos, only carrier females and normal females would result. Normal children have been born from this procedure (91).

The overall cellular mass in the human blastocyst reduces when biopsy is performed at the eight-cell stage (105). However, the reduction is only in proportion to the original loss of cell material. The important ratio of inner cell mass cells and trophectoderm was maintained. The general health of these embryos was also accessed by monitoring their ability to incorporate glucose and pyruvate. Metabolic processes of the biopsied blastocysts appeared to be reduced, but only in proportion to the number of blastomeres removed.

Polymerase chain reaction

Polymerase chain reaction (PCR) has opened a new frontier of genetic analysis. This method allows for the amplification of a specific sequence of DNA by as much as one million times, and now makes analysis of DNA from a single cell possible (91). The method capitalizes on the thermostability of *Thermicus aquaticus* (Taq), a thermophilic bacterium that can survive extended incubation at 95°C. The polymerase chain reaction requires thermal cycling through a series of reactions at a variety of temperatures.

PCR is divided into three separate components: the melting reaction, the primer-annealing reaction, and the primer-extension reaction. A thermal cycler allows for the orderly progression from each step to the next. In the first reaction, the double-stranded target DNA is denatured at 94°C into single-stranded DNA. In the primer-annealing step, the temperature is lowered to a level, usually between 37° and 60°C, at which the specific primers can anneal to the single-stranded DNA. Since the primers are in molar excess, they preferentially anneal to the DNA rather than reforming double-stranded DNA. The primers are chosen such that they recognize a specific sequence of DNA of fragment length 50 to 2000 base pairs. Any known sequence of DNA can have primers constructed that will flank the region of interest. Most primers are from 15 to 25 bases in length and are easily synthesized on a DNA synthesizer. Each primer recognizes one of the two complementary strands of DNA. After annealing has been

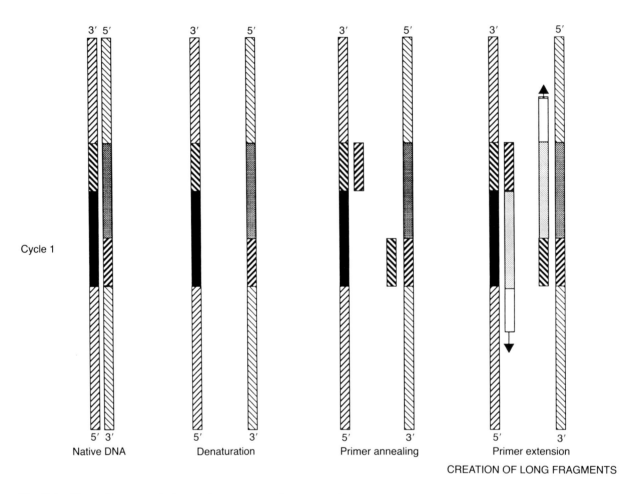

Fig. 7.2   The polymerase chain reaction occurs in three parts: denaturation, primer annealing, and primer extension. These steps comprise a cycle and are repeated many times. In the first cycle, the native template DNA is denatured, allowing the primers access to bind in the annealing step. Polymerization follows as Taq polymerase extends the sequence. Extension continues beyond the end of the sequence flanked by the primers, and thus long fragments are synthesized. This step occurs in each subsequent cycle. In cycle two, the long fragments also serve as template; however, when the end is reached, extension stops. Thus short fragments are created. These are the length that the primers flank. In cycle three, the short fragments serve as template, and primer extension results in the creation of a complementary short fragment. In every subsequent cycle the steps in cycle one, using native DNA as template, and in cycle two, using long fragments as template, are duplicated. However, short fragments are duplicated geometrically, long fragments arithmatically, and native DNA not at all. The result after many cycles is a population of DNA fragments mainly of short fragment length.

accomplished, the primer-extension reaction is started whereby the primer serves as the start point for the Taq polymerase to synthesize a complementary copy of the DNA template. This reaction is usually carried out at 72°C, but each specific template may have an optimum temperature, which is determined empirically. In the first cycle, the length of the newly synthesized DNA extends beyond the boundary set by the primer set (Fig. 7.2). At this point the denaturation step is repeated, making all of the DNA single-stranded. Now four single-strand copies of DNA containing the sequence of interest are present: the original double-stranded template and two newly synthesized fragments. All of these can now serve as templates for another round of annealing and primer extension. Thus, at the end of the second cycle of PCR, eight new single-stranded fragments of DNA are present; however, all are of varying length, the original template (two strands), a fragment

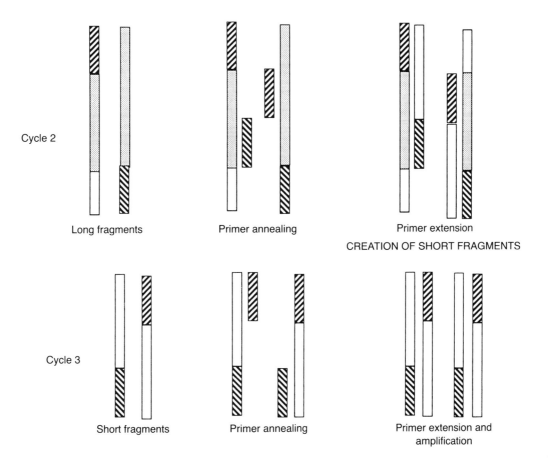

Cycle 2

Long fragments   Primer annealing   Primer extension

CREATION OF SHORT FRAGMENTS

Cycle 3

Short fragments   Primer annealing   Primer extension and amplification

Figure 7.2 *cont.*

of length defined by the region where the primers flank (two strands called short fragments), and a fragment with an ill-defined length, where polymerase was able to copy beyond the site where the primer flanks when the original DNA served as template (four strands called long fragments) (Fig. 7.2). As the reaction goes through a number of cycles, there is a logarithmic increase in the number of short fragments, there is an arithmetic increase in the number of long fragments, and, of course, there is no change in the original template DNA. Thus, at the end of many cycles, the predominant DNA contained in the reaction vessel is a fragment of DNA of length defined by the number of base pairs separating the primer pair.

This technology adds a new level of sensitivity to genetic analysis. For specific gene defect disorders, PCR allows one to amplify a sequence of DNA that contains the site of the defect (deletion, mutation). Further refinement strategies are being developed that allow a single gene from a single cell to be analyzed. Currently, the most useful application of PCR preimplantation genetics is embryo sexing using a single cell removed by biopsy. The strategy capitalizes on chromosome-specific repeat sequences on either the X- or Y-chromosome. The fact that these sequences are repeated many times on the chromosome of interest is a distinct advantage.

In particular, two Y-chromosome-specific primer sets have been utilized on blastomeres obtained from human embryo biopsy (91, 102, 104). Both primer pairs flank Y-chromosome-specific repeat sequences; thus amplification of DNA is enhanced by the fact that 800 to 1500 copies of the sequence of interest are contained in a single cell. In one instance, the additional strategy of utilizing nested primers also increases the level of sensitivity of the assay. This strategy involves a second amplification with a second primer set that flanks a sequence contained within the first amplification product. Thus, the second amplification increases the product by another order of magnitude, making visualization using ethidium bromide and ultraviolet light more feasible (91, 102, 104). The other Y-chromosome-specific primer pair described does not require nested primers to amplify DNA from a single cell (106).

Single gene defect disorders could also potentially be identified with PCR analysis of single cells. DNA from single human oocytes has been genetically analyzed (107). Gene markers have been identified closely linked to the genes affected in cystic fibrosis and Duchenne muscular dystrophy. Thus, it is feasible to amplify DNA from a haploid cell. The β-hemoglobin sequences have been amplified in single oocytes and polar bodies (108). A 680 base pair sequence was obtained by first amplifying a 725 base pair fragment and then amplifying a 680 base pair sequence present within the first fragment. The utilization of nested primers in this fashion offers a more sensitive method for analysis. Moreover, since the sickle cell mutation destroys the Dde-1 site, a method of distinguishing normal from sickle cell genotype is provided. Restriction analysis of the 680 base pair fragment amplified by this method and then digested by Dde-1 results in one 210 and one 180 base pair fragment when the normal gene is analyzed and a diagnostic 381 base pair fragment when the sickle cell mutation is present. In addition, allele-specific oligonucleotide probes offer a very sensitive and specific method for detecting the hemoglobin S, C, and A genotypes and could be coupled with PCR analysis of single cells to provide a preimplantation diagnosis (109). Drawbacks of these methods are that duration of analysis is prolonged and radioactively labeled probes are required.

Cystic fibrosis has been diagnosed in embryos by analyzing the first polar body and a blastomere (110). An embryo homozygous for the Δ508 deletion was thus identified and not replaced. Improvement of techniques for detection of single gene disorders will be necessary prior to wide-scale application to preimplantation genetics. Finally, in situ hybridization may provide a means for numerical chromosome analysis (111). It provides a direct analysis of a single cell using chromosome-specific probes. Contamination is less likely to occur, and the time span for analysis is such that it will be suitable for application in preimplantation diagnosis.

Gene transfer in the human

Benefactors and madmen have long dreamed of altering the human germ line for good or ill. As our understanding of the molecular biology of disease, health, and the human genome expands, scientists and ethicists are, for the first time, seriously considering practical human germ line modification. Recent developments in somatic gene therapy will surely act as a catalyst both to those for and to those against human germ line therapy research (112).

Mammalian germ line alteration has been a reality for more than 15 years (113). Transgenic animals, a term coined by Gordon and Ruddle (114), have been produced in the mouse, pig, sheep, and cow (114). However, the gene transfer techniques currently available are far from perfect, and experience with these techniques in the human is nonexistent.

Methodology

It has been 10 years since the first practical germ line gene transfer was accomplished in the mouse (115). The elegant method, employed in the first experiments, of injecting specific concentrated DNA into the pronuclei of zygote-stage embryos has been refined over the years and remains the method of choice despite the development of alternatives. Jaenisch proposed simply infecting early embryos with a modified retrovirus acting as a vector for the gene to be inserted (118,119). A third methodology involves the formation of chimeric embryos using embryonic stem (ES) cells previously transfected with the desired gene by either retroviral or chemicophysical means (120,121).

Each of these techniques has advantages, but the disadvantages of the latter two would probably preclude their use in the human. One disadvantage of retroviral vectors is that the size of the DNA to be inserted is limited to about 10 kilobases (kb) (122). Many genes of interest would be too large for transfer in this way. Also, the control of transgene expression in retroviral vectors can be problematic owing to the presence of viral control sequences. Moreover, since multicell embryos are used for transfection and viral integration is relatively inefficient, successful transfer occurs in only a fraction of the cells, and the resulting transgenic individuals are usually mosaics. Mosaicism is the major disadvantage of ES chimeras, as well. By the very nature of the technique used, offspring created in this way will be mosaic for the transgene. While mosaicism is only a slight drawback in animal experimentation (where selective breeding can easily produce a population of nonmosaic transgenic offspring), it would most likely be completely unacceptable in human treatment scenario.

Pronuclear injection can result in transgene mosaicism (probably due to delayed integration), but this occurs only 30% of the time (123). The overall integration efficiency for pronuclear injection is low, perhaps 25% at best (123). However, the ability to screen preimplantation embryos for genetic content would allow positive transgenic embryos to be identified (91,125). The main problem with pronuclear injection is that DNA integration occurs randomly, often involving substantial perturbations to both the transgene and the chromosomal DNA (126). Not only can insertional events result in serious immediate effects such as lethal mutations and chromosomal rearrangement, but also insertion site and orientation can cause a wide variation in the subsequent expression of the transgene (123). Even when positive integration could be verified by preimplantation diagnosis, the ambiguity resulting from random insertion would probably render pronuclear injection unacceptable as a technique for human clinical use at present. It is likely that improved DNA constructs will be developed in the future that will allow for controlled insertion in an efficient manner.

One advantage of ES cell gene transfer is that integration is obtained in a more stable fashion. In fact, techniques have been developed that allow for targeted gene replacement through homologous recombination (127). For instance, this technique was recently used successfully in mice to correct the genetic defect associated with Lesch-Nyhan syndrome (128).

This technique cannot be directly related to pronuclear injection since it relies on cell culture techniques for forcibly selecting the few successfully transformed cells (a few per thousand). Perhaps in the future some characteristics of homologous gene targeting could be incorporated into improved injection constructs or new methodologies.

A new method for DNA transfer has been discussed using sperm as the vector for the transgene. In the mouse, an experiment was carried out in which sperm were exposed to DNA and then used to fertilize oocytes. The resulting offspring were transgenic for the new gene with 30% efficiency (129). Unfortunately, this work cannot be reproduced despite efforts by several laboratories (130). However, the original workers continue to claim that the technique is successful in their hands and, in fact, allude to preliminary success using the technique in pigs (131).

Practical considerations for gene transfer in the human

The first step in any attempt at gene transfer is the identification, isolation, and characterization of the desired gene. This is a far from trivial matter. However, many genes of potential "clinical" interest are already available, and the future will no doubt provide an exponential expansion in gene characterization. Once a gene is available, a genetic construct must be devised and created for use in gene transfer. Obtaining a satisfactory level of expression with the desired tissue and/or temporal specificity would probably require the creation of a complex fusion construct. This can be a painstaking and laborious process involving the precise placement of the transgene in relation to regulatory DNA sequences. For instance, by including the promoter sequence from the elastase gene in the construct, expression of the transferred gene can be directed to the pancreas in a highly specific manner (132). Also, in this way expression can be modulated by factors such as hormones or environmental signals (133,134). It must be recalled that our understanding of gene expression (certainly one of the most complex regulatory systems in biology) is in its infancy. There have been several cases of incorrect and unexplained transgene expression patterns (135,136)

Once a construct is devised and created, pronuclear injection should be a relatively straightforward procedure in the human. In fact, recent experiments involving the microsurgical removal of pronuclei from polyspermic human zygotes indicate that success with the pronuclear injection procedure itself might even be superior in the human (78). Mouse zygotes are easily killed by the cytoplasmic insertion of a relatively large enucleation pipette while human zygotes survive the procedure quite well (H. E. Malter, personal observation). Also, the pronuclei of human zygotes are readily visualized by light microscopy.

The injection procedure would entail the use of a standard embryologic micromanipulation setup. The zygote would be held by a suction-holding pipette while a fine-pointed injection needle (preloaded with an aqueous solution of the DNA construct) was introduced into the target pronucleus until pronuclear expansion (perhaps 2×) was observed. A percentage of zygotes would be damaged by the procedure. Based on murine pronuclear injection, once the injection conditions (timing, size of needle, DNA concentration, etc.) were optimized, a success rate of 70% or more could be expected. Factors affecting the success of pronuclear injection in research animals have been discussed extensively elsewhere (124,137,138). Certainly there would be some embryonic loss from the injection technique itself, and this would have to be taken into account in its clinical application. Successfully injected zygotes would be cultured and then biopsied before transfer to determine their genetic component as discussed above.

Strategies for germ line gene therapy

One great advantage of germ line therapy would be that, if successful, it would phenotypically terminate the heredity of the genetic lesion. A transgenically corrected genome would be theoretically passed on to any future generations, although animal experiments have demonstrated some exceptions to this (134,139). Theoretically, any single gene defect could be corrected by the transfer of a functional transgene with (and perhaps, in some cases, even in the absence of) the correct expression pattern and control. Germ line therapy would be particularly indicated in treating genetic lesions associated with the central nervous system since the blood-brain barrier would probably preclude somatic cell gene therapy in this case (140). Several successful mouse models exist for using transgenes to circumvent deficiencies due to genetic lesions (128,141).

Gordon has suggested several novel treatment strategies for individuals with heritable cancers (125). Chemotherapy efficacy might be greatly improved if multiple drug resistance genes, providing protection from the toxic effects of chemotherapeutic agents, could be transferred through the germ lines of affected individuals. Expression could even be targeted, using the appropriate tissue-specific promoters, to organs that were particularly susceptible to chemotherapeutic toxicity. Preliminary mouse experiments have shown that this methodology can work (142). Alternatively, genes for tumor killing agents could be linked to promoters involved with atavistic expression in malignant cells to create an automatic "magic bullet" for curbing tumor growth (125). Certainly as our knowledge of human genetics expands, new treatment strategies as well as new treatment challenges will be defined that will be amenable to germ line genetic manipulation.

Considering the present state of knowledge about germ line gene transfer and gene regulation, it would be highly premature to proceed with human germ line alteration. A tremendous amount of research must be undertaken before we can open this Pandora's box and have a reasonable expectation of being satisfied with what we find. New methods must be devised to improve drastically the efficiency and control of transgene integration. New strategies for the manipulation of gene expression in the human system will be required. Eventually, direct experience with human embryos must be gained and evaluated.

The ability to alter the human genome will be attended by tremendous responsibility. Negative aspects, such as abusive uses of this technology for eugenic reasons, wait in the wings and will have to be dealt with by society. However, the potential to "cure" the multitude of genetic lesions that plague the health of millions would seem reason enough to pursue aggressively the goal of human germ line therapy.

Acknowledgments: Janet Trowbridge is gratefully acknowledged for editing the manuscript.

References

1. Austin CR. Sperm maturation in the male and female genital tracts. In: Metz CB, Monroy A, eds. Biology of fertilization, vol 2. Orlando, Fla: Academic Press, 1985.

2. Olson GE, Orgebin-Crist MC. Sperm surface changes during epididymal maturation. Ann NY Acad Sci 1982;383:372–391.

3. Oliphant G, Reynolds AB, Thomas TS. Sperm surface components involved in the control of the acrosome reaction. Am J Anat 1985;174:269–283.

4. Fraser LR, Quinn PJ. A glycolytic product is obligatory for initiation of sperm acrosome reaction and whiplash motility required for fertilization in the mouse. J Reprod Fertil 1981;61:25–35.

5. Fawcett DW. The mammalian spermatozoon. Dev Biol 1975;44:394–436.

6. De Vries JWA, Willemsen R, Geuze HJ. Immuno-cytochemical localization of acrosin and hyaluronidase in epididymal and ejaculated porcine spermatozoa. Eur J Cell Biol 1985;37:81–88.

7. Meizel S. Molecules that initiate or help stimulate the acrosome reaction by their interaction with the mammalian sperm surface. Am J Anat 1985;174:285–302.

8. Wassarman PM, Bleil JD, Florman HM, et al. The mouse egg's receptor for sperm: what is it and how does it work? Cold Spring Harbor Symp Quant Biol 1985;50:11–19.

9. Tesarik J. Comparison of acrosome reaction-inducing activities of human cumulus oophorus, follicular fluid and ionophore A23187 in human sperm populations of proven fertilizing ability in vitro. J Reprod Fertil 1985;74:383–388.

10. Yanagimachi R. Mammalian fertilization. In: Knobil E, Neill J, eds. The physiology of reproduction. New York: Raven Press, 1988.

11. Austin CR. Capacitation and the release of hyaluronidase from spermatozoa. J Reprod Fertil 1960;3:310–311.

12. Cummins JM, Yanagimachi R. Development of ability to penetrate the cumulus oophorus by hamster spermatozoa capacitated in vitro, in relation to the timing of the acrosome reaction. Gamete Res 1986; 15:187–212.

13. Talbot P. Sperm penetration through oocyte investments in mammals. Am J Anat 1985;174:331–346.

14. Bleil JD, Wassarman PM. Autoradiographic visualization of the mouse egg's sperm receptor bound to sperm. J Cell Biol 1986;102:1363–1371.

15. Bleil JD, Wassarman PM. Sperm-egg interactions in the mouse: sequence of events and induction of the acrosome reaction by a zona pellucida glycoprotein. Dev Biol 1983; 95:317–324.

16. Urch UA, Wardrip NJ, Hedrick JL. Limited and specific proteolysis of the zona pellucida by acrosin. J Exp Zool 1985;233:479–483.

17. Sato K, Blandau RJ. Time and process of sperm penetration into cumulus-free mouse eggs fertilized in vitro. Gamete Res 1979;2:295–304.

18. Yanagimichi R, Noda YD. Physiological changes in the postnuclear cap region of mammalian spermatozoa: a necessary preliminary to the membrane fusion between sperm and egg cells. J Ultrastruc Res 1970;31:486–493.

19. Gaddum-Rose P. Mammalian gamete interactions: what can be gained from observations on living eggs? Am J Anat 1985;173:347–356.

20. Shuel H. Functions of egg cortical granules. In: Metz CB, Monroy A, eds. Biology of fertilization, vol. 3. Orlando, Fla.: Academic Press, 1985.

21. Wassarman PM, Florman HM, Greve JM. Receptor-mediated sperm-egg interactions in mammals. In: Metz CB, Monroy A, eds. Fertilization, vol 2. Orlando, Fla.: Academic Press, 1985.

22. Jaffe LA, Sharp AP, Wolf DM. Absence of an electrical polyspermy block in the mouse. Dev Biol 1983; 96:317–323.

23. Gordon JW, Talansky BE. Assisted fertilization by zona drilling: a mouse model for correction of oligospermia. J Exp Zool 1986;239:347–354.

24. Talansky BE, Gordon JW. Cleavage characteristics of mouse embryos inseminated and cultured after zona pellucida drilling. Gamete Res 1988;21:277–287.

25. Malter H, Cohen J. Blastocyst formation and hatching in vitro following zona drilling of mouse and human embryos. Gamete Res 1989;24:67–80.

26. Talansky BE, Barg PE, Gordon JW. Ion pump ATPase inhibitors block the fertilization of zona-free oocytes by acrosome-reacted spermatozoa. J Reprod Fertil 1987; 79:447–455.

27. Conover JC, Gwatkin RBL. Fertilization of zona-drilled mouse oocytes treated with monoclonal antibody to the zona glycoprotein, ZP3. J Exp Zool 1988;247:113–118.

28. Talansky BE, Malter HE, Cohen J. A preferential site for sperm-egg fusion in mammals. Mol Reprod Dev 28:183–188,1991.

29. Gordon JW, Grunfeld L, Garrisi GJ, Talansky BE, Richards C, Laufer N. Fertilization of human oocytes by sperm from infertile males after zona drilling. Fertil Steril 1988;50:68–73.

30. Garrisi GJ, Talansky BE, Grunfeld L, Sapira V, Gordon JW. Clinical evaluation of three approaches to micromanipulation-assisted fertilization. Fertil Steril 1990; 54:671–677.

31. Depypere HT, McLaughlin FJ, Seamark RF, Warnes GM, Mathews CD. Comparison of zona cutting and zona drilling as techniques for assisted fertilization in the mouse. J Reprod Fertil 1988;84:205–211.

32. Odawara Y, Lopata A. A zona opening procedure for improving in vitro fertilization at low sperm concentrations: a mouse model. Fertil Steril 1989;51:699–704.

33. Cohen J, Malter H, Fehilly C, et al. Implantation of embryos after partial opening of oocyte zona pellucida to facilitate sperm penetration. Lancet 1988;2:162.

34. Cohen J, Edwards R, Fehilly C, et al. In vitro fertilization: a treatment for male infertility. Fertil Steril 1985;43:422–432.

35. Cohen J, Weber RFA, van der Vijver JCM, Zeilmaker GH. In vitro fertilizing capacity of human spermatozoa with the use of zona-free hamster ova: interassay variation and prognostic value. Fertil Steril 1982;37:565–572.

36. Aitken RJ, Ross A, Lees MM. Analysis of sperm function in Kartagener's syndrome. Fertil Steril 1983;40:696–698.

37. Ahmad T, Conover JC, Quigley MM, et al. Failure of spermatozoa from *T/t* mice to fertilize in vitro is overcome by zona drilling. Gamete Res 1989;22:369–373.

38. Gordon JW, Uehlinger J, Dayani N, et al. Analysis of the hotfoot (ho) locus by creation of an insertional mutant in a transgenic mouse. Dev Biol 1990;137:349–358.

39. Cohen J, Talansky BE, Malter HM, et al. Microsurgical fertilization and teratozoospermia. Hum Reprod 6:118–123,1991.

40. Bronson RA, Cooper GW, Rosenfeld DL. Sperm antibodies: their role in infertility. Fertil Steril 1984;42:171–183.

41. DeFelici M, Siracusa G. "Spontaneous" hardening of the zona pellucida of mouse oocytes during in vitro culture. Gamete Res 1982;6:107–113.

42. DeFelici M, Salustri A, Siracusa G. "Spontaneous" hardening of the zona pellucida of mouse oocytes during in vitro culture. II. The effect of follicular fluid and glyco-saminoglycans. Gamete Res 1985;12:227–332.

43. Barg PE, Wahrman MZ, Talansky BE, Gordon JW. Capacitated, acrosome-reacted but immotile sperm, when microinjected under the mouse zona pellucida, will not fertilize the oocyte. J Exp Zool 1986;237:365–374.

44. Mettler L, Yamada K, Kuranty A, Michelmann HW, Semm K. Microinjection of spermatozoa into oocytes. Ann NY Acad Sci 1988;541:591–600.

45. Yamada K, Stevenson AFG, Mettler L. Fertilization through spermatozoal microinjection: significance of acrosome reaction. Hum Reprod 1988;3:657–661.

46. Mann JR. Full term development of mouse eggs fertilized by a spermatozoon microinjected under the zona pellucida. Biol Reprod 1988;38:1077–1083.

47. Lacham O, Trounson A, Holden C, Mann J, Sathananthan H. Fertilization and development of mouse eggs injected under the zona pellucida with single spermatozoa treated to induce the acrosome reaction. Gamete Res 1989; 23:233–243.

48. Yang X, Chen J, Chen YQ, Foote RH. Improved development of rabbit oocytes fertilized by sperm microinjection into the perivitelline space enlarged by hypertonic media. J Exp Zool 1990;255:114–119.

49. Barros C, Gonzalez J, Herrera E, Bustos-Obregon E. Human sperm penetration into zona-free hamster oocytes as a test to evaluate the sperm fertilizing ability. Andrologia 1979;11:197–210.

50. Lassalle B, Testart J. Human sperm injection into the

perivitelline space (SI-PVS) of hamster oocytes: effect of sperm pretreatment by calcium-ionophore A23187 and freeze-thawing on the penetration rate and polyspermy. Gamete Res 1988;20:301–311.

51. Laws-King A, Trounson A, Sathananthan H, Kola I. Fertilization of human oocytes by microinjection of a single spermatozoon under the zona pellucida. Fertil Steril 1987; 48:637–642.

52. Mortimer D, Curtis EF, Dravland JE. The use of strontium-substituted media for capacitating human spermatozoa: an improved sperm preparation method for the zona-free hamster egg penetration test. Fertil Steril 1986;46:97–103.

53. Ng SC, Bongso A, Ratam SS, et al. Pregnancy after transfer of sperm under zona. Lancet 1988;2:790.

54. Bongso TA, Sathananthan AH, Wong PC, et al. Human fertilization by micro-injection of immotile spermatozoa. Hum Reprod 1989;4:175–179.

55. Cohen J, Alikani M, Malter, HE, Adler A, Talansky BE, Rosenwaks Z. Partial zona dissection or subzonal sperm insertion: microsurgical fertilization alternatives based on evaluation of sperm and embryo morphology. Fertil Steril 1991;56:696–706.

56. Thadani VM. A study of hetero-specific sperm-egg interactions in the rat, mouse, deer mouse using in vitro fertilization and sperm injection. J Exp Zool 1980;212: 435–453.

57. Uehara T, Yanagimachi R. Microsurgical injection of spermatozoa into hamster eggs with subsequent transformation of sperm nuclei into male pronuclei. Biol Reprod 1976;15:467–470.

58. Markert CL. Fertilization of mammalian eggs by sperm injection. J Exp Zool 1983;228:195–201.

59. Ng SC, Bongso A, Sathananthan H, Ranam SS. Micromanipulation: its relevance to human in vitro fertilization. Fertil Steril 1990;52:203–219.

60. Keefer CL. Fertilization by sperm injection in the rabbit. Gamete Res 1989;22:59–69.

61. Goto K, Kinoshita A, Takuma Y, Ogawa K. Fertilization by sperm injection in cattle [abstract]. Theriogenology 1990;33:238.

62. Keefer CL, Younis AI, Brackett BG. Cleavage development of bovine oocytes fertilized by sperm injection. Mol Reprod Dev 1990;25:281–285.

63. Keefer CL, Fayer-Hosken RA, Brown LM, Brackett BG. Culture of in vitro fertilized rabbit ova. Gamete Res 1988;20:431–436.

64. Hosoi Y, Miyake M, Utsumi K, Iritani A. Development of rabbit oocytes after microinjection of spermatozoa. Presented at the 11 Int Cong Anim Reprod A I, Dublin, 1988.

65. Lazendorf S, Maloney M, Ackerman S, Acosta A, Hodgen G. Fertilizing potential of acrosome-defective sperm following microsurgical injection into eggs. Gamete Res 1988;19:329–337.

66. Lazendorf SE, Maloney MK, Veeck LL, Slussler J, Hodgen GD, Rosenwaks Z. A preclinical evaluation of pronuclear formation by microinjection of human spermatozoa into human oocytes. Fertil Steril 1988;49:835–842.

67. Cohen J, Malter H, Wright G, Kort H, Massey J, Mitchell D. Partial zona dissection of human oocytes when failure of zona pellucida penetration is anticipated. Hum Reprod 1989;4:435–442.

68. Wolf DP. The block to sperm penetration in zona-free mouse eggs. Dev Biol 1978;64:1–10.

69. Malter H, Talansky BE, Gordon JW, Cohen J. Monospermy and polyspermy after partial zona dissection of reinseminated human oocytes. Gamete Res 1989;23:377–386.

70. Fishel S, Jackson P, Antinori S, Johnson J, Grossi S, Versaci C. Subzonal insemination for the alleviation of infertility. Fertil Steril 1990;54:828–835.

71. Tucker MJ, Bishop FM, Cohen J, Wiker SR, Wright G. Routine application of partial zona dissection for male factor infertility. Hum Reprod 6:676–681,1991.

72. Cohen J, Wright G, Malter H, et al. Impairment of the hatching process following in vitro fertilization in the human and improvement of implanattion by assisting hatching using micromanipulation. Hum Reprod 1990;5:7–13.

73. Cohen J, Malter H, Talansky B, Tucker M, Wright G. Gamete and embryo micromanipulation. In: Marrs RP, Speroff L, eds. The impact of IVF on the infertile couple. New York: Thieme, 1990.

74. Veeck LL. Atlas of the human oocyte and early conception. Baltimore: Williams and Wilkins, 1986.

75. Kruger TF, Acosta AA, Simmons KF, Swanson RJ, Matta JF, Oehninger S. Predictive value of abnormal sperm morphology in in vitro fertilization. Fertil Steril 1988; 49:112–121.

76. Aitken RJ. Evaluation of human sperm function. In: Edwards RG, ed. Assisted human conception. Edinburgh: Churchill Livingstone, 1990.

77. Gordon JW, Grunfeld L, Garrisi GJ, Navot D, Laufer N. Successful microsurgical removal of a pronucleus from tripronuclear human zygotes. Fertil Steril 1989;52(3): 367–372.

78. Malter HE, Cohen J. Embryonic development after microsurgical repair of polyspermic human zygotes. Fertil Steril 1989;52(3):373–380.

79. McGrath J, Solter D. Nuclear transplantation in the mouse embryo by microsurgery and cell fusion. Science 1983;220:1300–1302.

80. Willadsen S. Nuclear transplantation in sheep embryos. Nature 1986;320:63–65.

81. Rawlins RG, Binor Z, Radwanska E, Dmowski WP. Microsurgical enucleation of tripronuclear human zygotes. Fertil Steril 1988;50(2):266–272.

82. Wiker S, Malter H, Wright G, Cohen J. Recognition of paternal pronuclei in human zygotes. J In Vitro Fert Embroy Transf 1990;7(1):33–37.

83. Kane MT. Variability in different lots of commercial bovine serum albumin affects cell multiplication and hatching of rabbit blastocysts in culture. J Reprod Fertil 1983;69:555–558.

84. Boatman DE. In vitro growth of non-human primate pre- and peri-implantation embryos. In: Bavister BD, ed. The mammalian preimplantation embryo. New York: Plenum Press, 1987.

85. Fehilly CB, Cohen J, Simons RF, Fishel SB, Edwards RG. Cryopreservation of cleaving embryos and expanded blastocysts in the human: a comparative study. Fertil Steril 1985;44:638–644.

86. Lindenberg, Hyttel P, Sjogren A, Greve T. A comparative study of attachment of human, bovine and mouse blastocysts to uterine epithelial monolayer. Hum Reprod 1989;4:446–456.

87. Wiemer KE, Cohen J, Wiker SR, Malter HE, Wright G, Godke RA. Coculture of human zygotes on fetal bovine uterine fibroblasts: embryonic morphology and implantation. Fertil Steril 1989;52:503–508.

88. Willadsen SM. A method for culture of micromanipulated sheep embryos and its use to produce monozygotic twins. Nature 1979;77:298–301.

89. Cohen J, Malter H, Elsner C, Kort H, Massey J, Mayer MP. Immunosuppression supports implantation of zona pellucida dissected human embryos. Fertil Steril 1990; 53:662–665.

90. Dale B, Gualtieri R, Talevi R, Tosti E, Santella L, Elder K. Intercellular communication in the early human embryo. Mol Reprod Dev;29:22–28.

91. Handyside AH, Kontogianni EH, Hardy K, Winston RML. Pregnancies from biopsied human preimplantation embryos sex by Y-specific DNA amplification. Nature 1990;344:378–380.

92. Ozil JP. Production of identical twins by bisection of blastocysts in the cow. J Reprod Fertil 1983;69:463–468.

93. Nagashima H, Matsui K, Sawasaki T, Kand Y. Production of monozygotic twin mouse twins from microsurgically bisected morulae. J Reprod Fertil 1984;70:357–362.

94. Allen WR, Pashen RL. Production of monozygotic (identical) horse twins by embryo micromanipulation. J Reprod Fertil 1984;71:607–613.

95. Gardner RL, Edwards RG. Control of sex ratio at full term in the rabbit by transferring sexed blastocysts. Nature 1968;218:346–348.

96. Croxatto HB, Fuentealba B, Diaz S, Pastene L, Tatum H. A simple non-surgical technique to obtain unimplanted eggs from human uteri. Am J Obstet Gynecol 1972;112:662–665.

97. Buster JE, Bustillo M, Rodi IA, et al. Biological and morphologic development of donated human ova recovered by non-surgical uterine lavage. Am J Obstet Gynecol 1985; 153:211–217.

98. Verlinsky Y, Ginsberg N, Lifchez A, Valle J, Strom CM. Analysis of the first polar body: preconceptual genetic diagnosis. Hum Reprod (in press).

99. Monk M, Handyside AH, Hardy K, Whittingham D. Preimplantation diagnosis of deficiency of hypoxanthine phosphoribosyl transferase in a mouse model for Lesch-Nyhan syndrome. Lancet 1987;2:423–425.

100. Monk M, Muggleton-Harris AL, Rawlings E, Whittingham DG. Pre-implantation diagnosis of HPRT-deficient male and carrier female mouse embryos by trophoectoderm biopsy. Hum Reprod 1988;3:377–381.

101. Summers PM, Campbell JM, Miller MW. Normal in vivo development of marmoset monkey embryos after trophoectoderm biopsy. Hum Reprod 1989;3:389–393.

102. Wilton LJ, Trounson AO. Biopsy of preimplantation mouse embryos: development of micromanipulated embryos and proliferation of single blastomeres in vitro. Biol Reprod 1989;40:145–152.

103. Wilton LJ, Shaw JM, Trounson AO. Successful single cell biopsy and cryopreservation of preimplantation mouse embryos. Fertil Steril 1989;51:513–517.

104. Handyside AH, Penketh RJA, Winston RML, et al. Biopsy of human preimplantation embryos and sexing by DNA amplification. Nature 1989;1:347–349.

105. Hardy K, Martin KL, Leese HJ, Winston RML, Handyside AH. Human preimplantation development in vitro is not adversely affected by biopsy at the 8-cell stage. Hum Reprod 1990;5:708–714.

106. Grifo JA, Tang YX, Kogelman L, Pratten MK, Sanyal MK, Fenton W. Characterization of a new human Y-chromosome specific primer pair for polymerase chain reaction (pcr). J In Vitro Fert Embryo Transf 1990;7:192–196.

107. Coutelle C, Williams C, Handyside A, Hardy K, Winston R, Williamson B. Genetic analysis of DNA from single human oocytes: a model for preimplantation diagnosis of cystic fibrosis. Br Med J 1989;299:22–24.

108. Monk M, Holding C. Amplification of a β haemoglobin sequence in individual human oocytes and polar bodies. Lancet 1990;335:985–988.

109. Saiki RK, Bugawan TL, Horn GT, Mullis K, Erlich HA. Analysis of enzymatically amplified β-globin and HLA-Δ DNA with allele-specific oligonucleotide probes. Nature 1986;324:163–166.

110. Strom CM, Verlinsky Y, Milayeva S, et al. Preconception genetic diagnosis of cystic fibrosis. Lancet 1990; 336:306–307.

111. Grifo JA, Boyle A, Fischel E, et al. Preembryo biopsy and analysis of blastomeres by in situ hybridization. Am J Obstet Gynecol (in press).

112. Bank A. Prospects for gene therapy. J In Vitro Fert Embryo Transf 1990;7:185.

113. Jaenisch R. Infection of mouse blastocysts with SV40 DNA: normal development of the infected embryos and persistence of SV40 specific DNA sequences in the adult animals. Cold Spring Harbor Symp Quant Biol 1974;39:375–380.

114. Gordon JW, Ruddle FH. Germ line transmission in transgenic mice. In: Burger MB, Weber R, eds. Embryonic development, part B: cellular aspects. New York: Alan R. Liss, 1982.

115. Gordon JW, Scangos GA, Plotkin DJ, Barbosa JA, Ruddle RH. Genetic transformation of mouse embryos by microinjection of purified DNA. Proc Natl Acad Sci USA 1980;77:7380–7384.

116. Hammer RE, Pursel VG, Rexroad CE, et al. Production of transgenic rabbits, sheep and pigs by microinjection. Nature 1985;315:680–683.

117. Birry KA, Bondioli KR, DeMayo FJ. Gene transfer by pronuclear injection in the bovine. Theriogenology 1988; 29:224.

118. Van der Putten H, Botteri FM, Miller AD, et al. Efficient insertion of genes into the mouse germ line via retroviral vectors. Proc Natl Acad Sci USA 1985;82:6148–6152.

119. Jaenisch R, Fan H, Croker B. Infection of preimplantation mouse embryos and of newborn mice with leukemia virus: tissue distribution of viral DNA and RNA and leukemogenesis in the adult animal. Proc Natl Acad Sci USA 1972;72:4008.

120. Lovell-Badge RH, Bygrave AE, Bradley A, Robertson E, Evans MJ, Cheah KSE. Transformation of embryonic stem cells with the human type II collagen gene and its expression in chimeric mice. Cold Spring Harbor Symp Quant Biol 1985;50:707–711.

121. Stewart CL, Vanek M, Wagner EF. Expression of foreign genes from retroviral vectors in mouse teratocarcinoma chimeras. EMBO J 1985;4:3701–3709.

122. Shimotohno K, Temin HM. Formation of infectious progeny virus after insertion of herpes simplex thymidine kinase gene into DNA of an avian retrovirus. Cell 1981;26:67–77.

123. Palmiter RD, Brinster RL. Germ-line transformation of mice. Annu Rev Genet 1986;20:465–499.

124. Brinster RL, Chen HY, Trumbauer ME, Yagle MK, Palmiter RD. Factors affecting the efficiency of introducing foreign DNA into mice by microinjecting eggs. Proc Natl Acad Sci USA 1985;82:4438–4442.

125. Gordon JW. Approaches to germinal cell gene therapy. J In Vitro Fert Embryo Transf 1990;7:191–193.

126. Covarrubias L, Nishida Y, Mintz B. Early development mutations due to DNA rearrangements in transgenic mouse embryos. Proc Natl Acad Sci USA 1986;83:6020–6022.

127. Smithies O, Gregg RG, Sallie SB, Koralewski MA, Kucherlapati RS. Insertion of DNA sequences into the human chromosomal β-globin locus by homologous recombination. Nature 1985;317:230–234.

128. Thompson S, Clarke AR, Pow AM, Hooper ML, Melton DW. Germ line transmission and expression of a corrected HPRT gene produced by gene targeting in embryonic stem cells. Cell 1989;56:313–321.

129. Lavitrano M, Camaioni A, Fazio VM, Dolci S, Farace MG, Spadafora C. Sperm cells as vectors for introducing foreign DNA into eggs: genetic transformation of mice. Cell 1989;57:717–723.

130. Brinster RL, Sandgren EP, Behringer RR, Palmiter RD. Letter. No simple solution for making transgenic mice. Cell 1990;59:239–240.

131. Lavitrano M, Camaioni A, Fazio VM, Dolci S, Farace MG, Spadafora C. Response to letter. No simple solution for making transgenic mice. Cell 1990;59:240.

132. Ornitz DM, Palmiter RD, Hammer RE, Brinster RL, Swift G, MacDonald RJ. Specific expression of an elastase–human growth hormone fusion gene in pancreatic acinar cells of transgenic mice. Nature 1985;313:600–603.

133. Mayo KE, Palmiter RD. Glucocorticoid regulation of metallothionein gene expression. Biochem Act Hormones 1985;12:69–88.

134. Palmiter RD, Chen HY, Brinster RL. Differential regulation of metallothionein–thymidine kinase fusion genes in transgenic mice and their offspring. Cell 1982;29:701–710.

135. Wanger EF, Stewart TA, Mintz B. The human β-globin gene and a functional thymidine kinase gene in developing mice. Proc Natl Acad Sci USA 1981;78:6376–6380.

136. Swanson LW, Simmons DM, Arriza J, Hammer R, Brinster RL. Novel developmental specificity in the nervous system of transgenic animals expressing growth hormone fusion genes. Nature 1985;317:363–366.

137. Gordon JW, Ruddle FH. Gene transfer into mouse embroys: production of transgenic mice by pronuclear injection. Methods Enzymol 1983;101:411–433.

138. Walton JR, Murray JD, Marshall JT, Nancarrow CD. Zygote viability in gene transfer experiments. Biol Reprod 1987;37:957–967.

139. Chisari FV, Pinkert CA, Milich DR, Filippi P, McLachlan A. A transgenic mouse model of the chronic hepatitis B surface antigen carrier state. Science 1985;230:1157–1160.

140. Walters L. The ethics of human gene therapy. Nature 1986;320:225–227.

141. Constantini F, Chada K, Magram J. Correction of murine β thalassemia by gene transfer into the germ line. Science 1986;233:1192–1194.

142. Isola LM, Gordon JW. Systemic resistance to methotrexate in transgenic mice carrying a mutant dihydrofolate reductase gene. Proc Natl Acad Sci USA 1986;83:9621–9625.

8

Third-Party Involvement in Assisted Reproductive Technologies

Richard P. Marrs

Introduction

The development of in vitro fertilization and embryo transfer (IVF-ET) almost one and one-half decades ago opened the door for the assisted technologies to expand so that most forms of reproductive failure can now be treated. Whether a couple is treated with IVF-ET, gamete intrafallopian transfer (GIFT), frozen embryo transfer (FET), zygote intrafallopian transfer (ZIFT), or any of the associated procedures that have commonly come to be called the assisted reproductive technologies (ARTs), inherent within the treatment modality is the need for a normal male and female gamete. In situations of gamete abnormality, donor gametes can now be substituted in any of the ARTs to proceed with reversal of the couple's infertile state. Reproductive failure had persisted in cases in which gamete production was normal but uterine function was either abnormal or absent. Recently, the use of surrogate gestational carriers has become a helpful clinical tool in assisting couples in having their own genetic offspring when the female has no uterine function.

The focus of this chapter will be to review, in detail, oocyte donation as it exists today, to look at sperm donation in the context of ARTs, and to report results of using gestational surrogate carriers for couples utilizing ARTs.

The use of donor oocytes in ART

In 1984, Lutjen et al. (1) reported the successful establishment and delivery of a pregnancy in a woman with ovarian failure after oocyte donation and in vitro fertilization (IVF). Since that time, numerous reports of successful pregnancy establishment after oocyte donation, IVF, and either gamete intrafallopian transfer, uterine transfer, or cryopreserved embryo transfer have been reported (2–11).

Indeed, the use of donated oocytes for women without ovarian function or with abnormal ovarian function has extended the use of the assisted reproductive technologies to patients who have no gametes (egg production) or have a genetic abnormality limiting normal reproductive function. Inherent in the success of donor oocyte procedures is the appropriate timing of embryo transfer to a well-prepared endometrium. Moreover, the selection of appropriate healthy, fertile donors is of major importance, as well as the stimulation and cycle synchronization of that individual with the recipient. Risks to the oocyte donor and to the recipient appear to be minimal but must be looked for and observed as these procedures continue to be more widely utilized in the treatment of the infertile couple.

Indications for oocyte donation

The most common reason for oocyte donation is ovarian failure. Premature ovarian failure is defined as secondary amenorrhea and elevated gonadotropin levels occurring before the age of 35. This entity occurs in approximately 3% to 4% of all women. It may be related to autoimmune disorders or to ovarian destruction caused by surgical procedures, radiation, or chemotherapy. The mechanism involved in premature ovarian failure remains unclear but most likely is related to an autoimmune phenomenon. Primary ovarian failure due to gonadal dysgenesis, or Turner syndrome, occurs in a smaller percentage of the population; approximately one out of every 10,000 women will have some type of gonadal dysgenesis causing primary ovarian failure.

A secondary indication for the use of donated oocytes is to reduce or eliminate transmission of genetic disorders. Women with sex-linked or autosomal recessive diseases may opt to use donated oocytes to avoid the alternatives of prenatal diagnosis and possible pregnancy termination. A further indication for egg donation is the occurrence of repeated failed attempts at

IVF in women who are thought to have abnormal or poor quality oocytes. Most often these are women who are either approaching 40 years of age or are over 40 and have not become pregnant with multiple cycles of conventional IVF or GIFT therapy.

Donor selection

Donor oocytes can be obtained in various ways. Originally, reports of donor egg use came from infertile women undergoing ovarian stimulation for IVF who allowed their excess eggs to be donated to unrelated recipients. In that type of approach, the infertile women donating the egg may or may not conceive, and the recipient of the extra eggs may or may not conceive. In situations in which the recipient conceives and the donor does not, ethical discomfort for the treating physician or group may be a concern.

After the initial use of infertile women as egg donors, either unrelated or related donors were then utilized on a volunteer basis. Currently the vast majority of donor oocytes are from unrelated volunteers who are either openly or anonymously matched with a recipient. The egg donors undergo individual cycles of ovarian hyperstimulation for the sole purpose of oocyte production for donation to the matched recipient. The risk associated with ovarian hyperstimulation, anesthesia, and surgical recovery of the oocytes has to be balanced with the necessity for oocyte donation to the recipient for pregnancy occurrence.

The selection of oocyte donors is based on primarily medical findings, but also social and psychological considerations have to be included. Egg donors should be in general good health and have no history of significant medical problems or of difficulty in conceiving. For the most part, donors are chosen if they are under age 35 and have at least one live birth of their own. All oocyte donors should be screened for sexually transmitted diseases and for a history of any type of hereditary disorder. The partner of the egg donor is screened in a similar fashion. In most programs of oocyte donation, the donor and the recipient undergo independent psychological testing and screening and separate discussion of the risks and benefits of the oocyte donation process. Moreover, since most states do not have distinct legislation concerning oocyte donation procedures, individual contracts are used for the protection of the donor, the recipient, and the medical team. These documents are usually prepared by each individual center or practitioner offering oocyte donation. Since standards have yet to be established to either qualify the type of relationship that the donor may or may not have with the recipient couple and/or offspring, or identify the risk with repetitive treatment of individuals for multiple cycles of egg donation, the legal and ethical policies have to be established on a center-by-center, state-by-state basis. Robertson (12) has reviewed the status of the legal issues in human egg donation. For the most part, no guidelines have been agreed upon, and therefore individual approaches are the norm.

Donor stimulation

Initially, donor oocytes were selected from infertile patients who were undergoing controlled ovarian hyperstimulation for in vitro fertilization. Individuals would volunteer to donate any eggs in excess of a certain number that would be for their own use. The difficulty in this type of situation from an ethical standpoint has been mentioned. From a clinical standpoint, the use of donor eggs from a woman known to be infertile may also decrease the odds of pregnancy outcome in an unrelated recipient. Therefore, for the most part, volunteer donors are selected, screened, and purposely stimulated for oocyte donation to a matched recipient. These individuals are stimulated in a similar fashion to infertile women undergoing controlled ovarian hyperstimulation for oocyte collection for any of the ARTs. The type

of stimulation the donor undergoes is based upon either synchrony with the recipient's natural cycle and the donor's cyclicity or a preselected stimulation regimen to synchronize with a hormonal replacement cycle for a recipient who has ovarian failure. For the most part, any of the standard stimulation regimens for controlled ovarian hyperstimulation can be utilized (13). The most commonly used stimulation protocols involve the combination of leuprolide acetate (Lupron; TAP Pharmaceuticals, Chicago, Ill.) and human menopausal gonadotropin (hMG: Pergonal; Serono Pharmaceuticals, Braintree, Mass.). Depending upon the natural synchrony between the egg donor and the recipient, one of two regimens is utilized. The "flare-up" regimen is utilized if approximate synchrony between the recipient and the donor is already evident. The "flare-up" regimen utilizes Lupron on day 2 and/or day 3 of the cycle followed by either purified follicle-stimulating hormone (FSH: Metrodin; Serono Laboratories, Braintree, Mass.) or hMG (Fig. 8.1). An alternative regimen that can be utilized to allow synchrony for the donor to the recipient cycle is the Lupron "down-regulation" scheme. In this case, if the donor's cycle and the recipient's natural cycle

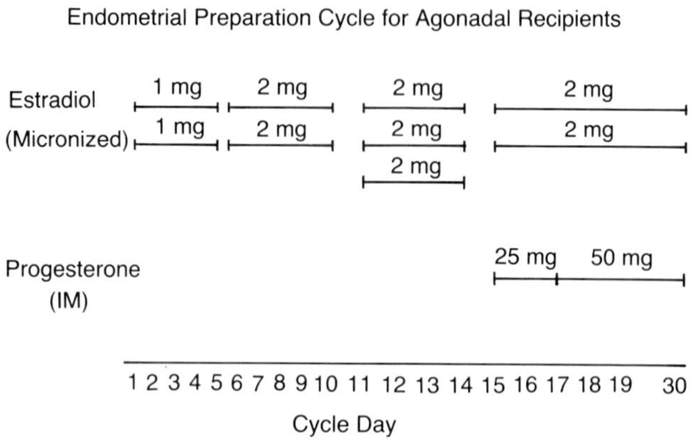

Fig. 8.1

are not synchronous (i.e., are more than 2–4 days apart), the donor is placed on Lupron, 1 mg administered subcutaneously per day beginning day 24 of the cycle, and is down-regulated and held until stimulation with hMG is started approximately 12 days before the recipient's expected time of natural cycle ovulation. By utilizing down-regulation, optimal synchronization can occur between the donor and the recipient (Fig. 8.2). Since the donor is selected because of normal fertility and is in a young age range, conventional stimulation with hMG alone can be utilized if synchrony is optimal in a natural state with the donor and the recipient. The difficulty in utilizing regimens of stimulation without Lupron is that any asynchrony that may develop during the stimulation phase between the donor and the recipient cannot be adjusted. With the use of Lupron, a one- or 2-day asynchrony can be adjusted for by delaying hCG administration for a period of time. Therefore, in the majority of egg donation cycles, the donor will be stimulated with either the flare-up or down-regulation scheme utilizing Lupron.

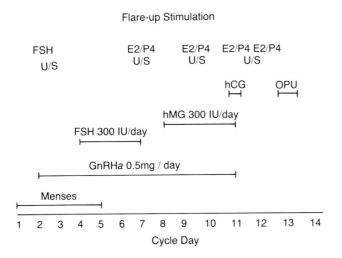

Fig. 8.2

The optimal synchronization between donor and recipient should be viewed as administration of hCG to the stimulated donor at the same time the recipient is having a luteinizing hormone (LH) surge in her natural cycle, or if in a fixed regimen replacement cycle with estrogen and progesterone, it should correspond to the first day of progesterone administration in the estrogen/progesterone replacement cycle for the recipient. The difficulty in optimal synchronization when a natural cycling recipient is used is obvious; however, in those individuals who have regular ovulatory cycles, a natural cycle can be used without any reduction in pregnancy outcome. For those women receiving transfers of donated oocytes/embryos, the natural cycle must be evaluated prior to an egg donor cycle. This evaluation includes preovulatory estradiol levels, LH monitoring, ultrasound visualization of endometrial growth and development, postovulatory estrogen and progesterone measurement in the luteal phase, and timed endometrial biopsy performed 7 to 10 days after ovulation. If all testing and evaluation including an in phase endometrial biopsy have been performed, the natural cycle can be utilized for the recipient. In cases where the ovum donor is stimulated and the recipient, in her natural cycle, fails to ovulate in a timely and synchronous fashion, the option to collect oocytes from the donor and fertilize and freeze all embryos is available and should not decrease overall pregnancy outcome in the recipient.

One of the potential risks to women volunteering to be oocyte donors is that of ovarian hyperstimulation. This risk includes not only ovarian hyperstimulation syndrome (OHSS) but also potential risks from the ovarian stimulatory drugs. For the most part, ovulation induction drugs have been viewed to be safe for treatment of ovulatory disorders in infertile women. In fact, a review and long-term follow-up study by Ron et al. (14) demonstrated no evidence of an increased incidence of cancer in infertile women receiving hMG stimulation. Other studies have shown that ovarian cancer risks and exposure to ovarian stimulation drugs are unchanged (15,16). Recently an article by Whittemore et al. (17) concluded in a metanalysis that nulligravid women who used fertility drugs were 27 times more likely than infertile control subjects to develop ovarian cancer. They also found that infertile women using fertility drugs who conceived had no increased risk of ovarian cancer. This study certainly has serious implications, if it is substantiated, for the use of ovulation induction drugs in fertile women for the purpose of inducing egg donation cycles. However, a major problem in the Whittemore study is that only 4% of the infertile controls in that study had used fertility drugs, yet it is estimated that 28% to 30% of infertile women in the United States use fertility drugs. Therefore, if the controls had reflected a 28% to 30% frequency of fertility drug use, there would be no significant increased risk of ovarian cancer in those published data. Therefore, it is the feeling that the Whittemore study is flawed in its appraisal of the purported association between fertility drug use and ovarian cancer occurrence and does not support the hypothesis of an increased risk of ovarian cancer in fertility drug users. However, the risks of using drugs in a fertile population of women who are volunteering to be egg donors must continue to be assessed and the information passed along to the volunteer donor population group.

Recipient replacement cycle for the oocyte donation

In patients who have no ovarian function, hormonal preparation of the endometrium is necessary prior to embryo transfer either to the fallopian tube or to the uterine cavity. Various regimens of hormonal replacement therapy have been used successfully from different centers (18–20). The primary focus of hormonal replacement therapy in the recipient is to mimic a natural cycle ovula-

tory event and normal luteal phase. Various estrogen preparations have been used to proliferate and prepare the endometrium for a progesterone conversion. For the most part, either micronized estradiol (Estrace) or estradiol valerate is taken orally in incremental doses prior to the initiation of progesterone. The use of the transdermal estrogen patch also has been shown to be effective (18). Recipients who are agonadal and are placed on a hormonal replacement regimen must undergo a "test cycle" in which the regimen is administered, serum levels of estrogen and progesterone are measured at various times, and an endometrial biopsy is performed prior to synchronization of the donor and recipient for transfer cycle (Fig. 8.3). After either oral or parenteral estradiol preparation of the endometrium, intramuscularly administered progesterone has been used in most cases. Even though endometrial biopsies have been reported to have an asynchronous gland-to-stromal consistency (19), this glandular asynchrony does not appear to interfere with implantation of donated embryos.

It is apparent from several authors that the dose,

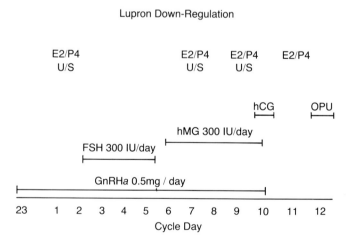

Fig. 8.3

or the time, of estrogen administration prior to progesterone initiation has little effect on implantation rates (20,21). Because there is variability in the time of estrogen priming of the endometrium, synchronization with the stimulated donor can be accomplished with this regimen. It has also been demonstrated that women who require egg donation but have ovarian function may have improved clinical pregnancy success if they are made functionally or artificially agonadal and then receive estrogen/progesterone therapy (20). This regimen utilizes Lupron to down-regulate ovarian activity followed by replacement with Estrace and progesterone as in an agonadal individual receiving estrogen/progesterone replacement therapy. This type of artificial agonadism can be utilized for difficult synchronization cycles or for individuals who have abnormal ovulatory cycles or have failed to achieve pregnancy in previous egg donation cycles in which their natural cycle was utilized.

Time of transfer to the recipient

Whether the recipient is naturally cycling or is on a prepared estrogen/progesterone replacement, the window of transfer time for optimal endometrial receptivity is thought to be relatively large. A study that was performed in 1989 by Navot et al. (21) demonstrated that the window of receptivity was most likely optimal between cycle days 17 and 19 of a prepared estrogen/ progesterone replacement cycle. Day 15 in that regimen is the first day of progesterone administration after estrogen priming. In Navot's report, 37 transfers were performed between days 17 and 19 of the recipient cycle, of which 15 (40.5%) produced pregnancies, and 12 of the 15 delivered live babies. In patients who received transfers from day 20 to day 24 of the prepared cycle, no pregnancies occurred out of 11 transfers. Moreover, recipients of transfers on cycle day 16 of the prepared regimen had no pregnancies in 4 transfers. It is

therefore believed that the optimal time for embryo transfer is day 17 to 19 of the prepared endometrial cycle. The pregnancy success utilizing a hormonal replacement cycle in an agonadal woman ranges between 30% and 40% of transfer cycles.

All agonadal recipients of donor eggs must be hormonally maintained into early pregnancy until the luteal-placental shift takes place. It has been our experience that the supplementation with estradiol can be reduced and stopped early in pregnancy as serum estradiol levels begin to climb at a stationary dose of estrogen replacement. This most commonly will occur approximately 4 to 5 weeks after embryo transfer. Progesterone supplementation is maintained until the eighth to the twelfth week of pregnancy. At that time, progesterone is tapered off over several weeks' time, and serum levels are observed to make sure that serum progesterone is maintained in an adequate range by the placental production of progesterone.

Transfer of donated oocytes

In a report published in 1989, Borrero et al. suggested that higher pregnancy success and clinical outcome could be obtained when oocyte donation was combined with gamete intrafallopian transfer (22). In this report, a series of 19 patients with premature ovarian failure underwent GIFT utilizing donated oocytes. All recipients were on a replacement protocol with oral micronized estradiol and progesterone. GIFT was performed between day 12 and day 15 of the prepared cycle. In this report, 9 pregnancies out of 19 treatment cycles resulted in delivery. This report alluded to a higher pregnancy outcome; however, in subsequent reports, transfers of fresh embryos to the uterus have produced similar results, and therefore GIFT, or ZIFT, has not been a procedure that has been utilized extensively for oocyte donation protocols. Furthermore, a report published in 1989 by Abdalla et al. (23) demonstrated that the transfer of cryopreserved embryos either to the fallopian tube or to the uterine cavity produced similar birth outcomes. In their comparison there was no difference between fresh or frozen transfers to the uterine cavity or the fallopian tube with donated eggs. Overall, the pregnancy rate was 30% per transfer in the uterine transfer group and 40% in the tubal transfer group. Therefore, uterine transfer currently is utilized in virtually all egg donor recipient cycles, and fresh or cyropreserved thawed embryos can be used equally well in oocyte donation programs.

Clinical outcome with oocyte donation

Since the first report of a live birth with a donated oocyte (1), the clinical results have seemingly improved with this technique. In an article published by Leeton et al. (24), a clear separation and difference was seen between utilization of volunteer egg donors who were IVF patients and of volunteers who were stimulated for recovery of eggs for the primary purpose of oocyte donation. In their results the pregnancy rate per transfer more than doubled when a known volunteer donor was used for egg collection compared with the use of extra oocytes obtained at the time of IVF treatment of an infertile woman. These differences were true whether a sequential estrogen/progesterone protocol was used or a variable length of constant low-dose estrogen was used. It is evident that for egg donation to be highly successful, the best approach is to use a young woman of proven fertility who stimulates easily and can be utilized for an individual recipient and synchronized appropriate to that recipient.

The overall clinical pregnancy results that have been reported with the use of donor oocytes vary from center to center. Published reports have demonstrated clinical pregnancy rates ranging from 25% to 60% (25). In the annual report from the Society for Assisted Reproductive Technology (SART) and Medical Re-

search International (MRI), the results of donor oocyte usage in the United States during the calendar year 1990 was tabulated (26). In the SART report, 67 clinics in the United States reported utilizing donated oocytes in IVF-ET procedures: 498 patients were matched and participated in 547 donor oocyte transfer cycles; 160 (29%) of the transfer cycles produced a clinical pregnancy, which resulted in 122 (22%) live deliveries. There were 36 sets of twins, 3 sets of triplets, and one set of quadruplets out of the 122 deliveries. This pregnancy/birth rate of 22% per transfer is marginally different from the birth rate per embryo transfer in the same time period with in vitro fertilization. The live birth rate per embryo transfer in the 1990 report for IVF-ET in infertile women was 16%. Therefore, even though selected series of donor oocyte reports list very high pregnancy success overall, the live birth rate per embryo transfer is marginally better than IVF transfer with the infertile woman. The true live birth statistics will be stabilized when more centers record more cycles in a 12-month period.

In summary, the use of donated oocytes, especially in the agonadal woman, provides a 1-in-4 to 1-in-3 chance of having a live birth result after a transfer of embryos from oocyte donation. In infertile women who have had multiple failed cycles with assisted reproductive technologies, the use of donor oocytes as an alternative, especially in the women in the upper age range (over 39 years of age), will have a significant improvement of pregnancy outcome if donor oocytes are utilized in their treatment protocols.

Donor sperm

The use of donor sperm to treat the infertile couple became clinically established approximately four decades ago, yet historically, use of donor sperm dates back hundreds of years. Clinical reports demonstrated reproducible pregnancy rates with sperm donation by several different investigators as early as 1975 (27–29). With current legal and public acceptance of artificial insemination with donor sperm, the usefulness has been expanded. In 28 states, the law provides that the child conceived from artificial insemination with donor sperm is the legal child of the sperm recipient and her recipient husband (*People v. Sorensen*, 66 Cal RPTR 7, 437, P2d 495 [1968]).

The most common indication for use of donor sperm in treatment of infertile couples is the husband's lack of ability to produce functional sperm. Another factor that would necessitate or allow the use of artificial insemination with donor sperm is the husband's having a known hereditary or genetic disorder, such as Tay-Sach's, Huntington's disease, or hemophilia. In these situations, the desire of the couple to avoid the passage of an inherited disorder to its offspring would be reason enough for donor sperm usage. Moreover, in selected situations where a single woman desires pregnancy and a child, insemination with frozen or donor sperm for producing a viable pregnancy is reasonable.

Donor selection and screening

The American Fertility Society has provided guidelines for medical requirements for donor screening in the United States (30). Historically, any type of birth defect such as cleft lip or cleft palate or family history of hereditary diseases such as hemophilia or Huntington's disease would exclude an individual from being a sperm donor. Moreover, a complete screening for infectious disease, excluding syphilis, gonorrhea, *Chlamydia, Mycoplasma,* and herpes, must be obtained. The screening for Rh factor, Tay-Sach's disease in Jewish donors, and sickle cell anemia in black donors is another requirement. Most importantly, screening for human immunodeficiency virus (HIV) antibodies is done on a routine and frequent basis, as well as screening for hepatitis A,

B, and C. Currently, donor specimens are obtained, frozen, and quarantined for a minimum of 6 months before retesting the donor for HIV and hepatitis, and if the donor is cleared, the frozen specimens can be released from quarantine for use.

Clinical outcome

Prior to the use of frozen/thawed semen for donor insemination, most reports demonstrated that approximately 60% to 70% of women undergoing donor insemination with fresh sperm conceived during treatment. These pregnancies usually occurred within the first 6 months of insemination with an average time to conception of 3 to 4 cycles of insemination. Since the use of frozen/thawed semen has been a requirement to protect against serious infectious disease transmission, the length of time to conception is approximately double that which was achieved with fresh semen, and fewer patients overall who utilize frozen donor insemination will conceive ultimately. This outcome, most likely, is due to variability in frozen/thawed semen for donor insemination use.

Donor embryos

An embryo that results from in vitro fertilization and is not utilized by the genetic parents can be utilized by an infertile couple who do not produce eggs or embryos of their own. In this situation, the embryo has no lineal genetic relation to either party of the recipient couple. This has been used on an extremely limited basis in the human due to the fact that human embryos are rarely available for donation to an unrelated couple. In the past 10 to 12 years of experience with in vitro fertilization, it has been a rare occurrence for embryos to be donated from one infertile couple to a recipient infertile couple. At our institution, this has occurred on four occasions in the past 12 years. The indication for transfer, or donation, occurred as a result of an excess of embryos being produced during the stimulated cycle of the infertile couple—excess embryos having been frozen and stored after fresh embryo transfer was accomplished. These four couples had a resultant live birth of a multiple pregnancy and desired to have no more children. The decision to make their embryos available for donation to an unrelated couple was their own. They chose this alternative rather than allowing their embryos to thaw and be destroyed.

The screening between the donor and recipient couple was done anonymously. The donors, prior to the release of their embryos, underwent hepatitis and HIV screening. These embryos had been frozen, in all cases, for approximately 2 to 4 years. Once they were found to be free of any infectious disease, the recipient couple was matched to the donor couple on the basis of physical characteristics. The recipient couple asked for embryo donation to overcome problems with either egg production or sperm production. The donor couple was asked to file a statement through their attorney releasing all rights to their embryo. This statement was placed on file in their medical records. The recipient couple filed a similar statement through their attorney accepting all risks of receiving an anonymously donated frozen embryo if a child resulted. The recipient woman was then prepared for embryo transfer, with either hormonal replacement therapy if no ovarian function was present, or merely a natural cycle of ovulation timing for embryo replacement after embryo thawing. One of the four couples did conceive and carried to term and currently has a healthy, live baby from an anonymously donated embryo. With the more widespread use of egg donation, embryo donation is certainly something that is used very rarely. However, it is an alternative when couples have achieved their desires for a family and have excess cryopreserved embryos that they cannot use themselves. The ability to be able to donate embryos to an accepting, unrelated couple certainly allows use of the embryo, which is a potential life, rather than having the embryo thawed and destroyed.

Surrogate gestational carrier

The use of an unrelated or related surrogate to carry a genetically unrelated embryo was first reported by Utian et al. in 1985 (31). Subsequently, the same group reported results of 39 cycles of surrogate gestational carriers following in vitro fertilization in women who had no functional uterus (32). The primary indications for an infertile couple seeking third-party involvement by a surrogate gestational carrier are a surgically or congenitally absent uterus or a uterus that is nonfunctional either due to surgical damage or to developmental abnormalities. The use of a surrogate gestational carrier for other purposes such as convenience is not an acceptable indication for this type of medical treatment.

By definition a gestational surrogate carrier procedure is one whereby the infertile couple can produce the egg and sperm and embryo and the embryo is then transferred to an unrelated third party for gestation and delivery. The conventional surrogate mother alternative is much different in that the surrogate woman not only provides the uterus for gestation, but she also provides the egg, or gamete, which is fertilized by the male of the infertile couple, and the offspring is then a mix of the genetic makeup of the surrogate and the infertile couple's male. Gestational surrogate alternatives have no genetic relationship to the surrogate carrier, only a gestational or biologic relationship.

Because a distinction between a gestational surrogate and a conventional surrogate mother is based on the oocyte, the legal and ethical responsibilities and recognition of parental rights are less complicated in the surrogate gestational carrier situation. This is primarily due to the fact that the surrogate has no genetic relationship to the embryo or offspring, and merely provides a host uterus for development to viability and then delivery of the offspring. In several states, this form of reproductive technology has been acceptable in that the state legal systems have recognized the genetic parents as the true parents and do not recognize the surrogate carrier as a parent of the offspring. However, in some states, the woman who delivers the child is guaranteed by state law that she is the rightful parent of that offspring (33).

In a recent report from our institution, the use of a surrogate carrier program was described in detail (34). A prospective trial was undertaken randomizing surrogate carriers into either a uterine transfer modality or, upon agreement with the surrogate, a laparoscopic zygote intrafallopian transfer of pronuclear-stage embryos to the fallopian tube. The legal contracts for the surrogate gestational carrier and the infertile couple were provided by an outside organization. All surrogate selections, as well as preparation, psychological screening, and psychosocial support throughout the treatment cycle and the pregnancy, were performed by the surrogate organization. The legal contracts were developed by the same surrogate organization.

From September 1988 through August 1992, 45 infertile couples applied for a treatment cycle in the gestational surrogate carrier program. These 45 infertile couples underwent 81 cycles of assisted reproductive technologies to achieve a pregnancy. None of these individuals has previously produced a live offspring within their marriage. The women ranged in age from 31 to 45 years with a mean age of 38.8 years. All individuals were rendered infertile due to surgical removal of their uterus or an uncorrectable problem with uterine function; that is, congenital malformation or absence of the uterus. All couples had a complete infertility evaluation. Because these women had no uterine function, ovulatory function was determined by

baseline FSH and LH, and cyclicity was determined by a combination of basal body temperature charts, urinary LH monitoring, and serum hormonal monitoring. An established pattern of ovulatory function was determined in each woman before matching or synchronizing with a surrogate gestational carrier.

The male was evaluated by routine semen analysis and semen culture and sensitivity. If abnormalities were evident, a sperm penetration assay (hamster test) was performed to determine sperm function. Full serum screening of the infertile couple for syphilis, hepatitis, HIV, cytomegalovirus (CMV), as well as serum titers for herpes virus, were performed.

The surrogates had to demonstrate a normal medical and obstetrical history, to be less than 35 years of age, and to have at least one natural born child. The surrogates also had a full psychological evaluation and testing. If the surrogate was felt to be psychologically sound by the clinical psychologist, she was then referred to the medical practitioner, who obtained a complete medical history, including genetic pedigree history and full obstetrical history. The risks involved in the surrogate gestational carrier program were fully discussed. Tubal patency of the surrogate either was evaluated from history alone or, if no history of previous surgical sterilization was evident, hysterosalpingogram was performed. These screening procedures were conducted despite their uncomplicated fertility history and ease of conception. The surrogates also underwent evaluation of their ovulatory cycles by hormal monitoring, ultrasound, and endometrial biopsy.

The surrogate medical evaluation included serum testing for hepatitis, HIV, CMV, syphilis, herpes titers, and drug screen. The surrogates were also screened for *Chlamydia* and *Mycoplasma*. The surrogate's partner was also screened for HIV, hepatitis, and CMV. If the surrogate was cleared in her medical screening, then a conference was held between the infertile couple and the potential surrogate. A review of ovulatory cycles was performed at that time, with determination of the stimulated cycle synchronization to the surrogate's natural cycle. The contractual arrangement between the surrogate and the infertile couple was effected through independent legal counsel, and all legal contracts were outside of the medical team's responsibility.

The type of stimulation utilized for the infertile woman (egg donor) was based on the natural synchrony of the two individual cycles. If spontaneous cycle synchrony was close, the flare-up protocol was used (35). The Lupron down-regulation protocol (36) was utilized if synchrony required holding the donor for one to two weeks of synchrony with the surrogate. Ovulatory synchrony was satisfied when hCG administration to the stimulated donor occurred within 24 hours of the spontaneous LH surge of the surrogate in her natural cycle. If an LH surge did not occur within 24 hours of the hCG administration, hCG was administered to the surrogate provided follicle maturation was evidenced by ultrasound and hormonal evaluation. The transfer of embryos to the uterus or to the fallopian tubes of the surrogate occurred within 24 or 48 hours of egg recovery from the donor. If the LH surge and hCG timing were more than 48 hours out of synchrony, all eggs were collected, fertilized, and frozen, and subsequent frozen embryo cycles were performed according to the natural ovulation timing of the surrogate. In these instances, frozen embryos were transferred 3 days after the initiation of the LH surge in the natural cycle of the surrogate.

The monitoring methods utilized for timing the surrogate cycle are similar to the methods used for frozen embryo transfer, as previously reported (37). That is, once embryos were transferred to the surrogate gestational carrier, serum samples were obtained every 4 to 5 days for measurement of estradiol and progesterone. If any fluctuation in the progesterone and estradiol ration was seen in the luteal phase of the surrogate's cycle, appropriate support with progesterone and/or estradiol was undertaken. Serum β-hCG levels were determined on day 14 from embryo transfer. Once pregnancy was established, ultrasound analysis was performed approximately 3 weeks following the transfer of embryos, or when the serum hCG level exceeded 2,000 mIU/ml. Pregnancies were monitored by our medical team through the tenth week of gestation, after which the surrogate was referred to an obstetrician of her choice for routine obstetrical care. Amniocentesis was scheduled, as previously determined and agreed upon as part of the contract with the surrogate prior to initiation of treatment cycle. Amniocentesis was only performed based on the maternal age of the infertile woman (egg donor).

Forty-five (45) infertile couples underwent 81 cycles of ART utilizing a surrogate gestational carrier in our program. The infertile women ranged in age from 30 to 45 years with a mean of 38.8 $\pm$ 3.7 years (mean $\pm$ SD). Nineteen clinical pregnancies occurred during the 81 treatment cycles (19/81, 23.5%). Fifteen cycles produced an ongoing or delivered pregnancy (15/81, 18.5%). Thus 15 (33%) of the 45 patients have an ongoing or delivered pregnancy.

Of the 81 treatment cycles, 18 were randomized to a ZIFT procedure, and 29 underwent a uterine transfer of fresh embryos. Subsequently, 34 cycles of embryo transfer with frozen/thawed embryos were performed. No difference was demonstrated in clinical outcome between the ART procedures, even though the patients randomized to ZIFT were a significantly older group (40.5 $\pm$ 2.0 years vs. 38.0 $\pm$ 3.8 years, $p < 0.05$).

Of the 45 infertile women in the study, 17 (38%) were under age 39 at the time of treatment, while 28 (62%) were age 39 or over. Forty cycles of ART were performed in the women under 39, resulting in 9 clinical pregnancies (23%) compared with 10 clinical pregnancies (24%) in 41 cycles in women 39 or older. There was no statistical difference in the numbers of eggs collected, fertilized, or transferred in patients undergoing IVF-ET or ZIFT or in the two age groups.

The data from our gestational surrogate program study demonstrate several extremely important factors related to the use of surrogate gestational carriers in ART. First, even though the average age of the group of infertile women was near 39 years, a very satisfactory live birth rate (18.5%) per procedure was observed. Moreover, 62% of the infertile women were over age 39, yet the clinical pregnancy rate per procedure in those women was 24% (10/41). This figure is substantially higher than the clinical outcome reported with ART according to the most recent MRI Registry Report (26). It is possible that the use of the uterine environment of a younger ($<$ 35 years of age) surrogate gestational carrier of proven fertility may offset the negative impact of the infertile woman's age. More cycles of this nature are necessary to validate this theory.

A second important observation from these data relates to the location to which the embryo is transferred. The clinical outcome was not different when embryos (fresh or frozen) were transferred to the surrogate's uterus as opposed to the fallopian tubes. In both of these groups, the numbers of transferred eggs and embryos were similar, as were the fertilization rates. The only confounding issue between the ZIFT and IVF-ET groups was the higher age of the ZIFT group. This difference in age may be responsible for similar outcomes between groups. This observation of similar clinical outcome with IVF-ET and ZIFT with surrogate gestational carriers is similar to the report of equal outcome with GIFT/ZIFT and IVF-ET with egg donation (38). Again, the receptive uterine environment of the fertile surrogate carrier may provide a more appropriate environment for embryo implantation, irrespective of the location of initial transfer.

In conclusion, the use of a surrogate gestational carrier to support growth of embryos from women without uterine function provides an acceptable clinical outcome. Even though the economic issues of surrogate carrier use are restrictive, the simplicity of uterine embryo transfer and its resultant clinical outcome make it an acceptable alternative for infertile women without uterine function to have a genetically related offspring.

Conclusion

Assisted reproductive technologies have changed dramatically over the last one and one-half decades. The most recent developments that have been of tremendous significance are the use of donated gametes, specifically oocytes, and the use of a carrier uterus or a surrogate gestational carrier. These two additions to the basic IVF technology have opened doors for couples who heretofore had no option for carrying, gestating, or having an offspring biologically or genetically related to them. In the case of oocyte donation, women who have premature loss of ovarian function or, in a normal aging process, have lost the ability to conceive and carry a child can become a biologic parent. In most cases, use of donor oocytes will enhance the overall odds of pregnancy with the assisted technologies and certainly will allow a woman without ovarian function to gestate and deliver a biologic, although genetically unrelated child of her own. In a similar set of circumstances, women who have lost uterine function, or were born without uterine function, can produce a genetic offspring with their male partner, and that genetic embryo can be carried to term by a surrogate gestational carrier. Prior to the use of gestational carriers, or a host uterus situation, women without uterine function were destined to have no way to gestate their own pregnancy even though their ovarian function and egg production were normal. In the rare circumstance in which excess embryos were available, these embryos have been donated and transferred to infertile couples who have no ability to generate embryos of their own, and again, through the use of the IVF technology and third-party involvement, whether it be a uterine host, or a sperm or egg or gamete donor, the third-party involvement in the ARTs has broadened the ability of these technologies to allow previously childless couples to have children and families of their own. For the most part, the legal and ethical proscriptions have been well detailed and well identified and worked out, and few, if any, complications from a legal or ethical standpoint have resulted from third-party involvement in the ARTs. In the future, as more and more approaches are taken, and as comfort within the lay population increases, third-party involvement in reproductive function will become a more commonplace practice rather than an unusual, and reportable, occurrence.

References

1. Lutjen PJ, Trounson A, Leeton JF, Findlay J, Wood EC, Renou P. The establishment and maintenance of pregnancy using in vitro fertilization and embryo donation in a patient with primary ovarian failure. Nature 1984;307:174–175.

2. De Ziegler D, Frydman R. Different implantation rates after transfers of cryopreserved embryos originating from donated oocytes or regular in vitro fertilization. Fertil Steril 1990;54:682–688.

3. Abdalla HI, Baber R, Kirkland A, Leonard T, Power M, Studd JWW. A report on one hundred of oocyte donation; factors affecting the outcome. Hum Reprod 1990; 5(8):1018–1022.

4. Navot D, Scott RT, Droesch K, Veeck LL, Liu HC, Rosenwaks Z. The window of embryo transfer and the efficiency of human conception in vitro. Fertil Steril 1991;55: 114–118.

5. Kennard EAD, Collins RL, Blakstein J, et al. A program for matched anonymous oocyte donation. Fertil Steril 1989;51:655.

6. Serhal PF, Craft IL. Ovum donation—a simplified approach. Fertil Steril 1987;48:265–269.

7. Kogosowski A, Yovel I, Lessing JB, et al. The establishment of an ovum donation program using a simple fixed dose estrogen/progesterone replacement regimen. J In Vitro Fert Embryo Transf 1990;7(5):244–248.

8. Asch RH, Balmaceda JP, Ord T, Borrero C, Cefalu E, Gastaldi C, Rojas F. Oocyte donation and gamete intrafallopian transfer and premature ovarian failure. Fertil Steril 1988;49:263–267.

9. Sauer MV, Paulson RJ, Macaso TM, Francis MM, Lobo RA. Oocyte and pre-embryo donation to patients with ovarian failure: an extended clinical trial. Fertil Steril 1991; 55:39–43.

10. Abdalla HI, Baber RJ, Kirkland A, Leonard T, Studd JWW. Pregnancy in women with premature ovarian failure using tubal intrauterine transfer of cryopreserved zygotes. Br J Obstet Gynaecol 1989;96:1071–1074.

11. Devroey P, Camus M, Van Den Abbeel E, Waesberghe LV, Wisanto A, van Steirteghem AC. Establishment of twenty-two pregnancies after oocyte and embryo donation. Br J Obstet Gynaecol 1989;96:900–902.

12. Robertson JA. Ethical and legal issues in human egg donation. Fertil Steril 1989;52(3):353.

13. Vargyas JM, Morente C, Shangold G, Marrs RP. The effect of different methods of ovarian stimulation for human in vitro fertilization and embryo transfer. Fertil Steril 1984; 42:745–749.

14. Ron E, Lunenfeld B, Menczen J, et al. Cancer instance in a cohort of infertile women. Am J Epidemiol 1987;125:780–790.

15. Booth M, Beral V, Smith P. Risk factors for ovarian cancer; a case controlled study. Br J Cancer 1989;60:592–598.

16. Harlow BL, Weiss NS, Roth GJ, Chu J, Daling JR. Case controlled study of borderline ovarian tumors: reproductive history and exposure to exogenous female hormones. Cancer Res 1988;48:5849–5852.

17. Whittemore AS, Harris P, Itnryre J. And the collaborative ovarian cancer risk: collaborative analysis of 12 U.S. case controlled studies. II. Invasive epithelial ovarian cancers in white women. Am J Epidemiol 1992;136:1184–1203.

18. Droesch K, Navot D, Scott R, Kreiner D, Liu HC, Rosenwaks Z. Transdermal estrogen replacement and ovarian failure for ovum donation. Fertil Steril 1988;50:931–934.

19. Navot D, Laufer N, Kopolovic J, et al. Artificially induced endometrial cycles and establishment of pregnancies in the absence of ovaries. N Engl J Med 1986;314:806–811.

20. Meldrum DR, Wisot A, Hamilton F, Gutlay-Yeo AL, Marr B, Huynh D. Artificial agonadism and hormone replacement for oocyte donation. Fertil Steril 1989;52(3):509–511.

21. Navot D, Anderson TL, Droesch K. Hormonal manipulation of endometrial maturation. J Clin Endocrinol Metab 1989;68:801–807.

22. Borrero C, Remohi J, Ord T, Balmecedo JP, Rojas F, Asch RH. A program of oocyte donation and gamete intrafallopian transfer. Hum Reprod 1989;4(3):275–279.

23. Abdalla HI, Baber RJ, Kirkland A, Leonard T, Studd JWW. Pregnancy in women with premature ovarian failure using tubal and intrauterine transfer of cyropreserved zygotes. Br J Obstet Gynaecol 1989;96:1071–1075.

24. Leeton J, Rogers P, King C, Healy D. The comparison of pregnancy rates for 131 donor oocyte transfers using either a sequential or a fixed regimen of steroid replacement therapy. Hum Reprod 1991;6(2):299–301.

25. Sauer MV, Paulson RJ. Human oocyte and preembryo donation: an evolving method for the treatment of infertility. Am J Obstet Gynecol 1990;163:1421–1424.

26. Medical Research International and Society for Assisted Reproductive Technology. In vitro fertilization and embryo transfer (IVF-ET) in the United States: 1990 results from the IVF-ET registry. Fertil Steril 1992;57(1):15–24.

27. Sherman JK. Research on frozen human semen. Fertil Steril 1975;15:487–488.

28. Sherman JK. Clinical use of frozen human semen. Transplant Proc 1976;8:165s–168s.

29. Richardson DW. Organization of sperm banks on a national basis. In: David G, Price WS, eds. Human artificial insemination and semen preservation. New York: Plenum Press, 1980:65.

30. Ethical considerations in new reproductive technologies. Fertil Steril 1986;46(Suppl 1):85s–86s.

31. Utian WH, Sheean L, Goldfarb JM, Kiwi R. Successful pregnancy after in vitro fertilization–embryo transfer from an infertile woman to a surrogate. N Engl J Med 1985;313:1351–1352.

32. Utian WH, Goldfarb JM, Kiwi R, Sheean LA, Auld H, Lisbona H. Preliminary experience with in vitro fertilization–surrogate gestational pregnancy. Fertil Steril 1989;52:633–638.

33. Robertson JA. Procreative liberty in the states' burden of proof in regulating noncoital reproduction. Law Med Healthcare 1988;16(1–2):18–26.

34. Marrs RP, Ringler GE, Stein A, Vargyas JM, Stone BA. The use of surrogate gestational carriers for assisted reproductive technologies (ART). Am J Obstet Gynecol 1993 (in press).

35. Marrs RP, Brown J, Sato F, et al. Successful pregnancies from cryopreserved human embryos produced by in vitro fertilization. Am J Obstet Gynecol 1987;156:1503–1508.

36. Serafini P, Stone B, Kerin J, Batzofin J, Quinn P, Marrs RP. An alternative approach to controlled ovarian hyperstimulation (COH) in "poor responders": pretreatment with a GnRH analog (GnRHa). Fertil Steril 1988;48(1):90–95.

37. Borini A, Alam V, Ord T, Asch RH, Balmaceda JP. Embryo implantation rates in stimulated and hormonal replacement cycles: uterine versus tubal transfers. Presented at the 7th World Congress on In Vitro Fertilization and Assisted Procreation, Paris, France, 1991.

38. Marrs RP, Vargyas JM, Stein AL, Ringler GE, Greene J, Stone BA. Use of gonadotropin-releasing hormone (GnRH) agonist and its effects on outcome of assisted reproductive technologies (ARTs). In: Proceedings of the American Fertility Society, 1991; Orlando, Florida.

9

Anesthesia in Assisted Reproductive Technology

Anne E. Hood

Introduction

Anesthesia techniques utilized for the surgical procedures of assisted reproductive technology present a unique challenge for the anesthesiologist. An understanding of the events of fertilization and the molecular and cellular effects of anesthetic agents must be combined with the clinical skill needed to care appropriately for patients electing to undergo such procedures. A review of the process of fertilization is beyond the scope of this chapter; the reader is referred to an excellent summary by Yanagimachi (1).

Several studies have implied a detrimental effect of general anesthesia on oocyte quality and a tendency to an increase in detrimental effects with increased anesthetic exposure time (2–4). Virtually every anesthetic agent has the capacity to affect reproductive outcome by affecting calcium-regulating proteins such as calmodulin or protein kinase C, DNA or RNA synthesis, protein synthesis, and the hormonal status of the patient. However, comfortable and safe sedatives or anesthetics must be used for many of the patients undergoing assisted reproductive procedures.

Most of the data that the anesthesiologist must consider in formulating an anesthetic protocol are derived from work in nonmammalian models or small mammals; few clinical studies are available. Although much emphasis has been placed on teratogenicity in later gestational stages, there is no known applicability of teratogenic studies to the potential effect of any agent or combination of agents at the time of gamete exposure for assisted reproduction. Therefore, this chapter will be confined to the demonstrated effects of anesthetic agents on the gametes, fertilization, early cell division, and the clinical management of the patient undergoing an assisted reproductive technology (ART) procedure.

Physiology, pharmacology, and drug actions in the follicular fluid and fallopian tube

Many intravenously administered anesthetic drugs have been isolated from the follicular fluid of patients undergoing oocyte retrieval for in vitro fertilization, among them thiopental and thiamylal (5), fentanyl (6), alfentanil (7), propofol (8), and etomidate (9). A brief review of the pharmacokinetics of the commonly used drugs and the applicable follicular physiology follows to assist the reader in evaluating pharmacologic studies with regard to the follicular fluid.

Blood flow is a major determinant of the tissue uptake of an anesthetic drug. The ovarian follicle receives a blood flow per unit weight that is among the highest in the body (10). Follicular development is accompanied by the growth of a complex blood supply (11,12). At ovulation, and during the subsequent 5 to 7 days, the capillary blood supply to the fallopian tube on the ovulatory side increases, probably in response to the increased metabolic demands of fallopian tube motility (13). Therefore, at the time of oocyte retrieval and gamete or zygote transfer, drug passage into the ovary and the fallopian tubes is enhanced. The ovary and the fallopian tubes are clearly in the group of organs defined, for the purpose of discussing the uptake, distribution, and elimination of anesthetic drugs, as "vessel-rich." The vessel-rich organs receive a full intravenously administered dose of an anesthetic drug almost immediately after injection. This results in a tissue concentration that is in equilibrium with the blood. The observed clinical effects of an injected drug cease when the plasma level falls secondary to redistribution of the drug to the tissues. High levels of active drug, and in some cases active metabolites, persist in the body long after the apparent effect of the drug is gone.

Vessel-poor tissues (fat, muscle, etc.) serve as a drug reservoir. Active drug is continually released to the circulation, maintaining plasma levels as metabolism and elimination occur.

The ability of a drug to enter the follicular fluid is affected by the amount of protein binding of the drug and the pH difference between the plasma and follicular fluid. Most anesthetic drugs are highly protein bound, primarily to albumin. Although the total protein concentrations of follicular fluid and plasma are the same, the composition of the proteins in follicular fluid is quite different from plasma, with up to 30% more albumin in follicular fluid than in plasma (14). This may lead to a higher *total* concentration of drug in the follicular fluid than in plasma for anesthetic drugs. However, it is the non-protein-bound (free) drug that is both pharmacologically active and able to move across the cell membrane. Therefore, the total drug concentration in the follicular fluid or plasma may not reflect the active drug available to affect gamete function.

The pH of follicular fluid in humans has been found to be weakly alkaline compared with plasma; carbon dioxide insufflated for laparoscopy may decrease the pH of follicular fluid significantly (15). Any change in pH will change the degree of drug ionization. Most anesthetic drugs are weak acids and will therefore be more ionized in follicular fluid than in plasma. As only the unionized form of anesthetic drug can cross biological membranes and enter the gamete, ionization may complicate efforts to determine drug activity (or toxicity) based on total concentration of drug in the follicular fluid.

Inhalational anesthetics, which are highly lipid soluble, enter the blood via the alveoli as a result of partial pressure gradients between the alveoli, plasma, tissues, and site of action (e.g., capillaries, cell membranes, fallopian tube endothelium). The majority of any inhaled anesthetic is excreted through the lungs. Rapid equilibration occurs in all tissues, with vascularity a major determinant of the rate of tissue uptake of the anesthetic.

Despite the fact that inhalational anesthetics are seemingly short-acting, all commonly used agents (isoflurane, enflurane, halothane) and their metabolic products are detectable in blood up to at least 48 hours after administration (16–18). This has potential implications for use during both gamete intrafallopian transfer (GIFT) and zygote intrafallopian transfer (ZIFT). The degree of biotransformation of an anesthetic agent is proportional to both its ability to release calcium from sarcoplasmic reticulum and its potential for liver toxicity (19). Only comparative clinical studies can demonstrate the effect of low levels of anesthetic agents and metabolic products on the gamete or cell division, and determine if other agents, such as the intravenous sedatives and hypnotics, are superior for patients undergoing ART procedures.

Effects of anesthetic agents on gametes, fertilization, and cell division

Most evidence linking anesthetic agents to adverse reproductive outcome after gamete exposure is indirect. However, the potential that all drugs used for sedation, narcosis, or anesthesia (major hypnotics) may be harmful on a molecular basis is clear. Drugs capable of producing an anesthetic state (including sedatives, narcotics, and local anesthetics) "fluidize" cell membranes and cause conformational changes in membrane and cellular proteins (20–22). These changes have been demonstrated at clinically employed anesthetic concentrations (23). Not all of these effects are necessarily inhibitory; gamete membranes become more fluid (undergo lateral phase separations in the phospholipid bilayer) in preparation for cell fusion. Inhalational

anesthetics enhance fusion of phospholipid vesicles (24). Chloroprocaine, a halogenated local anesthetic of the ester class, has also been demonstrated to promote cell fusion (25). Specific negative effects of anesthetic agents on the gametes and on the processes of fertilization and cell division are summarized in Table 9.1. The effects in vivo on human gametes may differ significantly. A particular drug may inhibit one critical process and facilitate another. Only clinical studies can determine the net effect. Until the results of such studies are available, it is reasonable to anticipate some negative effect of anesthetic drugs on reproductive outcome in patients whose gametes are exposed to these agents. However, it cannot be assumed at this time that a particular local anesthetic or sedative combination is superior to an inhalational agent in terms of reproductive outcome.

Anesthetic drugs as calmodulin antagonists

It is probable that anesthetic agents affect, to some degree, all calcium-dependent events in the cell. Virtually every critical process involved in fertilization and cell division has been shown to involve calmodulin (39). A number of drugs used as anesthetics have been shown

Table 9.1 Potential and demonstrated anesthetic drug effects on gamete function

Parthenogenic activation of the oocyte (26)
"Fluidize" and disorder membranes (20,22)
Conformational and functional changes in regulatory proteins (21)
Membrane and intracellular ion fluxes (19,20)
Membrane fusion and cortical granule release (27–30)
DNA, RNA, and protein synthesis (31–33)
Abnormal spindle formation and unequal cleavage (34–36)
Activation of the acrosome reaction (37)
Decrease sperm motility (38)

References are in parentheses.

to reversibly inactivate calmodulin; these same drugs have been shown to inhibit some of the biological processes involved in fertilization and cell division. However, it must be stressed that a causal relationship between inhibition of calmodulin by anesthetic agents and negative effects on gamete functions has not been established.

The potency of calmodulin inactivation is best demonstrated by the phenothiazine derivatives (40). Local anesthetics have been shown to be weaker calmodulin antagonists than the phenothiazines (41). All classes of barbiturates have weak local anesthetic properties (42), and by their chemical structure they should similarly inhibit calmodulin. The action on calmodulin of the inhalational anesthetics halothane, enflurane, and isoflurane may be inferred by their action on intracellular calcium (19,43). Whether calmodulin is involved in the control of calcium channels is not yet certain. Benzodiazepines have calcium channel blocking properties and inhibit calmodulin (44). On the basis of the structure-activity relationships of the phenothiazines and other compounds inhibiting calmodulin, it can be postulated that the piperidine narcotics (meperidine, fentanyl, and derivatives) may also inhibit calmodulin and calmodulin-dependent processes (45,46).

Despite the demonstrated ability of local and general anesthetics to nonselectively inactivate calmodulin, the effect of these agents on in vivo biologic processes in fertilization and cell division may not be significant. Calmodulin is present in high concentrations in all tissues, particularly the testis, ovary, and the dividing cell (47). Only minute quantities of calmodulin are required by calmodulin-sensitive enzymes. Development of two-cell mouse embryos has been shown to be inhibited by weak calmodulin inhibitors but not by chlorpromazine and more potent calmodulin inhibitors (48). This may be because of the inability of these agents to penetrate the cellular membrane, or because the

inhibition of calmodulin by anesthetic agents is not the mechanism by which these drugs are embryotoxic.

Hormonal changes induced by anesthesia and stress

The hormonal response to surgical stress, as demonstrated by a rise in growth hormone, prolactin, luteinizing hormone (LH), follicle-stimulating hormone (FSH), cortisol, and β-endorphins, is well documented (49–52). Deep inhalational or high-dose narcotic anesthesia can blunt this response (53), but neither anesthetic technique is appropriate in ambulatory, and therefore reproductive, patients. Epidural and spinal anesthesia effectively inhibit the transmission of afferent stimuli to the hypothalamus from lower abdominal surgeries, preventing plasma increases in all stress-related hormones; however, they fail to do so without respiratory compromise in upper abdominal surgical procedures and laparoscopies (54). The importance of these hormonal fluctuations on outcome after ART procedures is unresolved. Research has concentrated primarily on two areas: the influence of prolactin on outcome following in vitro fertilization (IVF) and related procedures, and the effect of anesthetic intervention on the adequacy of the luteal phase.

Prolactin can be raised by stress, surgery, and certain anesthetic drugs including narcotics, barbiturates, metoclopramide, and droperidol. The induction of general anesthesia has been demonstrated to increase plasma prolactin by as much as 50-fold (55), reflecting probably both the stress of induction and specific drug effects. However, an increase in prolactin has not been correlated with a decrease in fertilization, embryo development, or pregnancy rate after IVF (56–59).

High prolactin levels have been shown in animals to interfere with capacitation of spermatozoa (60). This may have clinical significance when serum drawn from unpremedicated patients immediately before surgery (a time of high stress and usually prolactin levels) is used to culture gametes. It may also have implications in GIFT patients who continue to have high prolactin levels in the postoperative period secondary to pain, cold, or psychological stress.

The effect of anesthetics on the adequacy of the luteal phase has been another area of concern. Female patients who are unstimulated and undergo surgery in the late follicular phase demonstrate luteal phase inadequacy as evidenced by a decrease in plasma progesterone and a high incidence of irregular vaginal bleeding postoperatively unrelated to the operative procedure (61,62). However, in a study of 500 *stimulated* patients undergoing laparoscopic oocyte retrieval for IVF, no luteal phase defect was observed, possibly secondary to higher luteal phase progesterone levels in these patients (63,64).

Although the induction of anesthesia and follicular aspiration may result in a steep decline in plasma progesterone levels, plasma progesterone (and estradiol) in the luteal phase may not be related to the achievement of pregnancy (65). Lehtinen et al. have shown that luteal phase progesterone and ratios of progesterone to estradiol (P/E_2) are higher in patients receiving epidural anesthesia than in those receiving general anesthesia for oocyte recovery. However, this study did not demonstrate a correlation with pregnancy outcome (66). Surgical disruption of the granulosa cells alone may affect luteal phase progesterone levels (67). Luteal phase support with progesterone is currently common practice, making the significance of anesthetic-induced decreases in progesterone levels questionable.

Minimizing stress may be more important than the choice of anesthetic technique. Stress-induced increases in prolactin may alone affect luteal phase adequacy (68,69). Epidural anesthesia has been associated in 50% of patients in one study with an increase in prolactin and cortisol, presumably secondary to psychological stress and inadequate pain relief (70). An increase in cortisol is particularly undesirable because of the increase in blood glucose that may result (see below, osmolarity). Neurolept anesthesia directly increases prolactin by the effect of narcotics, particularly fentanyl (71,72), and droperidol. It indirectly increases both prolactin and cortisol (73) if an inadequate depth of anesthesia is achieved. Therefore, a neurolept anesthetic might be less desirable than other techniques.

Maintenance of homeostasis

Osmolarity

Changes in osmolarity may affect the oocyte and cell cleavage. Normal plasma osmolarity is 280 mosm/L. Cell cleavage will occur in an osmolarity ranging from 216 to 330 mosm/L; at the two-cell stage cleavage is maximal at an osmolarity that is below the physiologic range (74). Dextrose 5% in lactated Ringer's (D5/LR) has an osmolarity of 527 mosm/L.

Blood sugar levels in healthy women undergoing laparoscopy who received 1 L of D5/LR were found to be as high as 443 mg/dl and remained as high 258 mg/dl several hours after surgery (75). Patients who received 1 L of D5/½ normal saline (NS) became slightly hyponatremic and experienced similar blood sugar rises (76). Because of their potential for unpredictable changes in plasma and subsequently follicular fluid osmolarity, solutions containing glucose are undesirable during the operative period.

Acid-base balance

Changes in pH of the follicular fluid may be detrimental to gamete function (77). Alterations in the pH of the follicular fluid may markedly affect the ratio of ionized to unionized drug concentration, thereby changing the concentration of the active portion of the drug. Alterations in the drug activity on the oocyte will depend on the pKa of the injected drug. Therefore, changes in plasma pH produced by such factors as respiratory depression, ventilator-controlled hyperventilation, or hyperventilation produced by pain or anxiety must be taken into account when examining the effect of any drug in the follicular fluid based on total concentration alone.

Oxygen tension

The development of mouse oocytes has been shown to be progressively inhibited on days 1 to 4 of pre-implanattion when exposed to oxygen concentrations of greater than 5% (78). Maturation of the oocyte in the mouse (79) and hamster (80) and cleavage of sheep and cattle embryos (81) are optimal at 5%. Exposure of mouse one-cell preembryos to 20% oxygen (ambient air) for as short a period as 1 hour inhibited development. This inhibition was not apparent until four to five divisions later (82). Therefore, oxygen toxicity may not be apparent in laboratory studies of fertilization and early cleavage.

The oxygen concentration in the fallopian tube of mammals has been shown to range from 7% to 11.2% (15,83). This concentration supports embryo development in the laboratory. High partial pressures of oxygen cause a decrease in sperm motility, possibly by accelerating lipid metabolism with resultant oxygen free radicals (84). Work on human embryos is consistent with the above animal studies (85) and demonstrates that the greatest negative effect of excess oxygen is with male factor infertility.

Supplemental oxygen administration is a routine part of both general and intravenous anesthetic techniques, both intraoperatively and during the recovery time, this practice potentially raising the venous (and tubal) Pa_{O_2} to deleterious levels. The introduction of pulse oximetry and the ease of administering an acceptable anesthetic with air as the carrier gas allows a safe anesthetic and recovery course without routine excess supplemental oxygen.

Clinical studies

General anesthesia

General anesthesia can be performed using many agents and combinations of agents. By definition, patients are under a general anesthetic when they respond to neither verbal nor noxious stimuli, regardless of the type or dose of sedative or drug administered. All sedative drugs can induce a state of "general anesthesia," and major inhalational agents and nitrous oxide have long been used as analgesics. To properly evaluate reproductive outcome in studies comparing "general anesthesia" with sedation, regional, or local anesthesia, the specific anesthetic drugs and agents used must be known.

Hayes et al. retrospectively studied fertilization and cleavage data of laparoscopically retrieved oocytes and found a significant reduction in the cleavage rate of mature oocytes from the second ovary aspirated when compared with the first ovary (2). Boyers et al., using a prospective study design, found a decrease in fertilization rate, but not cleavage rate, with increasing anesthesia exposure time (3). The earliest retrieved oocytes exhibited no decline in either fertilization or cleavage.

General anesthesia has also been demonstrated to be detrimental to oocyte function when compared with epidural anesthesia for ultrasound-guided oocyte aspiration (4). Laparoscopically retrieved oocytes after general anesthesia have been shown to fertilize at a lower rate than those retrieved by ultrasound guidance after intravenous sedation (86).

None of the above reported studies employed well-controlled anesthetic protocols or corrected the data reports for anesthetic agents. They demonstrate only that *some* agent or factor during laparoscopy or general anesthesia may be detrimental to oocytes. The more difficult and pertinent task is to define which specific drugs, sedatives, anesthetic agents, or techniques are least detrimental to pregnancy outcome following ART procedures.

Nitrous oxide: Nitrous oxide has been the most frequently implicated anesthetic drug with regard to adverse reproductive outcome. Epidemiologic studies of operating room personnel and dentists have shown an increase in spontaneous abortions in women exposed to nitrous oxide (87,88). Nitrous oxide has been shown to be both teratogenic (89) and fetotoxic (90) when administered to animals in various stages of pregnancy. However, studies of anesthetics administered for cervical circlage during early human pregnancy have failed to demonstrate fetal toxicity (91).

Adverse reproductive outcome related to nitrous oxide has been commonly attributed to its ability to cause a decrease in DNA synthesis through the inactivation of the B_{12}-dependent enzyme methionine synthase, formerly termed methionine synthetase (92). Studies have demonstrated that folinic acid does not reverse the adverse reproductive effects of nitrous oxide in rats (93) and that nitrous oxide has markedly different effects when administered on different gestational days (94). The relationship of methionine synthase inactivation to adverse reproductive outcome is unclear.

Nitrous oxide, long thought to be relatively inert, has been shown by Hong et al. to undergo metabolism in the intestinal tract, resulting in the release of free radicals (95). The significance of these free radicals is unknown. However, nitrous oxide is an intermediate compound in the reduction of nitrite (HNO_2) and nitric oxide (NO) (96,97). These free radicals, resulting from nitrogen reduction, have been shown to be both teratogenic and carcinogenic to distant target organs (98).

The effects of nitrous oxide administration during anesthesia for ART procedures on gamete function has only recently been studied, and its toxicity and use in such procedures remains controversial; most anesthesi-ologists are reluctant to abandon its use in ART procedures without compelling evidence of toxicity.

Nitrous oxide and oocyte retrieval: When nitrous oxide is administered to a patient undergoing oocyte retrieval for in vitro fertilization (laparoscopically or by ultrasound guidance), the oocyte alone would be affected. Rosen et al. studied the effect of the addition of nitrous oxide to isoflurane in patients undergoing laparoscopic oocyte retrieval for IVF (99). No significant difference in fertilization rates or pregnancy rate occurred. The control group in this study received 100% oxygen as the anesthetic carrier gas; oxygen toxicity on the oocyte must be considered, and may have affected the sensitivity of detecting a difference in reproductive outcome.

Palot et al. found a significantly detrimental effect of nitrous oxide on oocyte function when combined with propofol for ultrasound-guided oocyte retrieval (100), an effect not seen when propofol was administered without nitrous oxide (101). The same authors have studied the effect of the addition of nitrous oxide to halothane and found the combination to decrease significantly the cleavage rate of fertilized oocytes (102).

Nitrous oxide and GIFT: We have studied the addition of nitrous oxide to enflurane and nitrous oxide with sufentanil for general anesthesia in patients undergoing laparoscopic GIFT (103).

Patients who received nitrous oxide combined with enflurane had a higher spontaneous abortion rate than patients anesthetized with enflurane and air, resulting in a higher live birth rate when nitrous oxide was omitted (Table 9.2). Fertilization and cleavage rates significantly improved in the absence of nitrous oxide (Table 9.3). The cleavage rate significantly declined with increasing exposure to nitrous oxide and enflurane (Table 9.4).

In a second study of patients undergoing GIFT, nitrous oxide was added to sufentanil in a balanced

Table 9.2 Clinical outcome after GIFT with enflurane and nitrous oxide anesthesia compared with enflurane and air anesthesia

	Enflurane/N$_2$O (n=62)	Enflurane/air (n=69)
Clinical pregnancy rate	17 (27.4%)	26 (38.2%)
Spontaneous abortion rate	7 (41.2%)	6 (23.1%)
Ectopic pregnancy rate	1 (5.9%)	1 (3.9%)
Delivery rate	9 (14.5%)	19 (27.9%)

Table 9.4 Fertilization and cleavage rates of residual oocytes with increasing anesthetic exposure time; enflurane/nitrous oxide versus enflurane/air

Enflurane/N$_2$0	Exposure < 32 min (n=88)	Exposure > 32 min (n=90)
Fertilization	21/88 (23.9%)	23/90 (25.6%)
Cleavage	13/88 (14.8%)	4/90 (4.4%)[a]
Enflurane/air	**Exposure < 32 min (n=168)**	**Exposure > 32 min (n=178)**
Fertilization	76/168 (45.2%)	79/178 (44.4%)
Cleavage	39/168 (23.2%)	38/178 (21.4%)

[a]$p < 0.05$

anesthetic technique. These results were compared with those for the patient group receiving enflurane and nitrous oxide. There were no statistically significant differences in fertilization or pregnancy rate. There was a significant decline in the cleavage rate of later retrieved oocytes exposed to enflurane and nitrous oxide compared with those exposed to sufentanil and nitrous oxide. Spontaneous abortions were most frequent when enflurane, rather than sufentanil, was combined with nitrous oxide. Although this may have clinical significance, it was not statistically significant (Table 9.5).

In comparing the above two studies, it is notable that fertilization, embryo development, and live birth rate were all improved in the absence of nitrous oxide. It is possible that a negative effect of nitrous oxide is potentiated by the addition of enflurane to nitrous oxide. This potentiation has been demonstrated on the two-cell mouse embryo to occur with nitrous oxide and isoflurane (104). Although it is possible that nitrous oxide is not detrimental in combination with other anesthetic agents, we have abandoned the use of this agent for ART procedures and have not found this to be a clinical disadvantage.

Table 9.3 Fertilization and cleavage rates of residual oocytes after anesthetic exposure to enflurane and nitrous oxide and enflurane and air

	Enflurane/N$_2$O (n=178)	Enflurane/air (n=436)
Fertilization	44/178 (24.7%)	155/346 (44.8%)[a]
Cleavage	17/178 (9.6%)	77/346 (22.3%)[a]

[a]$p < 0.05$

Table 9.5 Clinical outcome after GIFT anesthesia with sufentanil/N$_2$O compared with enflurane/N$_2$O

	Sufentanil/N$_2$O (n=61)	Enflurane/N$_2$O (n=62)
Clinical pregnancy rate	14/61 (22.9%)	17/62 (27.4%)
Spontaneous abortion rate	2/14 (14.3%)	7/17 (41.2%)[a]
Ectopic pregnancy rate	2/14 (14.3%)	1/62 (5.9%)
Live birth rate	10/61 (16.4%)	9/62 (14.5%)

[a]$p = 0.13$ (Fisher's exact two-tailed test)

Major inhalational agents: Different inhalation agents may have different effects on gamete function and zygote development. Predictions of reproductive toxicity cannot be made based on the potency of the agent. Hinkley and Wright, using the sea urchin, demonstrated variable effects of inhalational anesthetic agents on fertilization and embryo development (36). Halothane, enflurane, and isoflurane also differ in their ability to alter intracellular calcium (19,43).

Enflurane and isoflurane are the most commonly used major inhalational anesthetic agents in the United States; halothane remains popular in Europe. The effect of an inhalational anesthetic must be examined not only in single-cell studies in vitro, but also in studies in vivo, which include the effect of biotransformation on the gamete or zygote. Trace amounts of inhalational anesthetics are detectable in anesthesiologists up to 64 hours after occupational exposure (16); excretion of metabolites may take considerably longer. Patients are exposed for shorter periods of time but to much higher concentrations. About 20% of absorbed halothane is metabolized, resulting in the release of chloride and bromide ions (105). Enflurane is metabolized at a rate of 2.4% of the administered dose (17); isoflurane at 0.17% (106). Sevoflurane (not yet released in the United States) also undergoes significant biotransformation at a rate similar to enflurane (18).

Biotransformation of all three of these agents results in the release of organic fluorine and inorganic fluoride. Fluoride ions have been shown to inhibit motility in sperm, and this may be important in GIFT or ZIFT patients (107). Halothane is the most studied inhalational anesthetic with regard to gamete function and cell division. Mitosis is inhibited by halothane (108). Halothane has been shown to be deleterious to both the oocyte (34,109) and sperm (37,38). Halothane inhibits fertilization and cleavage in the sea urchin model, an effect not seen after exposure to enflurane (36). When halothane was compared with enflurane as a general anesthetic for embryo transfer, the use of halothane significantly reduced the incidence of implantation (86).

Isoflurane, both alone and in combination with nitrous oxide, has been shown to inhibit the development of two-cell mouse embryos (104). In the same study, embryos developed normally when exposed to nitrous oxide and fentanyl or meperidine.

Unfortunately, controlled comparative clinical studies using enflurane, isoflurane, or halothane for general anesthesia in patients undergoing oocyte retrieval (laparoscopic or ultrasound guided) or gamete or zygote intrafallopian transfer have not been reported. The above studies seem to indicate that halothane, among the three agents, would be the least desirable choice for patients undergoing ART procedures. There are currently no data indicating that there would be a difference in outcome after exposure to isoflurane or enflurane.

Intravenous sedation, analgesia, and anesthesia

Benzodiazepines: All benzodiazepines are calcium channel blockers and calmodulin inhibitors (47). Diazepam has been demonstrated to interfere with fertilization in mice (110); both diazepam and lorazepam have long-acting active metabolites (detectable up to 2 weeks after oral administration), making them less than desirable for acute ambulatory sedation. Midazolam, which is short-acting, has generally replaced diazepam and lorazepam in the practice of ambulatory anesthesia.

We prospectively studied the effect of the addition of midazolam to thiamylal in the induction protocol of 150 patients undergoing GIFT (unpublished data). No differences in pregnancy or spontaneous abortion rates were observed in patients receiving midazolam and thiamylal for general anesthetic induction compared with those receiving thiamylal alone. However, with prolonged exposure time, a significant decline in embryo development was observed in patients *not* receiving midazolam.

Deleting premedication in GIFT and IVF patients is commonly practiced to reduce oocyte drug exposure. Whether this is beneficial or necessary is questionable.

Phenothiazines: Detrimental effects of phenothiazines have been demonstrated on both the oocyte and sperm. Phenothiazines have been demonstrated to be parthenogenic, and chlorpromazine has been shown to inhibit sperm motility in vitro (108).

All classes of phenothiazines (chlorpromazine) and butyrophenones (droperidol) have been shown to inhibit calmodulin. The causal relationship of calmodulin inhibition to adverse gamete effects has not been established, nor has the relative potency of this inhibition compared with other anesthetics and sedatives. However, a safe and comfortable anesthetic can be administered without using these agents, and they might best be avoided in the absence of clinical data supporting their use in patients having ART procedures.

Barbiturates: As early as 1940 barbiturates were shown to inhibit cell respiration (111), a property not unique to barbiturates; it may be inherent in the mechanism of action of all anesthetic agents. Both thiamylal and thiopental, commonly used barbiturates, have been isolated from the follicular fluid (5). As might be anticipated from protein binding, the total concentration of drug was found to be higher in the follicular fluid than in simultaneously obtained plasma samples. Thiopental concentration in the follicular fluid peaked more rapidly after injection than thiamylal concentration, demonstrating some pharmacokinetic differences.

Methohexital (Brevital) has not been studied in the follicular fluid, but it would be expected to enter the follicular fluid similarly to thiopental and thiamylal. It has a clinical advantage in having a shorter duration of action. We compared methohexital with thiamylal for induction of general anesthesia for GIFT patients. The

Table 9.6 Outcome of oocytes not transferred for GIFT exposed to either methohexital or thiamylal

	Methohexital ($n=324$)	Thiamylal ($n=254$)
Fertilization excess oocytes	145/324 (44.7%)	125/254 (49.2%)
Development excess oocytes	82/324 (25.3%)	86/254 (33.8%)[a]

[a]$p < 0.025$

maintenance of anesthesia consisted of enflurane and air. No difference in reproductive outcome (pregnancy rate, spontaneous abortion rate, or live birth rate) was demonstrated. Total fertilization of oocytes not transferred for GIFT did not differ significantly; however, a decline in cleavage rate was seen in oocytes exposed to methohexital compared with those exposed to thiamylal (Table 9.6). Both fertilization and cleavage significantly declined with increasing anesthetic time in oocytes exposed to methohexital compared with thiamylal (Table 9.7).

We have also reviewed oocyte function after

Table 9.7 Fertilization and cleavage rates of residual oocytes with increasing anesthetic exposure time

Methohexital	**Exposure < 29 min** ($n=166$)	**Exposure > 29 min** ($n=158$)
Fertilization rate	90/166 (54.2%)	55/158 (34.8%)[a]
Cleavage rate	55/166 (33.1%)	27/158 (17.1%)[a]
Thiamylal	**Exposure < 29 min** ($n=146$)	**Exposure > 29 min** ($n=108$)
Fertilization rate	72/146 (49.3%)	53/108 (49.1%)
Cleavage rate	53/146 (36.3%)	33/108 (30.5%)

[a]$p < 0.001$

methohexital administration in patients undergoing transvaginal ultrasound–guided oocyte retrieval. Oocyte retrieval was initiated after patients were sedated with midazolam (a maximum of 5 mg) and sufentanil (maximum dose of 7.5 μg) administered intravenously. Patients who required further sedation were then given incremental boluses of methohexital. The relationship of each oocyte retrieved to the time of drug administered was recorded. The outcome of oocytes not exposed to methohexital was compared with that of those that were exposed. There was no difference in fertilization or development of embryos and those not exposed to methohexital, despite the fact that oocytes exposed to methohexital were retrieved later.

The clinical significance of these two studies is uncertain. Dosages of methohexital were greater when it was used as the anesthetic induction agent for GIFT than when administered after sedation for ultrasound aspiration. In GIFT patients, the oocytes judged to be the "best" or most mature were selected for transfer, so the effect of methohexital on oocytes not transferred for GIFT may be only on immature or poorer quality oocytes. Methohexital remains an important clinical agent in ambulatory patients, and further studies comparing methohexital with other major hypnotics should be performed before abandoning its use in IVF patients.

Propofol: Propofol has been studied for use in ART anesthetics by Palot et al. Follicular fluid concentrations of propofol do not rise with time as demonstrated with pentothal (100); this may be due to the more rapid metabolism and excretion of propofol or pharmacokinetic differences in the redistribution of propofol. Propofol has not been demonstrated to negatively affect oocyte performance when administered alone, or with midazolam or isoflurane as an anesthetic for oocyte retrieval. Cleavage is inhibited when propofol is administered with nitrous oxide (101).

The clinical advantages of its short duration and very low incidence of nausea make propofol valuable as an anesthetic induction agent and for use as a major hypnotic (intravenous general anesthetic) in patients needing more than narcotic or anxiolytic sedation. The effects of propofol on embryo development and sperm are unknown; further studies on the outcome of gamete and zygote intrafallopian transfer after propofol administration are warranted.

Etomidate: Etomidate is unique among anesthetic induction agents currently available in that it depresses adrenal function and decreases circulating cortisol for 24 hours after surgery, blunting the usual glycemic response (112). The significance of adrenal suppression on reproductive outcome is unknown. Follicular fluid levels of etomidate are relatively low, but rise over time; fertilization and cleavage rates are not affected by etomidate when administered for oocyte retrieval (9). Estradiol and progesterone do not change in follicular fluid after etomidate administration for oocyte retrieval, but slightly decrease in plasma during the perioperative period (5). Etomidate is not a popular major hypnotic for ambulatory work because of the related pain at the injection site and the high incidence of nausea and vomiting associated with its use.

Narcotics: Clinical studies demonstrating a negative effect on reproductive outcome after narcotic exposure of the gamete or zygote are few. As with barbiturates, narcotics have been shown to decrease cellular functions (113). Fentanyl and morphine have been shown to significantly raise prolactin (72,73); this may occur with other narcotics also.

Fentanyl, a synthetic narcotic, has been shown not to affect fertilization and cleavage in sea urchin oocytes (114). In a limited study, fentanyl was not isolated in significant amounts from the follicular fluid of patients undergoing laparoscopic oocyte retrieval (6). Alfentanil, a close derivative of fentanyl, has been isolated from human follicular fluid but has not been found to be deleterious to the oocyte (7).

Meperidine and fentanyl have been demonstrated not to inhibit mouse embryo development at the two-cell stage (105). Meperidine is widely used as a supplement to local anesthesia for ultrasound oocyte retrieval, and although comparative clinical studies have not been published demonstrating its effect on oocyte quality, it remains a very useful clinical agent.

The effects of these narcotics on spermatozoa and the zygote are unknown. However, methadone, which is structurally very similar to morphine, rapidly passes into spermatozoa in humans (115) and has been shown to negatively affect offspring in animal studies (116).

Local anesthetic agents

Local and regional (epidural or spinal) anesthetics offer viable and increasingly popular alternatives to general anesthesia for ART procedures. They are suitable in the ambulatory setting and allow the patient some degree of participation. It is possible, with a well-administered regional anesthetic, to deliver less anesthetic agent to the gamete than with either sedation or a general anesthetic, and the luteal phase may be less disturbed (66).

The most commonly used local anesthetic agent is lidocaine. The clinical significance of lidocaine toxicity on oocytes is unknown. A concentration of 1.0 μg/ml (an easily obtainable level in plasma under clinical conditions) has been demonstrated to inhibit mouse embryo development (117). Local anesthetics are calmodulin inhibitors (41). They have been demonstrated to affect the cortical granule release at fertilization and the block to polyspermy (28,29). Lidocaine inhibits sperm motility (118). Local anesthetics are parthenogenic (26) and may inhibit cell fusion (30).

Neither local anesthesia (paracervical block or infiltration) nor major regional block anesthesia ensures that anesthetic drugs do not reach the gametes in appreciable concentrations. They will not necessarily be less detrimental agents than specific general anesthetic agents. Significant blood levels are attained very quickly after the administration of paracervical, epidural, caudal, and spinal anesthesia. Paracervically administered lidocaine (up to 300 mg in premeasured kits) enters the bloodstream similarly to an intravenous injection. Serum and follicular fluid lidocaine levels have been measured after paracervical block (100 mg) (119) and caudal anesthesia (120) for ultrasonically guided vaginal oocyte retrieval and found to be significant (more than 1.0 μg/ml in follicular fluid). Peak blood levels of lidocaine after epidural administration occur at 18 minutes with blood concentrations as high as 6.0 μg/ml. Absorption patterns after spinal anesthesia are similar, although the volume and dose of agent will be lower (121).

Many of the toxicity problems of the local anesthetics can be avoided by choosing drugs of the ester class, such as procaine or tetracaine for spinal anesthesia and chloroprocaine for epidural anesthesia. Ester local anesthetic drugs are rapidly hydrolyzed in plasma by pseudocholinesterase and are not appreciably detectable in plasma after administration in regional anesthetics. Blood levels of chloroprocaine are only minimally detectable after epidural injection due to the rapid hydrolysis in the plasma (122). However, the incidence of severe spasmodic lumbar back pain following epidural anesthesia with chloroprocaine is unacceptably high (123,124).

Clinical management of assisted reproductive anesthetics

In general, patients presenting for assisted reproductive procedures are more anxious and emotional than similar patients presenting for elective ambulatory procedures. Studies of psychological factors causing stress in IVF patients have identified the fear of anesthesia as a significant source of stress (125,126). Most IVF patients have had prior, sometimes multiple, anesthetic exposures. Personal experiences and levels of acceptance vary with regard to minor morbidity (nausea and vomiting, sore throat, dizziness, dysphoria).

Some patients have a major fear of undergoing any anesthetic; often this is related not to an anxiety regarding potential risk or adverse outcome, but to a loss of control of the events in their immediate environment. This presents a unique challenge as even mild sedatives may be psychologically unacceptable. Despite this, some anesthesia may be necessary to accomplish the planned surgical procedure. Other patients may be equally upset by the perception that the surgical procedure, if performed with a local anesthetic or sedation, may be painful. An individualized approach to the patient is mandatory, and a consistent relationship between the reproductive team and anesthesiologists who understand the particular psychological needs and fears of IVF patients is desirable. In the event that an ART procedure is unsuccessful on one attempt, it may be desirable for the patient to return. A negative surgical or anesthetic experience can be enough to prevent this, thereby reducing the chance of individual success. Every attempt should be made to minimize the discomforts of the operative day *as the patient perceives them* by individualizing the approach to each patient and allowing patients maximum input (compatible with appropriate surgical conditions) into the conduct of their care. The time taken to accomplish this benefits the entire reproductive team.

Preoperative medical workup will vary with the institutional requirements. We perform only a hematocrit evaluation on healthy ambulatory patients. Other tests are done as indicated by individual medical conditions. They are performed and reviewed before the surgical date.

Cancellations of surgery the day of oocyte retrieval by the anesthesiologist cause great financial and emotional hardship for the patient. Every effort should be made to avoid them. A thorough history and physical examination and communication between the reproductive team and the anesthesiologist as early as possible in the workup of the patient are essential.

Occasionally patients will appear on the day of surgery with new medical problems. The most common are upper respiratory infections, influenza, and bronchitis. These patients are fully informed of the potential for respiratory complications postoperatively, a pertinent physical examination is performed, and surgery is performed as scheduled.

There are also patients who, despite all instructions, have eaten the morning of surgery. If a patient is known to have eaten, she is again informed of the risks, and surgery proceeds on schedule. Metoclopramide, 10 mg intravenously, is given preoperatively to increase gastric emptying. Rapid sequence induction and intubations are performed on patients receiving general anesthesia.

Proceeding with a general anesthetic in a patient with an acute upper respiratory infection or a full stomach may be contrary to what many anesthesiologists would consider appropriate management of elective surgical patients. However, considering the patient's input in terms of time, emotion, and finances into a stimulation for oocyte retrieval, and the necessity that oocytes be retrieved within a small window of time once the human chorionic gonadotropin is administered, the elective nature of oocyte retrievals is debatable.

Ultrasound-guided transvaginal oocyte retrieval

The introduction of transvaginal ultrasound-guided oocyte retrieval has been the greatest advance to date in increasing patient comfort and acceptance of oocyte retrieval.

Programs vary in the type of anesthetics offered for transvaginal oocyte recovery based on many factors, including availability of consistent and qualified anesthesiologists, cost considerations, and the location of service (office, radiology department, surgical or obstetrical suite).

The office setting offers the advantage of convenience to the surgeon and a lower cost to the patient. Although there may be some discomfort associated with oocyte aspiration performed with intravenous analgesia, it is acceptable to most patients if appropriate educational and psychological preparation is provided. The majority of the discomfort associated with transvaginal oocyte retrieval is from the initial ovarian puncture; a surgeon who minimizes the number of ovarian punctures will minimize both the time required for aspiration and the degree of discomfort to the patient. Oocytes in difficult or inaccessible positions present a greater challenge to patient tolerance. Some surgeons, particularly in institutions without an active embryo-freezing program, will elect not to aspirate these follicles. When aspiration is attempted, the patient will usually experience enough discomfort that a major hypnotic would be beneficial. This cannot be recommended in the office setting without the appropriate equipment and personnel to administer anesthesia.

Even if major hypnotic agents are not to be used, an office suite where oocyte retrievals are performed should be prepared with suction, oxygen, a defibrillator, appropriate resuscitative agents, emergency airway equipment, cardiac and blood pressure monitoring, pulse oximetry, and a staffed recovery area. Respiratory depression, apnea, and aspiration secondary to obtunded laryngeal reflexes after intravenous sedatives are unpredictable. Midazolam, alone or in combination with an opiate, has gained wide popularity in the office

surgical setting. In a controlled study the combination of midazolam (0.05 mg/kg) and fentanyl (2 μg/kg) produced hypoxemia in 92% of healthy volunteers (127). Half of these subjects experienced periods of apnea. Of the adverse reactions to midazolam reported to the U.S. Department of Health and Human Services, 96% of the deaths occurred outside the operating room; 75% involved oxygenation or ventilatory problems, and more than half of these patients had received both midazolam and a narcotic. The experience with diazepam combined with a narcotic has been similar (128).

The surgical suite offers the advantage of the availability of personnel who can individualize the approach to the patient's analgesia or anesthesia. We use almost exclusively total intravenous anesthesia for transvaginal ultrasound-guided retrievals. The patients are sedated with midazolam and a low dose of narcotic during the preparation; general anesthesia is induced with propofol or methohexital just before oocyte aspiration. The patients breathe spontaneously and are given oxygen by nasal cannula as indicated by pulse oximetry. This technique offers the patient maximum comfort with rare postoperative side effects such as nausea and offers the surgeon optimum conditions for retrieval. To avoid oxygen toxicity on the oocyte, oxygen is administered only as indicated by pulse oximetry. Using this technique, the total aspiration time is consistently less than 15 minutes. Our own analysis of oocyte outcome (see above, barbiturates) indicates that this technique is not more detrimental to oocyte outcome than sedation alone, and it has been exceptionally well accepted by the patients.

Epidural anesthesia offers an equally satisfactory analgesia. A study by LeFebvre et al. demonstrated a higher cleavage rate of oocytes retrieved under epidural anesthesia than under general anesthesia with halothane (4). Similarly, fertilization rates were improved when local anesthesia supplemented by sedation for transvaginal ultrasound aspiration was compared with laparoscopy with enflurane and nitrous oxide anesthesia (85). To date, a prospective study of regional anesthesia compared with intravenous sedation or total intravenous anesthesia has not been published. Until more information is available, the decision to use a regional anesthetic should be individualized to the patient's acceptance and expectations.

Laparoscopic GIFT and ZIFT

More than for any other procedure, the choice of a comfortable and safe anesthetic for laparoscopic GIFT or ZIFT demands that the anesthesiologist be knowledgeable and experienced in ambulatory anesthesia and postoperative care. Both regional and general anesthetics are acceptable for ambulatory ART procedures.

Regional anesthesia: Epidural and spinal anesthesia are both acceptable for ambulatory patients, particularly with the short-acting agents chloroprocaine, procaine, and lidocaine (129). Regional anesthetics offer the theoretical advantage of lower plasma and follicular fluid levels of anesthetic agents. Patients who prefer not to receive a general anesthetic find epidural anesthesia a welcome alternative.

There are some distinct disadvantages of regional anesthesia in laparoscopic ART surgeries. Spontaneous respiratory movement may hinder efficient laparoscopic surgery. Regional anesthesia in ART procedures can be clinically difficult for the anesthesiologist to manage, particularly if the surgical procedure is prolonged. Carbon dioxide is the safest insufflating gas for both the patient and the gamete. However, carbon dioxide, unlike air or nitrous oxide, is highly irritating to the peritoneum; this pain is referred to the C4 level from the diaphragm and therefore is not alleviated by safe regional anesthetic sensory levels. The addition of fentanyl to the epidural agent (up to 50 μg) helps to alleviate the shoulder discomfort associated with regional anesthesia for laparoscopies, but its use is associated with pruritus and nausea.

Neither air nor nitrous oxide is irritating to the peritoneum, and many centers where epidurals are popular for diagnostic laparoscopy employ nitrous oxide for peritoneal insufflation. The use of air for peritoneal insufflation presents the hazard of air emboli by absorption into multiple small veins that may be undetectable by the surgeon. Monitoring with a precordial Doppler stethoscope, continuous end-tidal carbon dioxide measurement, and the rapid ability to insert a central line for air aspiration should be available if air is used at any time during laparoscopy.

Unless heavy sedation is required or there is underlying pulmonary disease, respiratory function is not compromised during well-conducted regional anesthesia (130). Steinbrook and Conception have demonstrated a *decrease* in end-tidal carbon dioxide levels after spinal anesthesia in unpremedicated patients that positively correlates with the height of the sensory block (131).

Spinal headaches, often considered minor and treatable by anesthesiologists, may be perceived in patients having ART procedures as a major complication. The incidence of headache with a 27 gauge spinal needle ranges from 5% (132) to 11% (133) in ambulatory patients. Young women are more susceptible to postdural puncture headaches. Fluid shifts that accompany hyperstimulation for oocyte retrieval result in intravascular volume depletion. Both of these factors would make spinal headaches more common in patients having ART procedures.

After performing 30 consecutive ZIFT procedures with epidural anesthesia, and observing no difference in outcome between those and subsequent ZIFT procedures performed with total intravenous anesthesia supplemented with low-concentration inhalation agent, we

Table 9.8 Anesthetic protocol for patients undergoing GIFT and ZIFT (not on anesthesia study protocols)

Intravenous: Balanced electrolyte solution

Premedication (in operating room during monitor placement):
Midazolam 3.0–5.0 mg IV

Induction:
Propofol 2.0–3.0 mg/kg

Maintenance:
Air with oxygen added only to maintain Sa_{O_2} above 97%
Incremental boluses of propofol
Low-dose enflurane (0.5%) optional
Meperidine 50 mg IV (if given, delete meperidine from recovery orders)

Muscle relaxants:
Atracurium (for intubation and intraoperative relaxation) 0.4–0.5 mg/kg, supplemented in 5 mg increments as indicated by nerve stimulator

Reversal:
Atropine and edrophonium

have abandoned regional techniques for laparoscopic procedures. Surgical conditions were less than satisfactory, patient acceptance was low, and the shoulder pain secondary to the carbon dioxide was difficult to manage safely.

General anesthesia: The introduction of short-acting agents and the ability to perform a laparoscopy with total intravenous anesthesia (TIVA) or TIVA supplemented with subanesthetic concentrations of enflurane or isoflurane have dramatically decreased the incidence of minor morbidity, such as nausea and vomiting and shivering, after general anesthesia. Midazolam (5 mg) and propofol (induction dose and supplemental increments or infusion) with a 0.5% or less inspired

concentration of enflurane in air is the preferred general anesthetic protocol at this time in our program (see Table 9.8). We do not use any narcotics intraoperatively or antiemetics prophylactically; fewer than 10% of patients experience nausea, and rarely have patients required more than 25 mg of meperidine in the recovery area for pain. The intraoperative use of narcotics, particularly fentanyl, has been associated with an unacceptable incidence of urinary retention and nausea. Meperidine (12.5 mg intravenously) is highly effective when used for shivering postoperatively and has produced less nausea than fentanyl, sufentanil, or alfentanil in our program (see Table 9.9).

Pneumoperitoneum with carbon dioxide is associated with a decrease in the pH of the follicular fluid (134), which may be detrimental to oocyte function (77). Carbon dioxide diffuses rapidly and directly into the ovarian tissues and vascular system. The effect of controlled hyperventilation on follicular fluid pH during laparoscopy with carbon dioxide pneumoperitoneum has not been studied; therefore, we maintain end-tidal carbon dioxide in the physiologic range (32–35 mm Hg).

Adequate muscle relaxation is essential in lapa-

Table 9.9 Postanesthesia recovery orders: GIFT and ZIFT patients (laparoscopic)

1. Oxygen 1–4 L/min by nasal cannula PRN Sa_{O_2} below 97% only. Use minimal oxygen to maintain Sa_{O_2} of 97% or greater.
2. Meperidine 12.5 mg IV PRN pain. May repeat once in 10 minutes.
3. Darvocet N-100 or acetaminophen orally for pain.
4. Vistaril 25 mg and ephedrine 25 mg IM PRN nausea. May repeat once in 60 minutes.
5. Intravenous rate at 200 cc/hour. Follow surgical solution with 5% dextrose/½ normal saline.
6. Minimum recovery stay of 2 hours.

roscopic anesthesia, particularly at the time of trocar insertion. All laparoscopy patients are intubated at our institution. Except when contraindicated, nondepolarizing agents (atracurium, vecuronium) are used to aid intubation and provide surgical relaxation. This avoids postoperative myalgias from succinylcholine. Nerve stimulator monitoring is essential in these patients. There is great variability in the dose requirements for nondepolarizing relaxants in hyperstimulated patients, and we have had several unexplained incidences of difficulty in muscle relaxant reversal. This may be due to changes in distribution of body water or to a direct neuromuscular end plate effect of estrogen. Intubation and maintenance doses of muscle relaxants are reduced by about 30% from anticipated requirements, and every attempt is made to retain two twitches on train-of-four monitoring. We reverse the muscle relaxant in all patients. Patients are not extubated until full return of central muscular tone is demonstrated by intact cough reflexes with forward motion or positive head lift.

No topical, lubricant, or intravenous lidocaine is used during general anesthesia; this avoids potential lidocaine toxicity on the gamete and interference with muscle relaxant reversal. Endotracheal 4% lidocaine sprays (used before intubation) introduce as much as 200 mg of lidocaine with a peak blood level of lidocaine as early as 5 minutes after administration (135).

Premedication remains controversial. During either GIFT or ZIFT the gametes will eventually receive full anesthetic exposure; therefore, it is difficult to justify the omission of a premedicant such as low-dose midazolam. The practice of preparing and draping patients without sedation and then rapidly inducing anesthesia warrants study. It is an anxiety-provoking practice for the patient and is inherently less safe than a slow, controlled anesthetic induction with full nursing and physician attention.

Nitrous oxide is omitted from all reproductive procedures in our program. Besides avoiding potential toxicity, bowel distention is reduced. All anesthesia machines used for patients undergoing ART procedures are equipped with compressed air. We use the Drager Narkomed, which has an obligatory oxygen flow of 200 cc per minute. To avoid oxygen toxicity, this 200 cc flow is diluted with 6 to 8 L per minute of air, giving a fractional concentration of O_2 in inspired gas close to that of room air. Patients are monitored by pulse oximetry, and the oxygen is increased only as necessary. Oximeter monitoring is continued throughout the recovery period, and supplemental oxygen is minimized in both amount and time of exposure.

Nausea is a frequently reported complication of laparoscopy (136), and every effort is made to avoid its occurrence and minimize the severity if it occurs. Cimetidine or ranitidine is administered in two oral doses the night before surgery and again in the morning. Fluids (non-dextrose-containing balanced electrolyte solutions) are liberally administered. Narcotics are avoided if compatible with patient comfort. Patients who have a history of postoperative nausea have an oral gastric tube placed and suctioned during the procedure. The combination of these measures has reduced the incidence of nausea in stimulated laparoscopic patients to below 10% in our program.

All anesthesiologists working in our reproductive program cooperate in following prewritten anesthetic protocols. Every effort is made to maximize both patient comfort and reproductive outcome. We have an ongoing analysis of anesthetic protocols in relation to fertilization, embryo development, pregnancy, and spontaneous abortion rates. Postoperative minor morbidity and discomfort (pain, nausea, etc.) are recorded by the recovery staff for all patients. Patients are also contacted by telephone the morning after oocyte retrieval. Every significant change in anesthetic administration is followed by a review of both patient acceptance and reproductive outcome. An outline of our current general anesthesia protocols (for patients not participating in research studies) for GIFT and ZIFT can be found in Tables 9.8 and 9.9.

Electroejaculation

Electrical stimulation to obtain semen samples in nonejaculatory males (after spinal cord injury or testicular carcinoma resection) is becoming more common as the availability and success of this technique for previously infertile couples becomes more well known. Brindley (137) and Bennett et al. (138) have reported pregnancies after electroejaculation and insemination. Electroejaculation therapy and in vitro fertilization and embryo transfer have been successfully combined (139). In our program electroejaculation has been successfully utilized in combination with insemination, GIFT, ZIFT, and embryo transfer.

Electroejaculation requires an anesthetic in paraplegic patients with residual sensation or low sensory deficits and in all nonparaplegic patients. Little information is available on drug entry into semen.

Testicular plasma differs from blood plasma in having a very low protein content, and the existence of a partial blood-testis barrier has been proposed (140). However, it is unlikely that any effective barrier exists to the passage of pharmacologically active drugs. Antibiotics (141), salicylates (142), alcohol (143), and methadone (115) are among the drugs that have been isolated from semen.

Both spinal and general anesthesia are used in our program. Spinal anesthesia has been exceptionally well received by these patients, and is preferable in spinal cord injury patients to avoid the problems of autonomic hyperreflexia. Epidural anesthesia has been less than satisfactory in providing analgesia when chloroprocaine is used; lidocaine results rapidly in a potentially toxic blood level for the spermatozoa.

Spinal anesthetics are administered with a 25 or 27 gauge needle, and 5% lidocaine or 5% procaine is used to achieve a sensory level of T4. If this sensory level is not reached, supplementation or conversion to general anesthesia may be necessary due to the peritoneal stimulation that accompanies the procedure. Despite adequate analgesia and a voluntary motor block, strong muscle contractions may occur in the lower extremities, resulting in significant postoperative myalgias. These frequently require therapy with analgesics and muscle relaxants for 1 to 3 days.

General anesthesia is performed using total intravenous anesthesia and atracurium or vecuronium. Patients who are completely paralyzed during the stimulation and therefore do not experience the involuntary lower-extremity muscle contractions are more comfortable postoperatively and are easier to manage during the procedure. We are currently using midazolam, propofol, and a narcotic agent for the anesthetic; we avoid nitrous oxide and inhalational agents because of the potential for toxicity to the sperm (37,38). Similarly, oxygen administration is kept as low as possible, and patients are ventilated with compressed air, given minimal supplemental oxygen, and monitored with pulse oximetry.

Perioperative patient management

Nausea and vomiting

Nausea and vomiting, although generally minor in consequence, constitute the most frequent and aggravating problem that occurs in the postoperative period following ambulatory anesthesia. The hormonal changes and hyperstimulation preceding oocyte retrieval cause several physiological and psychological changes that precipitate a higher incidence of nausea and vomiting in ART patients than in other patients having similar surgeries. The incidence and severity of nausea and vomiting have been shown to be increased as the serum estrogen level increases in the menstrual cycle (144) and to correlate with peak estrogen levels in patients undergoing oocyte retrieval (145).

Mild hypotension at the chemoreceptor zone (emetic center) of the brainstem is thought to be responsible for some of the nausea and vomiting in ambulatory patients; indeed, most occurs when patients begin to ambulate. An increase in estrogen causes a decrease in peripheral vascular resistance (146). Both estrogen (147) and increased renin activity (148) associated with ovarian stimulation cause an increased capillary permeability and decreased intravascular colloid osmotic pressure (149). This results in a variable degree of third spacing. The additional decrease in vascular tone that persists for some time after an anesthetic or sedation will potentiate this problem.

Bleeding after oocyte retrieval may result in nausea and vomiting secondary to hypotension and must be considered in any patient having prolonged nausea and vomiting or dizziness.

Laparoscopies have been reported to be associated with an incidence of nausea and vomiting that is as high as 43% in patients receiving a fentanyl-based anesthetic. The same study reported a 25% incidence when isoflurane was the primary anesthetic agent (150). We compared the incidence of nausea in three anesthetic protocols for laparoscopic GIFT. One group of patients received enflurane and air, a second enflurane and nitrous oxide, and a third sufentanil and nitrous oxide. Results are shown in Fig. 9.1. The incidence and severity of nausea and vomiting were unacceptably high with a narcotic-based technique.

The management of nausea and vomiting in the postoperative period begins before the patient arrives at the facility to undergo a procedure. The basis for treatment relies on decreasing gastric acidity and output, managing the relative intravascular fluid deficit secondary to the effects of estrogen, and the use of minimal narcotics.

Outpatients have been shown to be at an increased risk of aspiration because of the lack of anxiolytic premedication the night before and morning of surgery. This problem is magnified in ART patients. In vitro fertilization patients are generally more anxious than patients arriving for most other elective surgical procedures.

The administration of H_2 blockers (cimetidine or ranitidine) the night before surgery and the morning of surgery is effective in reducing the acidity and volume of gastric secretions the day of surgery (151,152). The addition of metoclopramide, a gastric kinetic, reduces gastric volume and offers further protection (153,154). Psychological and extrapyramidal side effects have been demonstrated with the acute intravenous administration of metoclopramide; therefore, it should be reserved for carefully selected patients (e.g., in cases of obesity or intractable vomiting). If necessary, both the psychological and extrapyramidal reactions can be rapidly and reliably treated with the administration of 50 mg of benadryl intravenously.

Droperidol has been a popular antiemetic in ambulatory patients for many years. It is most effective against nausea and vomiting secondary to the administration of narcotics. Acute extrapyramidal reactions and severe dysphoria have been reported after discharge in patients receiving low-dose droperidol (155,156). Furthermore, the decrease in peripheral resistance seen with even small doses of droperidol may aggravate estrogen and anesthetic-induced vasodilatation, limiting the overall effectiveness of droperidol in ART patients.

Hydroxyzine (Vistaril; 25 mg) administered in-

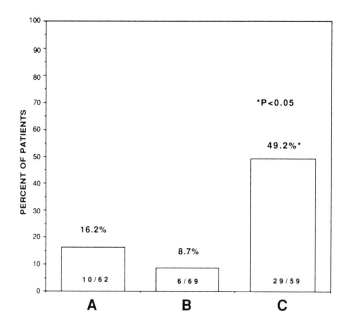

(A) enflurane and nitrous oxide; (B) enflurane and air; (C) sufentanil (0.5 μg/kg) and nitrous oxide. Induction in all groups by methohexital.

Fig. 9.1 Effect of anesthetic protocol on the incidence of severe nausea and vomiting.

tramuscularly with ephedrine (25 mg), as reported by Freeman (157), has proved to be the most effective antiemetic we have yet used, and it is a rare patient that does not respond to two doses an hour apart. Patients who have experienced vomiting in the recovery room and continue to have some nausea at the time of discharge can be given a prescription for hydroxyzine and ephedrine (25 mg each) to be taken orally at home every 4 to 6 hours.

The importance of fluids cannot be overemphasized. Dehydration exacerbates subtle hypotension and nausea. In our facility, patients receive an average of 1800 cc of fluid in the total perioperative period, and fluid challenges are tried on all patients who experience nausea.

Bleeding

Bleeding in the postoperative period may be deceptively subtle in its presentation, after both ultrasound aspiration and laparoscopy. Most bleeding occurs from small veins, is steady, slow, and gradual, and does not result in a sudden decompensation in vital signs. Bleeding may not be noticeable at the time of laparoscopy owing to venous tamponade by the insufflation gas. Because mild orthostatic changes and dizziness are commonly attributed to sedation and anesthesia, it may be difficult to diagnose with certainty clinically significant bleeding in the recovery area in less than 2 hours. It is therefore advisable that patients remain under observation for at least this period of time and be totally free of orthostatic changes upon discharge.

Pain

With few exceptions, patients do not experience significant pain after either laparoscopy or transvaginal ultrasound-guided oocyte retrieval. We use low doses (12.5–25 mg) of meperidine in the recovery room for pain management. Darvocet or acetaminophen are used as oral analgesics. Prostaglandin inhibitors such as ibuprofen, aspirin, and injectable ketorolac are avoided. Patients who require high doses of pain medication should be examined by a physician. An unusual amount of pain in the recovery room after either laparoscopic or ultrasound-guided oocyte retrieval may be associated with bleeding (abdominal wall or retroperitoneal) or bladder irritation.

Urinary retention

Urinary retention is most commonly associated with the use of narcotics intraoperatively. However, bladder irritation secondary to catheterization or the surgical procedure may also contribute to urinary retention.

If a patient is unable to void and the bladder is distended, an in-and-out catheterization is unavoidable. When patients are not distended and have no urge to void, we allow them to be discharged home with instructions to return if bladder distention or discomfort occurs.

The patient with systemic disease

Most patients undergoing ART procedures are in good health. A few will have underlying systemic diseases that require attention through the perioperative period. It is important to the smooth function of a busy program and the maximum reduction of patient risks that the potential seriousness of medical problems be recognized by the nurses and physicians of the reproductive team and brought to the attention of an appropriate anesthesiologist as early as possible.

Although all oocyte retrievals are performed in our program in a free-standing ambulatory surgery unit, the full resources of the hospital are readily available. Our unit is attached to the hospital, and admission is rapid and straightforward. Full emergency and monitoring equipment is available on site. The following are some of the situations we have encountered; the management outlined is not meant to be comprehensive.

Asthma: Asthma is one of the more common systemic problems encountered in ART patients. As anxiety may rapidly precipitate an attack, premedication is usually given, and many patients are placed on anxiolytic medications (i.e., Xanax) for one or two days preoperatively. A reassuring preoperative visit with the anesthesiologist is particularly helpful. Patients are asked to take all their morning medications and to bring both their medications and inhalers with them. A patient who appears for surgery with some wheezing is managed preoperatively with appropriate sedation and bronchodilators before anesthetic induction.

Cardiac disease: Mitral valve prolapse is fairly common in the population of patients undergoing ART procedures. Anesthesia-related problems are usually minor and amenable to treatment, and consist of ventricular arrhythmias and tachycardic episodes. A baseline electrocardiogram is advisable. Most patients are already well aware of their diagnosis and are under the care of an internist or cardiologist. Patients who have been placed on beta-blockers for rate or cardiac rhythm control should take their usual morning dose.

Antibiotic prophylaxis against bacterial endocarditis is recommended in patients with mitral valve prolapse (158). A single dose of ampicillin (2 g intravenously) with gentamycin (1.5 mg/kg intravenously) 30 minutes preoperatively is the current American Heart Association recommendation; Vancomycin (1 g *infused slowly*) should be substituted for ampicillin in penicillin-allergic patients.

Nongenetically related surrogate gestation has made it possible for a woman medically unable to safely tolerate pregnancy to have a child. A few patients with severe, surgically uncorrectable, cardiac disabilities will present for oocyte retrieval in programs participating in surrogate work. These situations demand early and close communication between the reproductive team, cardiologists, and anesthesiologist. This should occur before the patient begins to cycle, so that all the risks can be presented before stimulation is begun. The same patients who, for cardiac reasons, may be unable to withstand the physiologic changes of pregnancy also may not tolerate severe ovarian hyperstimulation if it occurs. As the risk of ovarian hyperstimulation is significantly increased if oocytes are not retrieved once stimulation has been completed, it is imperative that any decision not to undergo oocyte retrieval based on the risks of the sedation, anesthetic, or surgery be made before injection of human chorionic gonadotropin.

If oocyte retrieval is planned, then full and appropriate monitoring as dictated by the patient's underlying condition, including invasive monitoring and pacemaker standby, is warranted.

Insulin-dependent diabetes mellitus:

There are almost as many "routines" for managing the insulin-dependent diabetic in the perioperative period as there are anesthesiologists, endocrinologists, and surgeons. In our center, a regimen described by Natof (159) has been very successful in diabetics undergoing ambulatory surgery. He uses the phrase "Moving the sun in the sky" to describes the process, which makes it very easy to remember. The entire day's clock with regard to insulin and food intake is pushed back. Patients have surgery as the first scheduled case in the morning. Postoperatively, when they are awake and able to eat, they have a meal that is similar to their normal breakfast, and take their full dose of insulin. Meals are then spaced normally through the day, but pushed back by whatever delay occurred between the time they had breakfast and the time they usually eat in the morning. Afternoon insulin is similarly pushed later in the day. The following morning, to avoid hypoglycemia from late insulin administration, additional protein is added to their breakfast.

All diabetic patients bring their own insulin with them the day of surgery. Assisted reproductive patients are usually highly educated about their disease and their normal control, and working closely with the patient can be very helpful. Educated patients become quite anxious if they feel that their insulin needs are not being as specifically tailored as they usually keep them at home. In addition, hyperglycemia has some potential to be detrimental to the oocyte. Intravenous dextrose solutions are avoided, and frequent blood sugar determinations are made. Every effort is made to keep patients' blood sugar as close to their best control as possible.

The success of this management is totally dependent on the patient's being able to take nourishment, and exceptional care must be exercised to avoid nausea.

Malignant hyperthermia susceptibility:

It is the standard of care that any area where anesthesia is administered has the capability to treat an episode of malignant hyperthermia.

Patients susceptible to malignant hyperthermia can be cared for on an ambulatory basis after they are known to the anesthesiologist, have been followed through at least one perioperative course, are appropriately educated on the disorder, and can easily return to the hospital if necessary. A preoperative baseline creatinine phospokinase (CPK) level is obtained, at least three hourly postanesthetic CPKs are performed. Patients remain at the facility at least 6 hours after surgery. Postoperative CPK levels have been examined in patients without this susceptibility after laparoscopy in our center and found to be normal. Therefore, no patient is discharged home with an abnormal CPK or temperature. The anesthesiologist who actually administered the anesthetic should be available to the patient for the first 24 hours. Patients are instructed to take their temperature hourly for at least 6 hours after returning home and to call if they experience muscle cramping or fatigue, dysphoria, or hyperventilation.

Pretreatment with dantrolene remains controversial, but increasingly anesthesiologists are electing to omit pretreatment in selected patients. If an appropriate nontriggering anesthetic is administered, the anesthesia machine has been properly prepared, end-tidal carbon dioxide and temperature monitoring are performed, and dantrolene is available, a general anesthetic is not contraindicated.

Ovarian hyperstimulation syndrome: The incidence of severe ovarian hyperstimulation varies with stimulation protocols. The overall incidence is not known, but the occurrence is not rare and has been reported to vary from 0.4% to 4% of treatment cycles (160,161). Oocyte retrieval usually avoids or lessens the severity of hyperstimulation, but at least one case of hyperstimulation has been reported after all follicles have been aspirated (162). Clinical manifestations include severe third spacing secondary to increased vascular permeability, intravascular volume deficits, ascites, pleural effusions, electrolyte imbalances, hemoconcentration, prerenal oliguria, coagulopathies, and liver function abnormalities (163).

Ovarian hyperstimulation syndrome becomes apparent several days after oocyte retrieval. Conception increases the severity of the clinical course and can cause rapid deterioration, so pregnancy termination may be indicated as a life-saving measure. Therefore, anesthesiologists working closely with an ART program should be aware of the presentation and management of this syndrome. It requires aggressive early management to avoid serious adverse outcome, including invasive monitoring and intensive care unit supervision.

References

1. Yanagimachi R. Mechanisms of fertilization in mammals. In: Mastroianni L, Biggers JD, eds. Fertilization and embryo development in vitro. New York: Plenum Press, 1981.

2. Hayes MF, Sacco AG, Savoy-Moore RT, Magyar DM, Endler GC, Moghissi KS. Effect of general anesthesia on fertilization and cleavage of human oocytes in vitro. Fertil Steril 1987;48(6):975–981.

3. Boyers SP, Lavy G, Russell JB, DeCherney AH. A paired analysis of in vitro fertilization and cleavage rates of first- versus last-recovered preovulatory human oocytes exposed to varying intervals of 100% CO_2 pneumoperitoneum and general anesthesia. Fertil Steril 1987;48(6):969–974.

4. LeFebvre G, Vauthier D, Seebacher J, Henry M, Thormann F, Darbois Y. In vitro fertilization: a comparative study of cleavage rates under general anesthesia—interest for gamete intrafallopian transfer. J In Vitro Fert Embryo Transf 1988;5(5):305–306.

5. Endler GC, Stout M, Magyar DM, et al. Follicular fluid concentrations of thiopental and thiamylal during laparoscopy for oocyte retrieval. Fertil Steril 1987;48(5):828–833.

6. Schoeffler PF, Levron JC, Jany L, Brenas FJ, Pouly JL. Follicular concentration of fentanyl during laparocopic oocyte retrieval. Correlation with in vitro fertilization results. Anesthesiology 1988;69(3A):A663.

7. Palot M, Levron JC, Gabriel R, Gillery P, Rendoing J. Follicular concentration of alfentanil during ultrasonically guided oocyte retrieval. Influence on cleavage rate. Anesthesiology 1989;71(3A):A888.

8. Palot M, Harika G, Pigeon F, Lamiable D, Rendoing J. Propofol in general anesthesia for IVF (by vaginal and transurethral route)—follicular fluid concentration and cleavage rate. Anesthesiology 1988;69(3A):A573.

9. Palot M, Harika G, Levron JC, Larbre H, Rendoing J. Follicular fluid concentration of etomidate during general anesthesia for oocyte retrieval—hormonal status of follicular fluid and cleavage rate. Anesthesiology 1989;71(3A):A904.

10. Bruce NW, Moor RM. Bibliography (with review) on ovarian blood flow and function. J Reprod Fertil 1976;46:299–304.

11. Bassett DL. The changes in the vascular pattern of the ovary of the albino rat during estrous cycle. Am J Anat 1943;73:251–292.

12. Ellinwood WE, Nett RM, Niswender GD. Ovarian vasculature: structure and function. In: Jones RE, ed. The vertebrate ovary. New York: Plenum Press, 1978:583–614.

13. Maas DHA, Storey BT, Mastroianni L. Oxygen tension in the oviduct of the rhesus monkey (*Macaca mulatta*). Fertil Steril 1976;27(11):1312–1317.

14. Shalgi R, Kracer PF, Soferman N. Human follicular fluid. J Reprod Fertil 1972;31:515–516.

15. Daya S. Follicular fluid pH changes following intraperitoneal exposure of graafian follicles to carbon dioxide: a comparative study with follicles exposed to ultrasound. Hum Reprod 1988;3(6):727–730.

16. Corbett TH. Retention of anesthetic agents following occupational exposure. Anesth Analg 1973;52(4):614–617.

17. Chase RE, Holaday DA, Fiserova-Bergerova V, Saidman LJ, Mack FE. The biotransformation of Ethrane in man. Anesthesiology 1971;35:262–267.

18. Holaday DA, Smith FR. Clinical characteristics and biotransformation of sevoflurane in healthy human volunteers. Anesthesiology 1981;54:100–106.

19. Iaizzo PA, Seewald M, Powis G, Van Dyke RA. The effects of halothane, enflurane, and isoflurane on Ca^{2+} mobilization on rat hepatocytes. Anesthesiology 1989;71(3A):A319.

20. Seeman P. The membrane actions of anesthetics and tranquilizers. Pharmacol Rev 1972;24(4):583–655.

21. Richards CD, Martin K, Gregory S, et al. Degenerate perturbations of protein structure as the mechanism of anesthetic action. Nature 1978;276:775–779.

22. Dluzewski AR, Halsey MJ, Simmonds AC. Membrane interactions with general and local anaesthetics: a review of molecular hypotheses of anesthesia. Molec Aspects Med 1983;6:461–573.

23. Sturrock JE, Nunn JF. Mitosis in mammalian cells during exposure to anesthetics. Anesthesiology 1975;43:21–33.

24. Simmonds AC, Halsey MJ. General and local anesthetics perturb the fusion of phospholipid vesicles. Biochim Biophys Acta 1985;813:331–337.

25. Seravalli EP, Lear E, Cottrell JE. Cell membrane fusion by chloroprocaine. Anesth Analg 1984;63:985–990.

26. Sircusa G, Whittingham DG, Codonesu M, DeFelici M. Local anesthetics and phenothiazine tranquilizers induce parthenogenic activation of the mouse oocyte. Dev Biol 1978;65:531–535.

27. Stapleton CL, Mills LL, Chandler DE. Cortical granule exocytosis in sea urchin eggs is inhibited by drugs that alter intracellular calcium stores. J Exp Zool 1985;234:289–299.

28. Ahuja KK. In-vitro inhibition of the block to polyspermy of hamster eggs by tertiary amine local anesthetics. J Reprod Fert 1982;65:15–22.

29. Hylander BL, Summers RG. The effect of local anesthetics and ammonia on cortical granule–plasma membrane attachment in the sea urchin egg. Dev Biol 1981;86:1–11.

30. Poste G, Reeve P. Inhibition of cell fusion by local anesthetics and tranquilizers. Exp Cell Res 1972;72:556–560.

31. Hansen D, Billings R. Effects of nitrous oxide on macromolecular content and DNA synthesis in rat embryos. J Pharmacol Exp Ther 1986;238:985–989.

32. Fujinaga M, Mazze RI, Baden JM, Fantal AG, Shepard TH. Rat whole embryo culture: an in-vitro model for testing nitrous oxide teratogenicity. Anesthesiology 1988;69:401–404.

33. Mazze RI, Wilson AI, Rice SA, Baden JM. Reproduction and fetal development in rats exposed to nitrous oxide. Teratology 1984;30:259–265.

34. Hinkley RE, Chambers EL. Structural changes in dividing sea-urchin eggs induced by the volatile anesthetic halothane. J Cell Sci 1982;55:327–339.

35. Kusyk CJ, Hsu TC. Mitotic anomalies induced by three inhalation halogenated anesthetics. Environ Res 1976;12:366–370.

36. Hinkley RE, Wright BD. Comparative effects of halothane, enflurane, and methoxyflurane on the incidence of abnormal development using sea urchin gametes as an in vitro model system. Anesth Analg 1985;64:1005–1009.

37. Hinkley RE, Wright BD, Greenberg CA. Induction of the acrosome reaction in sea urchin spermatozoa by the volatile anesthetic halothane. Biol Reprod 1986;34:119–125.

38. Hinkley RE. Inhibition of sperm motility by the volatile anesthetic halothane. Exp Cell Res 1979;121:435–437.

39. Cheung WY. Biologic functions of calmodulin. Harvey Lect 1985;79:173–216.

40. Levin RM, Weiss B. Specificity of the binding of rifluoperazine to the calcium-dependent activator of phos-

phodiesterase and to a series of other calcium-binding proteins. Biochim Biophys Acta 1978;540:197–204.

41. Tanaka T, Hidaka H. Interaction of local anesthetics with calmodulin. Biochem Biophys Res Commun 1981;101; 447–453.

42. Krupp P, Bianchi CP, Suarez-Kurtz G. On the local anesthetic effect of barbiturates. J Pharm Pharmacol 1969;21: 763–768.

43. Murat I, Ventura-Clapier R, Vassort G. Halothane, enflurane, and isoflurane decrease calcium sensitivity and maximal force in detergent-treated rat cardiac fibers. Anesthesiology 1988;69;892–899.

44. Winkler MA, DeWitt LM, Cheung WY. Calmodulin and calcium channel blockers. Hypertension 1987;9:217–223.

45. Weiss B, Sellinger-Barnette M, Winkler JD, Schecter LE. Calmodulin antagonists: structure-activity relationships. In: Hidaka H, Hartshorne DJ, eds. Calmodulin antagonists and cellular physiology. Orlando, Fla.: Academic Press, 1985:41–62.

46. Weiss B, Levin RM. Mechanism for selectively inhibiting the activation of cyclic nucleotide phosphodiesterase and adenyl cyclase by antipsychotic agents. Adv Cyclic Nucleotide Res 1978;9:285–304.

47. Klee CB, Vanaman TC. Calmodulin. Adv Protein Chem 1982;35:213–321.

48. Lenz RW, Hart R, Ax RL, Cormier MJ. Inhibition of mouse embryonic development by calmodulin antagonists. Gamete Res 1984;9:253–260.

49. Aono T, Kurachi K, Miyata M, et al. Influence of surgical stress under general anesthesia on serum gonadotropin levels in male and female patients. J Clin Endocrinol Metab 1976;42:144–148.

50. Charters AC, Odell WD, Thompson JC. Anterior pituitary function during surgical stress and convalescence. Radioimmunoassay measurement of blood TSH, LH, FSH, and growth hormone. J Clin Endocrinol Metab 1969;29:63–71.

51. Noel GL, Suh HK, Stone JG, Frantz AG. Human prolactin and growth hormone release during surgery and other conditions of stress. J Clin Endocrinol Metab 1972;35: 840–851.

52. Wang C, Chan V, Yeung RTT. Effect of surgical stress on pituitary-testicular function. Clin Endocrinol (Oxf) 1978;9:255–266.

53. Kehlet H. The modifying effect of general and regional anesthesia on the endocrine-metabolic response to surgery. Reg Anaesth Suppl 1982;7:38–48.

54. Hagen C, Brandt MR, Kehlet H. Prolactin, LH, FSH, and cortisol response to surgery and the effect of epidural analgesia. Acta Endocrinol 1980;94:151–154.

55. Forman R, Fishel SB, Edwards RG, Walters E. The influence of transient hyperprolactinemia on in vitro fertilization in humans. J Clin Endocrinol Metab 1985;60(3):517–522.

56. Gonen Y, Casper RF. The influence of transient hyperprolactinemia on hormonal parameters, oocyte recovery, and fertilization rates in in vitro fertilization. J In Vitro Fert Embryo Transf 1989;6(3):155–159.

57. Taylor PJ, Trouson A, Besanko M, Burger HG, Stockdale J. Plasma progesterone and prolactin changes in superovulated women before, during, and immediately after laparoscopy for in vitro fertilization and their relation to pregnancy. Fertil Steril 1986;45(5):680–686.

58. Messinis IE, Templeton AA. Relationship between intrafollicular levels of prolactin and sex steroids and in-vitro fertilization of human oocytes. Hum Reprod 1987;2(7): 606–607.

59. Boyers SP, Lavy G, Russell JB, Polan ML, DeCherney AH. Serum prolactin response to embryo transfer during human in vitro fertilization and embryo transfer. J In Vitro Fert Embryo Transf 1987;4:269–272.

60. Fukuda A, Noda Y, Mori T, Mori C, Hashimoto H, Hoshino K. Effects of prolactin on gametes and zygotes during in vitro fertilization in mice. J In Vitro Fert Embryo Transf 1988;5(1):25–30.

61. Braunsberg H, Reed MJ, Short F, Dias VO, Baxendale PM. Changes in plasma concentrations of oestrogens and progesterone in women during anaesthesia and gynecological operations. J Steroid Biochem 1981;14:749–755.

62. Soules MR, Sutton GP, Hammond CB, Haney AF. Endocrine changes at operation under general anesthesia: reproductive hormone fluctuations in young women. Fertil Steril 1980;33(4):364–371.

63. Gronow MJ, Martin MJ, Hay D, Moro D, Brown

JB. The luteal phase after hyperstimulation for in vitro fertilization. Ann N Y Acad Sci 1985;442:391–401.

64. Kemeter P, Feichtinger W, Neumark J, Szalay S, Bieglmayer CH, Janisch H. Influence of laparoscopic follicle aspiration under general anaesthesia on corpus luteum progesterone secretion in normal and clomiphene-stimulated cycles. Br J Obstet Gynaecol 1982;89:948–950.

65. Mausher S, Acosta AA, Garcia JE, Jones GS, Jones H. Luteal phase serum estradiol and progesterone in in vitro fertilization. Fertil Steril 1984;41(6):838–843.

66. Lehtinen AM, Laatikainen T, Koskimies AI, Hovorka J. Modifying effects of epidural anesthesia on the stress hormone response to laparoscopy for in vitro fertilization. J In Vitro Fert Embryo Transf 1987;4(1):23–29.

67. Garcia J, Jones GS, Acosta AA, Wright GL. Corpus luteum function after follicle aspiration for oocyte retrieval. Fertil Steril 1981;36(5):565–572.

68. Del Pozo E, Wyss H, Tolis G, Alcaniz J, Campana A, Naftolin F. Prolactin and deficient luteal function. Obstet Gynecol 1979;53:607–609.

69. McNeilly AS, Glasir A, Janassen J, Howie P. Evidence for direct inhibition of ovarian function by prolactin. J Reprod Fertil 1982;65:559–569.

70. Brandt M, Kehlet H, Binder C, Hagen C, McNeilly AS. Effect of epidural analgesia on the glucoregulatory endocrine response to surgery. Clin Endocrinol (Oxf) 1976;5:107–114.

71. Hoehe M, Duka T, Doenicke A. Human studies on the m-opiate receptor agonist fentanyl: neuroendocrine and behavioral responses. Psychoneuroendocrinology 1988;13(5):397–408.

72. Tolis G, Hickey J, Guyda H. Effect of morphine on serum growth hormone, cortisol, prolactin, and thyroid stimulating hormone in man. J Clin Endocrinol Metab 1975;41:797–800.

73. Szalay S, Kemeter P, Feichtinger W, Beck A, Janisch H, Neumark J. The behavior of LH, FSH, PRL, T, P, estradiol and cortisol under different kinds of general anesthesias during laparoscopic oocyte recovery for in vitro fertilization. Europ J Obstet Gynecol Reprod Biol 1982;14:37–48.

74. Brinster RL. Studies on the development of mouse embryos in vitro. 1. The effect of osmolarity on hydrogen concentration. J Exp Zool 1965;158:49–57.

75. Doze VA, White PF. Effect of fluid therapy on serum glucose concentrations in fasted outpatients. Anesthesiology 1985;63(3A):A262.

76. Glasser SA, Siler JN. Serum electrolyte and glucose changes with intravenous fluid administration of D5/½NS solution. Anesthesiology 1985;63(3A):A263.

77. Puissant F, Degueldre M, Buisson L, Leroy F. Effects of carbon dioxide on acidification of mouse oocytes before in vitro fertilization, culture, and transfer. Gamete Res 1986;13:223–230.

78. Quinn P, Harlow GM. The effect of oxygen on the development of preimplantation mouse embryos in vitro. J Exp Zool 1978;206:73–80.

79. Haidri AA, Miller IM, Gwatkin RBL. Culture of mouse oocytes in vitro, using a system without oil or protein. J Reprod Fertil 1971;26:409–411.

80. Gwatkin RBL, Haidri AA. Oxygen requirements for the maturation of hamster oocytes. J Reprod Fertil 1974;37:127–129.

81. Tervitt HR, Whittingham DG, Rowson LEA. Successful culture in vitro of sheep and cattle ova. J Reprod Fertil 1972;30:493–497.

82. Pabon JE, Findley WE, Gibbons WE. The toxic effect of short exposures to the atmospheric oxygen concentration on early mouse embryonic development. Fertil Steril 1989;51(5):896–900.

83. Mastrioianni L, Jones R. Oxygen tension within the rabbit fallopian tube. J Reprod Fertil 1965;9:99–102.

84. Mann T, Jones R, Sherins R. Oxygen damage, lipid peroxidation, and motility of spermatozoa. In: Steinberger A, Steinberger E, eds. Testicular development, structure and function. New York: Raven Press, 1980:497.

85. Dorfmann AD, Bender S, Robinson P, Fugger E, Bustillo JD, Schulman JD. Effects of reduced oxygen concentration on in vitro fertilization and cleavage of human oocytes [abstract P-112] Presented at the 43rd Annual Meeting of the American Fertility Society, Reno, Nev., September 28–30, 1987.

86. Lavy G, Restrepo-Candelo H, Diamond M, Shapiro B, Grunfeld L, DeCherney AH. Laparoscopic and trans-

vaginal ova recovery: the effect on ova quality. Fertil Steril 1988;49:1002–1006.

87. Cohen EN, Belville HW, Brown BW. Anesthesia, pregnancy and miscarriage: a study of operating room nurses and anesthetists. Anesthesiology 1971;35:343–347.

88. Cohen EN, Brown BW, Wu ML, et al. Occupational disease in dentistry and chronic exposure to trace anesthetic gases. J Am Dent Assoc 1980;101:21–31.

89. Fink BR, Shepard TH, Blandau RJ. Teratogenic activity of nitrous oxide. Nature 1967;214:146–148.

90. Lane GA, Nahrwold ML, Tait AR, Taylor-Busch M, Cohen PJ. Anesthetics as teratogens: nitrous oxide is fetotoxic, xenon is not. Science 1980;210:899–901.

91. Crawford JS, Lewis M. Nitrous oxide in early human pregnancy. Anesthesia 1986;41:900–905.

92. Koblin DD, Watson JE, Deady JE, Stokstad ELR, Eger EI II. Inactivation of methionine synthetase by nitrous oxide in mice. Anesthesiology 1981;54:318–324.

93. Mazze RI, Fujinaga M, Baden JM. Halothane prevents nitrous oxide teratogenicity in Sprague-Dawley rats; folinic acid does not. Teratology 1988;38:121–127.

94. Fujinaga M, Baden JM. Effects of nitrous oxide on rat embryos grown in culture. Anesthesiology 1989;71:991–992.

95. Hong K, Trudell JR, O'Neil JR, Cohen EN. Metabolism of nitrous oxide by human and rat intestinal contents. Anesthesiology 1980;52:16–19.

96. Hardy RWF, Knight E Jr. Reduction of N_2O by biological N_2-fixing systems. Biochem Biophys Res Commun 1966;23:409–414.

97. Matsubara T, Mori T. Studies on denitrification. IX. Nitrous oxide, its production and reduction to nitrogen. J Biochem (Tokyo) 1968;64:863–871.

98. Mason RP, Holtzman JL. The mechanism of microsomal and mitochondrial nitroreductase. Electron spin resonance evidence for nitroaromatic free radical intermediates. Biochemistry 1975;14:1626–1632.

99. Rosen MA, Roizen MF, Eger EI II, et al. The effect of nitrous oxide on in vitro fertilization success rate. Anesthesiology 1987;67:42–44.

100. Palot M, Harika G, Pigeon F, Lamiable D, Rendoing J. Propofol in general anesthesia for IVF (by vaginal and transurethral route)—follicular fluid concentration and cleavage rate. Anesthesiology 1988;69(3A):A573.

101. Palot M, Harika G, Visseaux H, et al. Is it necessary to give nitrous oxide during general anesthesia for retrieval of oocytes? Presented at the XXXI Congress of the French Anesthesia Society, 1989 Paris, France.

102. Palot M, Visseaux H, Harika G, Carre-Pigeon F, Rendoing J. Effects of nitrous oxide and/or halothane on cleavage rate during general anesthesia for oocyte retrieval. Anesthesiology 1990;73(3A):A930.

103. Hood AE, Greene JM, Haddy SM, Quinn K, Marrs RP. The addition of nitrous oxide to enflurane anesthesia: effect on reproductive outcome following gamete intrafallopian transfer (GIFT). Anesthesiology 1988;69(3A):A662.

104. Chetkowski RJ, Nass TE. Isoflurane inhibits early mouse embryo development in vitro. Fertil Steril 1988;49(1): 171–173.

105. Rehder K, Forbes J, Alter H. Halothane biotransformation in man: a quantitative study. Anesthesiology 1967;28:711–715.

106. Eger EI II. The pharmacology of isoflurane. Br J Anaesth 1984;56:71S–99S.

107. Mann T. Biochemical basis of spermicidal activity. Proc Soc Study Fertil 1958;9:3–27.

108. Bruce DL, Taurig HH. The effect of halothane on the cell cycle in rat small intestine. Anesthesiology 1969;30: 401–405.

109. Hinckley RE, Webster DR, Rubin RW. Further studies on dividing sea urchin eggs exposed to the volatile anesthetic halothane. Exp Cell Res 1982;141:492–497.

110. Williamson RA, Stenchever MA. The effect of diazepam on rates of fertilization in the CF-1 mouse. Am J Obstet Gynecol 1981;139(2):178–181.

111. Clowes GH, Keltch AK, Krahl ME. The role of changes in extracellular and intracellular hydrogen-ion concentration and the action of local anesthetic bases. J Pharmacol Exp Ther 1940;68:312–329.

112. Lacoumenta S, Paterson JL, Myers MA, Hall GM.

Effects of cortisol suppression by etomidate on changes in circulating metabolites associated with pelvic surgery. Acta Anaesthesiol Scand 1986;30:101–104.

113. Cardasis C, Schuel H. The sea urchin egg as a model system to study effects of narcotics on secretion. In: Ford DH, Clout DH, eds. Tissue responses to addictive drugs. New York: Spectrum, 1976:631–640.

114. Bruce DL, Hinckley R, Norman PF. Fentanyl does not inhibit fertilization or early development in sea urchin eggs. Anesth Analg 1985;64:498–500.

115. Gerber N, Lynn RK. Excretion of methadone in semen from methadone addicts. Life Sci 1976;19:787–791.

116. Joffe JM, Peterson JM, Smith DJ, Soyka LF. Sublethal effects on offspring of male rats treated with methadone before mating. Res Commun Chem Pathol Pharmacol 1976; 13:611–621.

117. Schnell V, Ataya K, Sacco A, Moore R. Lidocaine decreases mouse in vitro fertilization and embryo cleavage [abstract P-153]. Presented at the 44th Annual Meeting of the American Fertility Society, Atlanta, Ga., October 10–13, 1988.

118. Thorneycroft IH, Wun WSA, Ewell M, Wheeler C, McFarland C. The effects of local anesthetics on sperm motility [abstract O22]. Presented at the 44th Annual Meeting of the American Fertility Society, Atlanta, Ga., October 10–13, 1988.

119. Bailey-Pridham DD, Reshef E, Drury K, Cook CL, Hurst HE, Yussman MA. Follicular fluid lidocaine levels during transvaginal oocyte retrieval. Fertil Steril 1990;53(1): 171–173.

120. Benhamou D, Labaille T, Benlabed M, Lamour O, Mazoit JX. Follicular and plasma concentrations after caudal anesthesia for IVF. Anesthesiology 1989;71(3A):A900.

121. Giasi RM, D'Agnostino E, Covino BC. Absorption of lidocaine following subarachnoid and epidural administration. Anesth Analg 1979;58:360–363.

122. Kuhnert BR, Kuhnert PM, Prochaska BS, Gross TL. Plasma levels of 2-chloroprocaine in obstetric patients and their neonates after epidural anesthesia. Anesthesiology 1980; 53:21–25.

123. Orkin FK, Bogetz MS. Back pain following uncom-

plicated epidural anesthesia with chloroprocaine. Anesthesiology 1989;71:A716.

124. Hynson JM, Sessler DI, Glosten B. Back pain in volunteers after epidural anesthesia with chloroprocaine. Anesth Analg 1991;72:253–256.

125. Callan VJ, Henessey JF. Emotional aspects and support in in vitro fertilization and embryo transfer programs. J In Vitro Fert Embryo Transf 1988;5(5):290–295.

126. Nero FA, Diamond MP, Greenfield DA, Greenfield DG, Stronk J, DeCherney AH. Sources of stress in an in-vitro fertilization (IVF) program. Presented at the Fifth World Congress IVF/ET, Norfolk, Va., 1987.

127. Bailey PL, Pace NL, Ashburn MA, Moll JWB, East KA, Stanley TH. Frequent hypoxemia and apnea after sedation with midazolam and fentanyl. Anesthesiology 1990; 73:826–830.

128. Tucker MR, Ochs MW, White RP. Arterial blood gas levels after midazolam or diazepam administered with or without fentanyl as an intravenous sedative for outpatient surgical procedures. J Oral Maxillofac Surg 1986;44:688–692.

129. Bridenbaugh LD, Soderman RM. Lumbar epidural block anesthesia for outpatient laparoscopy. Reprod Med 1979;23(2):85–86.

130. Ciofolo MJ, Clergue F, Seebacher J, LeFebvre G, Viars P. Ventilatory effects of laparoscopy under epidural anesthesia. Anesthesiology 1988;69(3A):A400.

131. Steinbrook RA, Conception M. Respiratory effects of spinal anesthesia: resting ventilation and single-breath CO_2 response. Anesth Analg 1991;72:182–186.

132. Burke RK. Spinal anesthesia for laparoscopy, a review of 1063 cases. Reprod Med 1978;21(1):59–62.

133. Perz RR, Johnson DL, Shinozaki T. Spinal anesthesia for outpatient surgery. Anesth Analg 1988;67:S168.

134. Daya S. Follicular fluid pH changes following intraperitoneal exposure of graafian follicles to carbon dioxide: a comparative study with follicles exposed to ultrasound. Hum Reprod 1988;3(6):727–730.

135. Bromage PR. Concentrations of lignocaine in the blood after intravenous, intramuscular, epidural and endotracheal administration. Anaesthesia 1961;16(4):461–478.

136. Metter SE, Kitz DS, Young ML, Baldeck AM, Apfelbaum JL. Nausea and vomiting after outpatient laparoscopy: incidence, impact on recovery room stay and cost. Anesth Analg 1987;66:S116.

137. Brindley GS. The fertility of men with spinal cord injuries. Paraplegia 1984;22:337–348.

138. Bennett CJ, Ayers JWT, Randolph JF Jr, et al. Electroejaculation of paraplegic males followed by pregnancies. Fertil Steril 1987;48:1070–1072.

139. Ayers JWT, Moinipanah R, Bennett CJ, Randolph JF, Peterson EP. Successful combination therapy with electroejaculation and in vitro fertilization–embryo transfer in the treatment of a paraplegic male with severe oligoasthenospermia. Fertil Steril 1988;49(6):1089–1090.

140. Setchell BP, Waites GMH. The blood-testis barrier. In: Greep RO, Astwood EB, eds. Handbook of physiology, sect 7. Endocrinology, vol 5. Washington, D.C.: American Physiological Society, 1975:143.

141. Malmborg AS, Dornbusch K, Eliasson R, Lindholmer C. Concentrations of various antibacterials in human seminal plasma. In: Proc symp genital infections and their complications. London: Wellcome Foundation, 1974:307.

142. Collier JG, Flower RJ. Effect of aspirin on human seminal prostaglandins. Lancet 1971;2(729):852.

143. Van Thiel DH, Gavaler JS, Cobb CF, Sherins RJ, Lester R. Alcohol-induced testicular atrophy in the adult male rat. Endocrinology 1979;105:888–895.

144. Beattie WS, Forrest JB, Buckley DN, Lindblad T. Nausea and vomiting correlates with estrogen levels and alters dose response for droperidol. Anesthesiology 1989;71(3A):A957.

145. Lindblad T, Forrest JB, Buckley DN, Beattie WS. Anesthesia decreases a hormone mediated threshold for nausea and vomiting. Anesth Analg 1990;70:S1–S450.

146. Slater AJ, Gude N, Clarke IJ, Walters WA. Haemodynamic changes and left ventricular performance during high-dose oestrogen administration to male transsexuals. Br J Obstet Gynaecol 1986;93:532–538.

147. Polishuk WZ, Schenker JG. Ovarian overstimulation syndrome. Fertil Steril 1969;20:443–450.

148. Navot D, Margalioth EJ, Laufer N, et al. Direct correlation between plasma renin activity and severity of the ovarian hyperstimulation syndrome. Fertil Steril 1987;48:57–61.

149. Tollan A, Holst N, Forsdahl F, Fadnes HO, Oian P, Maltau JM. Transcapillary fluid dynamics during ovarian stimulation for in vitro fertilization. Am J Obstet Gynecol 1990;162(2):554–558.

150. Metter SE, Kitz DS, Young ML, Baldeck AM, Apfelbaum JL, Lecky JH. Nausea and vomiting after outpatient laparoscopy: incidence, impact on recovery stay and cost. Anesth Analg 1987;66:S1–S191.

151. Manchikanti L, Colliver JA, Marrero TC, Roush JR. Ranitidine and metoclopramide for prophylaxis of aspiration pneumonitis in elective surgery. Anesth Analg 1984;63:903–910.

152. Stoelting RK. Gastric fluid pH in patients receiving cimetidine. Anesth Analg 1978;57:675–677.

153. Dimich I, Katende R, Singh PP, Mikula S, Sonnenklar N. The effects of intravenous cimetidine and metoclopramide on gastric pH and volume in outpatients. J Clin Anesth 1990;3:40–44.

154. Manchikanti L, Marrero TC, Roush JR. Preanesthetic cimetidine and metoclopramide for aspiration prophlaxis in elective surgery. Anesthesiology 1984;61:48–54.

155. Melnick BM. Extrapyramidal reactions to low-dose droperidol. Anesthesiology 1988;69:424–426.

156. Melnick B, Sawyer R, Karambelkar D, Phitayakorn P, Lim Uy NT, Patel R. Delayed side effects of droperidol after ambulatory general anesthesia. Anesth Anagl 1989;69:748–751.

157. Freeman LA. Ephedrine and hydroxyzine as treatment for post-operative nausea and vomiting. A study of 40 problem patients. Presented at the Society for Ambulatory Anesthesia, 3rd Annual Meeting, 1988 Scottsdale, Arizona.

158. Clemens JD, Horwitz RI, Jaffe CC Feinglein AR, Stanton BF. A controlled evaluation of the risk of bacterial endocarditis in persons with mitral valve prolapse. N Engl J Med 1982;307:776–781.

159. Natof HE. Anesthesia for ambulatory surgery. Wetchler BV, ed. Philadelphia: JB Lippincott, 1985:338.

160. Zosmer A, Katz Z, Lancet M, Konichezky S,

Schwartz-Shoham Z. Adult respiratory distress syndrome complicating ovarian hyperstimulation syndrome. Fertil Steril 1987;47:524–526.

161. Navot D, Relou A, Birkenfeld A, Rabinowitz R, Brezezinski A, Margalioth J. Risk factors and prognostic variables in the ovarian hyperstimulation syndrome. Am J Obstet Gynecol 1988;159:210–215.

162. Friedman CI, Schmidt GE, Chang FE, Kim MA. Severe ovarian hyperstimulation following follicular aspiration. Am J Obstet Gynecol 1984;150:436–437.

163. Schenker JG, Weinstein D. Ovarian hyperstimulation syndrome: a current survey. In: Wallach EE, Kempers RD, eds. Modern trends in infertility and conception control, vol 1. Philadelphia: Harper & Row, 1979:177.

10

Ethical and Legal Issues in Assisted Reproduction

John A. Robertson

Introduction

The use of noncoital or assisted reproductive techniques to overcome infertility is now widely accepted as a matter of both ethics and law, though a number of controversies remain. This chapter reviews the main legal and ethical issues, with an emphasis on assisted reproductive techniques involving in vitro fertilization (IVF).

As an ethical matter, the desires of an infertile married couple to have children biologically related to one or both rearing partners deserves great respect. The use of medical assistance to overcome infertility is generally regarded as an ethically acceptable and worthwhile enterprise. Although some religions oppose any separation of sex and reproduction, the use of noncoital techniques of conception is widely accepted. Concerns about interfering with the natural process have been raised; however, there is no sound ethical basis for finding medical assistance in conception and reproduction more problematic or less acceptable than other medical interventions.

The main ethical concerns that arise from assisted reproduction relate to the effects of the means used on the parties, on offspring, on donors of gametes and surrogates, on women generally, and on society. Although persons might differ in their evaluation of particular techniques, a close examination of the competing concerns reveals that use of particular noncoital techniques to treat infertility can usually be ethically justified as long as informed consent and adequate professional competence are demonstrated.

After describing the constitutional basis for legal regulation of assisted reproduction, this chapter will examine legal issues arising from IVF and manipulations of the preembryo. A final section will discuss legal issues that arise with use of donor gametes and surrogacy.

Constitutional aspects of procreative liberty

Currently, there is little direct regulation of IVF and donor-assisted reproduction in the United States, although it is likely that further regulation will occur. Regulation of noncoital reproduction raises questions of the constitutional power of the state to intervene in procreative choice.

The right to procreate—to do those things that will lead to biologic descendants—is of great significance to persons, but it has not received explicit legal recognition because the state has never attempted to restrict married couples from having children when and how they can. Noncoital conception and donor-assisted reproduction raise questions that require a more precise definition of a constitutional right to procreate. Although there are few precedents directly on point, there is good reason to expect the courts to recognize a constitutional right to procreate by noncoital and donor-assisted means. Such a right will not prevent regulation, but it will protect individual procreative choice unless there is a compelling need for state intervention (1).

On several occasions the United States Supreme Court has indicated strong support for procreative liberty, particularly of married persons. These statements suggest that the Court would recognize such a right if it were ever faced with a direct limitation on a married couple's desire to reproduce by sexual intercourse.

The language in these cases is broad and presumably would extend to both coital and noncoital reproduction, even if the latter were not contemplated at the time. In *Skinner vs. Oklahoma,* the Court struck down a mandatory sterilization law for habitual criminals because it interfered with marriage and procreation, which are among "the basic rights of man" (316 U.S. 535, 541 [1942]). In *Meyer vs. Nebraska,* the Court stated that constitutional liberty includes "the right of an individual to marry, establish a home and bring up children" (262 U.S. 390, 399 [1923]). Finally, Justice Brennan, in *Eisenstadt vs. Baird,* stated: "If the right of privacy means anything, it is the right of the individual, married or single, to be free of unwarranted governmental intrusion into matters so fundamentally affecting a person as the decision whether to bear or beget a child" (405 U.S. 438, 453 [1972]).

The argument for the right to reproduce coitally is clearest in the case of married persons but can also be made for unmarried persons. Although most of the Supreme Court dicta cited above apply explicitly to married persons, a strong argument can be made that unmarried persons also have a right to reproduce coitally, because they also have needs to have and rear biologic descendants, may be as competent parents as married couples, yet may be unable or unwilling to marry to satisfy this desire.

Noncoital and donor-assisted reproduction and the right to reproduce

The Supreme Court's statements supporting a couple's right to marry and found a family generally assume that reproduction will occur only as a result of sexual intercourse, because the statements were made before IVF and widespread use of donor sperm occurred. However, the couple's interest in reproducing is the same, no matter how reproduction occurs. The values and interests underlying a right to coital reproduction strongly suggest a married couple's right to noncoital reproduction as well and, arguably, to the assistance of donors and surrogates, as needed (2).

Coital reproduction is legally protected not for the coitus but for what the coitus makes possible: it enables the couple to unite egg and sperm in order to acquire the possibility of rearing a child of their own genes and gestation. The use of noncoital techniques, such as IVF or artificial insemination, to unite egg and husband's sperm, necessitated by the couple's infertility, should then also be protected.

The married couple's right to reproduce should thus extend to noncoital means of conception, which include the wide range of choices made possible by developments in IVF. The couple would then have the right to create, store, and have transferred to them extracorporeal preembryos created by their egg and sperm. They would have the right to determine whether their gametes would be used for reproduction and determine the disposition of preembryos created with their gametes, which would include a right to donate preembryos to other couples. Indeed, the right might also be found to extend to posthumous reproduction, which might occur with stored sperm or preembryos after the death of a spouse (3).

A strong legal argument can also be made that a married couple's procreative liberty would include the right to enlist the assistance of a third-party donor or surrogate to provide the gametes or uterine function necessary for the couple to beget, bear, or otherwise acquire for rearing a child genetically related to one of the partners. Although not as directly entailed as the right of noncoital conception, the logic and values behind protecting marital procreation suggest that the need for assistance of a third-party collaborator should be similarly treated. The donor is essential if the couple is to rear a child who has a gametic or gestational connection to them. Because the couple would be free, if fertile, to reproduce as often as they wanted to, they should be free to procreate with the help of gamete donors or the uterus of a willing surrogate gestator.

If this argument is accepted, couples attempting to reproduce would have the right to engage in a wide range of activities involving donors and extracorporeal preembryos. They would have the right to contract with others for the provision of gametes or preembryos, with the contract settling the parties' rearing rights and duties toward resulting offspring. A contractual approach would also extend to contracts with surrogates for them to gestate the couple's preembryo and to return it to them for rearing. Strictly analyzed, the logic of marital procreative liberty would require the state to enforce such contracts and would allow fees to be paid to donors for the various services provided. States might then regulate the circumstances under which parties would enter into reproductive contracts, but they would not ban such transactions altogether.

In short, the interests and values supporting the right to reproduce by sexual intercourse apply equally to noncoital activities involving the extracorporeal preembryo. Although the case is strongest for a couple's right to reproduce noncoitally, a strong argument can also be made for their right to enlist the aid of gamete donors and surrogates. Both methods enable a couple to rear a child who is the biologic descendant of, or who has been gestated by, one of them. Unmarried persons would also have the right to reproduce through extracorporeal fertilization and donor assistance if their right to coital reproduction were recognized.

Constitutional limits on noncoital reproduction

If the logic of procreative rights is strictly analyzed by the courts, the procreative rights of married couples would extend to noncoital activities that are essential for them to reproduce as described above. Constitutional rights, however, are no absolute, and restrictions might be imposed when necessary to serve important state interests. The question is whether noncoital and donor-assisted techniques pose harm to state interests sufficient to justify restriction of the procreative choices involving them.

Noncoital and donor-assisted reproduction raise a variety of concerns, from duties to extracorporeal preembryos to concern for the welfare of offspring, the family, and donors and surrogates. There are also more general societal concerns about dehumanizing or reifying reproduction through excessive technologizing and commercialization.

Although these are valid concerns that will influence individual choice, they may not be a constitutionally sufficient basis for preventing couples from using these techniques when the need for any particular restriction is scrutinized. Preembryo freezing and donation or contracts with gamete donors and surrogates may not risk sufficient tangible harm to the parties or the offspring to warrant state interference with the constitutional right to procreate. Their validity will have to be determined as disputes and efforts to limit access to noncoital assisted reproduction arise.

Existing laws that appear to limit noncoital reproduction by married persons are constitutionally dubious and may well be struck down if challenged in the courts. Fetal and preembryo research laws that appear to restrict a married couple's control of preembryos for reproduction are most vulnerable to attack. Also, existing legal presumptions about who is the rearing father or mother in situations of donor gametes and surrogacy may also fall when the full implications of marital procreative liberty are recognized. However, it should be noted that the New Jersey Supreme Court in the *Baby M* case (109 N.J. 396, 421–422, 537 A.2d 1227, 1240 [1988]) did not accept this constitutional argument. It held that neither could a surrogate mother's contract be enforced, nor could money be paid to a surrogate for her services. Other courts have also been inconsistent in recognizing the full implications of procreative liberty for noncoital and assisted reproduction. Still, a cogent argument for extending the couple's procreative liberty to include these activities should be recognized, for it will influence future cases and policy-making.

Two kinds of state restrictions, however, are constitutionally permissible: laws that prevent the couple, donors, and surrogates from maintaining anonymity if the offspring's welfare requires disclosure; and

regulations designed to ensure free, informed entry into donor and surrogate transactions in order to protect the autonomy of the parties.

Intangible religious, moral, or societal concerns about the nature of reproduction, family, the reproductive roles of women, and the power of science would not ordinarily justify interference with procreative liberty. Such deeply held religious or moral views about reproductive relations are of immense importance to individuals and to society, for these views represent value choices that constitute individual and societal moral commitment. However, moral, religious, or symbolic concerns that do not have direct, tangible effects on others are not sufficient constitutional grounds for interfering with fundamental rights of persons with different views.

Thus particular moral views of the rightness or wrongness of particular means of conception might properly animate individual and institutional choices to avoid, seek, or provide such services. Neither physicians nor institutions in the private sector are obligated to provide noncoital or extracorporeal reproductive services of any particular kind. Nor are persons obligated to use their reproductive capacity to assist the reproduction of others. The state is not constitutionally obligated to fund such services any more than it is obligated to fund abortions. But there is a limit to direct state interference with noncoital reproductive choice.

In sum, it appears that the constitutional status of procreative liberty requires that the legal system leave noncoital and donor-assisted reproduction largely to the moral decision of the physicians, patients, and institutions involved.

The moral and legal status of the preembryo

Many issues in noncoital reproduction concern the actions that may appropriately be taken with preembryos. In vitro fertilization is of great significance because it isolates the preembryo and makes it accessible to observation or intervention. The status of the preembryo must therefore be considered apart from the status of preembryos and fetuses at more advanced stages of development within the mother's body.

The moral and legal status of the preembryo will determine the limits of actions and omissions regarding preembryos and thus the freedom that physicians and patients have in activities concerning preembryos. The main issues that depend on preembryo status are these: what can be done to preembryos before transfer; whether all preembryos must be transferred; and, if not, what can be done to preembryos that are not transferred.

The questions raised are novel but not unanswerable. Although the extracorporeal preembryo has never had to be considered before, legal and moral principles exist to guide analysis and evaluation of this new situation. Indeed, precedents applying these principles to the situation of the extracorporeal preembryo are also emerging.

Different positions in the debate over preembryo status

Three major ethical positions have been articulated in the debate over preembryo status (4). At one extreme is the view of the preembryo as a human subject after fertilization, which requires that it be accorded the rights of a person. This position entails an obligation to provide an opportunity for implantation to occur and tends to ban any action before transfer that might harm the preembryo or that is not immediately therapeutic, such as freezing and some preembryo research.

At the opposite extreme is the view that the pre-embryo has a status no different from that of any other human tissue. With the consent of those who have decision-making authority over the preembryo, no limits should be imposed on actions taken with preembryos.

A third view—one that is most widely held—takes an intermediate position between the other two. It holds that the preembryo deserves respect greater than that accorded to human tissue but not the respect accorded to actual persons. The preembryo is due greater respect than other human tissue because of its potential to become a person and because of its symbolic meaning for many people. Yet, it should not be treated as a person, because it has not yet developed the features of personhood, is not yet established as developmentally individual, and may never realize its biologic potential.

Emerging consensus: special respect

An analysis of the question of preembryo status shows that there is considerably more consensus than is generally recognized (4). When law, ethical commentary, and the reports of official or professional advisory bodies are consulted, there is a wide consensus that the preembryo has a special moral status but not a status equivalent to that of a person.

The United States' Ethics Advisory Board, for example, unanimously agreed in 1979 that "the human preembryo [i.e., preembryo in this report] is entitled to profound respect, but this respect does not necessarily encompass the full legal and moral rights attributed to persons."

In 1984, the Warnock Committee in Great Britain took a similar position when it stated that "the human preembryo . . . is not under the present law of the United Kingdom accorded the same status as a living child or an adult, nor do we necessarily wish it to be accorded the same status. Nevertheless, we were agreed that the preembryo of the human species ought to have a special status."

The Ontario Law Reform Commission (Canada), which completed an extensive review of the issue in

1985, also took this view, as have nearly all other professional and official advisory bodies that have reviewed the question of preembryo status (5). Only groups holding the view that "personhood" begins at conception have taken a different position.

The advisory body conclusions parallel the traditional Anglo-American legal view of prenatal life. Given the legal precedents about fetuses of more advanced development, it is extremely unlikely that American law would assign to the preembryo the rights of persons (6). The law does not regard fetuses or preembryos as rights-bearing entities, although it has recognized that prenatal actions could affect the postnatal well-being of persons. In most states the preembryo is not a legal subject in its own right and is not protected by laws against homicide or wrongful death, nor is discard prohibited. However, three or four states have recently passed statutes that do protect extracorporeal preembryos from destruction. Aside from these few states, the preembryo generally has legal cognizance only if the interests of an actual person are at stake, such as when transfer occurs and offspring may be affected or when someone wrongfully interferes with the authority of another person to determine disposition of the preembryo.

The biology of early human preembryo development supports this legal status. Since the preembryo does not have differentiated organs, much less the developed brain, nervous system, and capacity for sentience that legal subjects ordinarily have, it cannot easily be regarded as a legal subject. Indeed, the preembryo is not yet individual, because twinning or mosaicism can still occur. Thus, it is not surprising that the law does not recognize the preembryo itself as a legal subject.

The widespread consensus that the preembryo is not a person but is to be treated with special respect because it is a genetically unique, living human entity that might become a person has certain implications. In cases in which transfer to a uterus is possible, special respect is necessary to protect the welfare of potential offspring. In such cases, the preembryo deserves respect because it might come into existence as a person. This viewpoint imposes the traditional duty of reasonable prenatal care when actions risk harm to prospective offspring. Research on or intervention with a preembryo, followed by transfer, thus creates obligations not to hurt or injure the offspring who might be born after transfer.

With regard to the questions of whether all preembryos must be transferred to a uterus and whether research can be conducted with nontransferred preembryos, the demands of special respect are less clear. Persons who view the preembryo itself as a human subject with the same rights as newborn infants would require that all preembryos be transferred and would greatly limit nontherapeutic research with nontransferred preembryos. Others may agree that preembryos should be transferred whenever reasonably possible but would allow discard and preembryo research in certain circumstances. These issues should be reviewed in advance by institutional review boards or other authorized and legitimate authorities.

Legal status of the preembryo

Legal status—position or standing in law—will define what rights, if any, early preembryos have and what duties are owed to them, thus determining what might be done with these entities and by whom. The main issues of legal status are who may properly exercise decisional authority over preembryos and what limits, if any, the state may or should place on that dispositional authority.

Although the legal status of early preembryos is still largely indeterminate, the main issues and trends in defining that status can be identified. At issue in determining legal status are several questions relating to the locus and scope of decisional authority over pre-embryos. With regard to decisional authority, the questions are what actors have decisional authority, whether they may exercise that authority in advance, and how decisional disputes will be resolved.

With regard to the scope of decisional authority, the issues of legal status concern whether early preembryos may or must be created, placed in a uterus, allowed to implant and continue to term, be frozen, be transferred among preembryo banks, be used in research, be donated to others, and be bought and sold, examined, and manipulated. While answers to some issues might depend on one's views of the preembryo's moral status, most answers will depend on one's evaluation of the importance of the interests sought through the pre-embryo activity in question.

A major legal status issue concerns who has decisional authority over fertilized eggs and early preembryos, a question analytically separate from the scope of that authority. "Who" has the right or authority to choose among available options for disposition of early preembryos is a question separate from "what" those dispositional options are.

The question of decisional authority is really the question of who owns or has a property interest in early preembryos. Applying terms such as "ownership" or "property" to early preembryos risks misunderstanding. Such terms do not signify that preembryos may be treated in all respects like other property. Rather, the terms merely designate who has authority to decide whether legally available options with early pre-embryos will occur, such as creation, storage, discard, donation, use in research, and placement in a uterus. Although the bundle of property rights attached to one's ownership of a preembryo may be more circum-scribed than for other things, it is an ownership or property interest nonetheless.

Each gamete provider separately, the couple jointly, their transferees, the physicians who create the pre-embryos, and the IVF program or preembryo bank that has actual possession are all possible candidates for decisional authority over early preembryos; however, the couple that provides the gametes to create the preembryos has the strongest claim to decisional author-ity or ownership of the preembryo (7). The more interesting questions concern whether and how they have exercised that authority, and whether advance instructions for disposition will be binding if their preferences or circumstances change.

Positive law has not yet explicitly recognized the gamete providers' joint property or decisional authority in external preembryos, but it is a reasonably safe assumption that the courts would so hold when confronted with disputes raising that issue.

The couple's joint ownership of preembryos cre-ated from their gametes, including a right of survi-vorship, is thus highly likely to be recognized as a matter of positive law. Since most IVF programs and preembryo banks are likely to honor the couple's ownership, the issue would be directly joined only if a program or bank refused to return or to release a stored preembryo. The question would also arise if the program intentionally or negligently destroyed the preembryo. For example, the couple's ownership of preembryos was implicitly recognized in *Del Zio vs. Columbia Presbyterian Hospital,* in which the couple was awarded $50,000 damages by a jury for intentional infliction of emotional distress when a doctor who objected to their efforts at IVF, without prior institu-tional review board approval, destroyed their incubat-ing preembryo (8).

Negligent or inadvertent destruction of preem-bryos, due to equipment malfunction or human error, is also likely to be actionable, or should be so because of the significant financial, physical, and emotional loss that it imposes. Only difficulties in calculating damages, and not doubts about the ownership rights of the couple, would stand in the way of tort remedies for negligent destruction of preembryos. However, except for the *Del Zio* case, no cases of damages for negligent destruction of preembryos have been reported.

York vs. Jones, a recent case involving two of the largest IVF programs in the United States, illustrates the question of ownership (9). A doctor and his wife living in New Jersey were infertile owing to problems with the wife's fallopian tubes. They sought IVF treatment at the Jones Institute in Norfolk, Virginia, the first and most successful IVF program in the United States. After moving to California, they returned to the Jones Institute three times for ovarian stimulation and egg retrieval (requiring a 3-week stay each time). The first two IVF attempts each produced three preembryos, which were placed in the wife's uterus, but no pregnancy resulted. The third attempt led to the placement of five preembryos in the wife, with a sixth preembryo frozen for later use.

After the third failure at an IVF pregnancy, the couple decided to pursue further efforts to achieve pregnancy at a leading IVF clinic in Los Angeles. They informed the Norfolk program that they wished to transport their frozen preembryo to California to be thawed and placed in the wife by their Los Angeles physician. Mr. York would travel to Norfolk and transport the preembryo in a sterile safe pack by commercial airliner to Los Angeles for thawing or further storage by their California physician.

The Norfolk program refused to release the frozen preembryo to the couple for shipment to California. It claimed that the couple had agreed to have the preembryo thawed for placement in the wife only in Norfolk, and that if they chose not to have thawing and placement occur in Norfolk, they could choose only to have the preembryo donated to another infertile couple, donated for research, or thawed, but not placed in a uterus. They also raised practical and legal objections to shipping preembryos from one program to another. Their objections included loss of refrigerant, theft or blackmail of the preembryo during shipment, the demeaning effect of shipping human embryos by air "ala [sic] cattle preembryos," lack of institutional review board approval, and liability risk of shipping to an unqualified program.

The couple then sued in federal district court in Norfolk for custody of their preembryo and damages for unlawful retention. The district judge denied the defendant's motion to dismiss for failure to state a claim (717 F. Supp. 421 [E.D. Va. 1989]). Shortly after this ruling the case was settled, and the Yorks were permitted to remove their frozen preembryo to Los Angeles.

York vs. Jones is significant because it is the first case directly dealing with a dispute between an IVF program and a couple over custody of a frozen preembryo. The court assumes without question that preembryos are the property of the gamete providers and finds that a transfer or relinquishment of their dispositional authority must be explicitly stated in the documents of participation provided by the program. It would strictly construe any documents purporting to effect such a transfer against the programs that drafted them. While a program could still insist that the preembryos that it creates not be transferred to other locations, such a restriction would be binding only if it clearly stated that the couple would have no right to remove their preembryos for placement elsewhere.

An important remaining legal question for gamete providers and for IVF programs and preembryo banks is whether joint advance instructions for disposition of preembryos will be legally binding. Binding advance instructions are important both to avoid and to resolve later disputes, and to give both gamete providers and physicians certainty about what disposition will occur in case of future contingencies such as death, divorce, passage of time, unavailability, or disagreement among the parties. If the gamete providers have joint dispositional control of external preembryos, their power to give advance binding instructions for disposition of their preembryos should also be recognized.

Such advance instructions would ordinarily be given at the time that preembryos are created or frozen. As part of the informed consent procedure, the gamete providers will be informed of the dispositional alternatives that are available at that program or bank—for example, whether preembryo discard or donation is permitted and the length of permissible storage. At that time, many programs may ask the couple to designate certain dispositional alternatives if contingencies such as divorce, death, disagreement, or unavailability occur. In some cases it may be possible for the couple to reserve the right to change their designated disposition at later times, but until they do, the options selected would be binding when the specified events occurred.

The legal question is whether those designated choices will be legally binding on the couple when the stated contingency occurs and one party at that time disagrees or wishes to make a different disposition, or when both partners wish to deviate from the conditions and restrictions of the IVF program to which they initially agreed.

The argument for recognizing the binding effect of joint advance instructions and acceptance of IVF program conditions rests on several grounds (10). The right to use preembryos to reproduce or to avoid reproduction should include the right to give binding advance instructions because certainty about consequences is necessary to exercise reproductive options. In addition, all parties gain from the ability to rely on prior instructions when future contingencies occur. Finally, it minimizes the frequency and cost of resolving disputes that arise over disposition of preembryos.

But arguments against binding oneself in advance also exist. Advance instructions may be issued at a time relatively early in the process of seeking pregnancy through IVF, when a person's needs and interests may not be as fully realized as they would be when later events occur. One's interests and preferences might change as future events unfold, in ways that cannot be foreseen when the instructions are given. Since preconception agreements to abort, not to abort, or to give up for adoption are not enforceable, one could argue that neither should preconception or preimplantation agreements for the disposition of preembryos be enforced. Also, there may be no easy way to ensure that the parties are fully informed and aware of the legally binding choices that they would be making. Finally, IVF programs and preembryo banks may have such monopoly power that the conditions they offer give couples little real choice, making them the equivalent of adhesion contracts.

The view most likely to prevail in such situations is to give binding effect to the parties' prior agreement for disposition of preembryos when they are unavailable or unable to agree between themselves (10). The advantages of such a position seem to outweigh the disadvantages and should be recognized by courts dealing with disputes on these issues. IVF programs and institutions directly involved with these matters should seek to have such agreements made and should inform the parties that they will be regarded as binding.

Divorce and disposition of cryopreserved preembryos

These principles may be illustrated by the widely publicized controversy that arose in 1989 in Tennessee over disposition of seven cryopreserved preembryos by a divorcing couple. The wife had insisted that the preembryos be available to her for thawing and placement in her uterus or that of a recipient. The husband objected to the idea of children from a marriage that had failed. The trial judge had awarded "custody" of the preembryos to the wife, on the ground that the preembryos were "children" whose best interests required the chance to implant and come to term (11). The couple had given no directions at the time of freezing as to disposition.

A Tennessee appellate court eventually reversed the trial court decision, requiring that any disposition of the preembryos be jointly agreed to by the husband and wife. The key point of the appellate decision was its reversal of the trial court's decision that preembryos are "children" whose best interests must be protected by implantation (12). The appeals court recognized that the dispute was not over an existing pregnancy, but over disposition of seven fertilized ova at the four- to eight-cell stage of development. At this stage "there is no development of the nervous system, the circulatory system, or the pulmonary system." It also noted that cryopreserved preembryos have a low chance of implanting and going to term.

Under Tennessee law preembryos had no legal status that required that implantation occur. Prenatal stages prior to quickening had never been legally recognized. The state's wrongful death statute did not permit recovery for the death of a viable fetus unless it is first born alive. Tennessee law also allowed abortion after viability to save the life of the mother. Nor do state murder statutes make abortion or the in utero death of a fetus by a third party a crime.

Given this recognition of the biologic status of preembryos, protecting them by giving them the chance to implant and come to term was not a sufficiently compelling justification for overriding the husband's "constitutionally protected right not to beget a child where no pregnancy has taken place."

The court thus concluded that the trial court had "ignored the public policy implicit in the Tennessee statutes, the case holdings of the Tennessee Supreme Court and the teachings of the United States Supreme Court" in treating preembryos as "children" whose interests must be protected. The court concluded: "On the facts of this case, it would be repugnant and offensive to constitutional principles to order Mary Sue to implant these fertilized ova against her will. It would be equally repugnant to order Junior to bear the pyschological, if not the legal, consequences of paternity against his will." (*Davis vs. Davis,* C/A No. 180, Tennessee Court of Appeals, September 13, 1990)

Since the parties share an interest in the seven preembryos, the court ruled in *Davis vs. Davis* that they should have "joint control of the fertilized ova and . . . equal voice over their disposition." Thus if both parties agree, the preembryos may be kept in storage, thawed and not transferred, donated to an infertile couple, or used by one or the other of them to initiate pregnancy. If they disagree, the preembryos will presumably remain in storage.

The appellate court's decision is a sound resolution of the dispute in the *Davis* case and should be a model for resolution of future disputes of this sort. The court is clearly correct in ruling that preembryos are not children. The lower court had ignored biologic reality in finding that preembryos are "in vitro children" because they are genetically unique. But genetic uniqueness and potential to implant and come to term do not mean that sufficient development has occurred to endow an entity with interests or rights. In so holding, the trial court gave preembryos a status that has been accepted only by persons who believe that personhood begins at fertilization.

A clear implication of the appellate court decision is that preembryos could be thawed and not transferred, or otherwise discarded. Since common law and Tennessee precedents give the preembryo no independent legal status, and Tennessee has not passed legislation requiring that all preembryos be placed in the uterus, nontransfer of preembryos, either before or after cryopreservation, is a legally available option. Unless a state has specifically prohibited preembryo discard (as Louisiana, New Mexico, and possibly Minnesota have done) or an IVF program requires that all preembryos be placed in a woman, persons undergoing IVF may request that unwanted preembryos not be transferred.

The court also correctly recognized that placing the disputed preembryos in the uterus over the objection of one partner would have the effect of making that partner a parent against his will. The appellate court, however, did not recognize the effect of its ruling against unwanted placement on the party wishing to use the disputed preembryos for reproduction. By giving priority to the husband's interest in not reproducing, the court implicitly interferes with the wife's interest in having children. Since a decision in either direction would interfere with the procreative liberty of one of the parties, it is not obvious why the wife's interest in reproducing should be subordinated to the husband's interest in avoiding reproduction, anymore than his interests should be subordinated to hers.

In the facts of this case, however, this apparent contradiction may not be serious. The wife has already remarried and appears to be a medically suitable candidate to produce other preembryos with her new spouse. Giving priority to the husband's desire not to have the disputed preembryos come to term does not prevent her from achieving parenthood with preembryos created with her new spouse.

In other cases in which there is no prior agreement on disposition, however, the courts should resolve such disputes according to whether the party wishing to preserve the preembryos has a realistic possibility of achieving his or her reproductive goals by other means. If there are no alternative opportunities to reproduce, it may be fairer to award the preembryos to the party for

whom they represent the last chance to have offspring, as might occur if the wife has lost ovarian function since the preembryos were preserved. In that case, the unconsenting party should also be relieved of child support obligations.

To avoid disputes such as occurred in *Davis vs. Davis* and give all participants (including the physicians and IVF program) certainty about future outcomes, the best solution would be for couples to designate at the time of cryopreservation the disposition they desire in case of divorce, dispute, or unavailability. Although the Tennessee court did not address the enforceability of such agreements (none had been signed in the *Davis* case), it is reasonable to assume that such agreements would be legally binding. This solution best serves the interests of all parties and minimizes the chance that litigation will occur.

In sum, the Tennessee decision is a much needed corrective to an inappropriate and poorly reasoned trial court decision and should be a model for resolving future disputes. It shows that the law is gradually arriving at a reasoned approach to the legal issues presented by assisted reproduction involving preembryos. IVF programs and couples should proceed with cryopreservation on the assumption that advance agreements for disposition of preembryos will be binding. They should also assume that the dispositional authority of couples includes choices for discard or for nontransfer of preembryos, except in those states that have specifically required that all preembryos be transferred or in programs that wish to limit that option.

Limits on the scope of authority over preembryos

Having seen that the gamete providers and their transferees have decisional authority over preembryos, we now consider the limits that the state may impose on exercise of that authority. Is their ownership of or property interest in early preembryos absolute, or may the state qualify or limit it in certain ways? As noted above, the answer to this question will depend on the reproductive interests implicated and the state's reasons for limiting the couple's ownership. Although some issues will turn on views of early preembryo moral status, most will turn on the reproductive interests at stake. The main questions that arise are whether the state could limit a couple's wishes to discard unwanted preembryos, to donate them to infertile couples, or to donate them for research.

Discard or nontransfer of preembryos

Cryopreservation avoids the dilemma of not inseminating or transferring all fertilized eggs; however, the question of discard or nontransfer of preembryos will inevitably arise even with cryopreservation. If the couple no longer wishes preembryos thawed for transfer to the egg source, they may want them to be discarded rather than donated to others.

Many IVF programs insist on transferring all fertilized eggs to the uterus, but this is not a legal requirement. Legally, the gamete providers, their transferees, and the storing facilities may discard preembryos that they do not want transferred to a uterus. Except in Minnesota, Louisiana, and possibly Illinois, destruction or discard of a preembryo is not covered by homicide or feticide laws (13).

Many persons would agree that the best solution to disposition of unwanted preembryos is to follow the couple's wishes. Some persons, however, will view preembryo discard or nontransfer as violating the rights of the preembryo, or so demeaning to human dignity and community that they will oppose granting couples this discretion. They may seek laws preventing discard and nontransfer, as Louisiana has done and as other states are likely to do, or they may seek laws prohibiting

insemination of more eggs (for example, four) than can safely be placed in the woman. An important question for IVF programs and couples undergoing IVF is whether laws that banned preembryo discard are within the constitutional power of the state.

The constitutionality of state laws that seek to prevent the discard or destruction of IVF preembryos does not depend on whether *Roe vs. Wade,* the case recognizing a woman's right to terminate pregnancy, is reversed. *Roe* protects a woman's interest in not having preembryos placed in her body, in not having preembryos inside her body implant in the walls of the uterus, or in terminating implantation (pregnancy) that has occurred. *Roe* would not directly apply to state restrictions on external preembryos that do not interfere with a woman's interest in bodily integrity. Under *Roe,* the state would be free to treat external preembryos as persons or give as much protection to their potential life as it chooses, as long as it did not trench on a woman's bodily integrity.

Are state laws that prevent preembryo discard or that require donation rather than destruction of unwanted preembryos then constitutionally valid? Although such laws do not infringe on the right of bodily integrity, they do interfere with decisions about having biologic offspring. A cogent argument, based on Supreme Court contraceptive cases, exists for finding a fundamental right to avoid biologic offspring. Even if parenthood entails only psychological burdens, as would occur with mandatory donation of unwanted preembryos, a person should still be free to decide whether an event of such paramount importance to personal identity will occur. If this argument were accepted, a state's desire to signify the importance of human life by giving preembryos the chance to implant and come to term would not constitute the compelling interest necessary to justify infringement of a fundamental right to avoid reproduction.

The counterargument (which I think is stronger) is that the Supreme Court is unlikely to recognize the right to avoid biologic offspring *tout court* as a fundamental right even if *Roe* remains intact (14). *Griswold, Roe,* and their progeny establish a right to avoid reproduction when reproduction is necessarily coupled with gestation or rearing burdens. Laws that prohibit preembryo destruction or that mandate preembryo donation can be written to protect preembryos without imposing any rearing duties on the persons who have provided the egg and sperm, thus imposing on them only the burden of having unknown biologic offspring.

It is unlikely that a Supreme Court disinclined to expand the menu of unwritten fundamental rights will accord the purely psychosocial interest in not having biologic offspring fundamental right status, even if *Roe* remains intact. If the Court found that no fundamental right to avoid genetic offspring *tout court* existed, then the state's interest in protecting preembryos by requiring donation of unwanted extras would easily meet the rational basis test by which such a statute would be judged. *Roe vs. Wade* presents no obstacle to such a law as long as the woman herself is not forced to accept the preembryos into her body.

It should be noted, however, that discussion applies to state restrictions on discard or nontransfer of preembryos. IVF programs are still free to refuse to participate in nontransfer or discard of preembryos, as long as they inform couples at the outset that they will not have this option. However, couples might still be free to remove their cryopreserved preembryos to other storage facilities at which such options exist.

Preembryo donation

Although preembryo donation for transfer to an infertile couple may occur independently of freezing, cryopreservation increases the likelihood of donation, because synchronization of menstrual cycles is facilitated.

Widespread preembryo banking with shipment to distant points will increase the choice of prospective recipients, just as sperm banking does. At present there appears to be no ethical or legal barrier to preembryo donations.

Preembryo donations enable preembryos that would otherwise have been discarded to be transferred and possibly brought to term. The separation of genetic from gestational and rearing parents that results is not so harmful to offspring that donation should be prohibited. But for the donation the offspring would never have existed. Indeed, preembryo donation provides a closer link with rearing parents than does postbirth adoption because the rearing mother will also have gestated.

Legally, states have no laws specifically regulating preembryo donations and few that apply by analogy. Although sometimes referred to as preembryo "adoptions," legal provisions applying to postbirth adoptions of children do not apply to donation of preimplantation preembryos. Thus no prior agency or court review of parental fitness is legally required. Preembryo donations are so close to sperm and egg donations that they should be treated similarly (15).

IVF programs and physicians, however, should use due care in arranging preembryo donations, as they would in using donor sperm. They should require the donating couple to execute a form relinquishing their rights and interests in the preembryo. The recipient should sign a form acknowledging the donation and agreeing to rear any children born as a result. Although the donating and recipient parties may strongly desire anonymity, confidential records of the transactions should be maintained in case the offspring at some later point is accorded a legal right to learn of his or her genetic roots.

As a legal transaction, the donating couple transfers their decisional authority over the preembryo and rearing rights and duties in resulting offspring to the recipient.

The recipient assumes rearing rights and duties in the preembryo that she gestates and brings to term. The genetic parents are eliminated as rearing or social parents, with the gestational parent and her consenting partner taking on rearing rights and duties. The offspring becomes the legitimate child of the recipient couple for all purposes unless specified otherwise.

Legislation specifying this result is probably desirable; however, it is likely that a preembryo donation agreement will be recognized by courts adjudicating disputes about custody, support, visitation, and inheritance even in the absence of legislation. Indeed, the Warnock Committee and other advisory groups have recommended a similar result in the case of preembryo donations for transfer.

An exception to the donor and recipient's right to settle rearing relationships in resulting offspring might arise from the offspring's interest in knowing his or her genetic roots. Because adopted children and offspring of donor sperm often have strong desires to learn their genetic roots, offspring born of preembryo donations might also wish to know their genetic parents. Although most states do not currently give adopted children this right, laws permitting offspring to learn their genetic identities would appear to be a valid ground for overriding promises of anonymity or confidentiality in the donation contract. In the meantime, IVF programs participating in preembryo donations should maintain records on donors so that such information is available if the right is later granted to offspring.

Preembryo donation for research

Cryopreserved preembryos may also be donated for research if the storing couple no longer wishes them transferred to initiate pregnancy. In most cases preembryos donated for research will be discarded after completion of the research. In a few cases, however,

transfer to a uterus may occur, in effect making it a donation for research and possible transfer.

The question of preembryo research has been controversial in Australia, Great Britain, and, to a lesser extent, the United States (16). To avoid controversy, many researchers are reluctant to conduct studies on human preembryos. However, developments in IVF and other fields will increasingly draw researchers to human preembryos as vehicles for research in infertility, contraception, genetics, cancer, and other fields.

Despite the cautious approach taken to preembryo research, a consensus recognizing the ethical and legal acceptability of preembryo research can be identified. Official and advisory bodies in the United States, Great Britain, Canada, and Australia have considered preembryo research and found it acceptable in well-designed studies approved by institutional review boards. Most of these bodies would limit extracorporeal preembryo research to 14 days. They would also permit transfer to a uterus when there is reasonable ground for thinking that the resulting offspring will be healthy. With the exception of Victoria in Australia, they would even permit research on preembryos created solely for that purpose.

Thus there is no question that stored preembryos created to treat infertility may be donated for research before discard. Such research does not harm preembryos and thus does not raise the ethical problems of research with nonviable abortuses and dying persons. If done for valid purposes, it is as consistent with respect for preembryos as is research with human subjects generally. A few American states have broadly drawn fetal research laws that might appear to prohibit any preembryo research. However, unless narrowly interpreted, such laws are vulnerable to constitutional challenge as an interference with first amendment and procreative rights.

IVF programs that offer cryopreservation should therefore inform couples storing preembryos of their right to donate them for research if they do not wish them thawed and transferred to a uterus. This option should be explored at the time of initial storage and when later decisions are made. By analogy to organ donation, request for donation of preembryos for research should be considered in all cases in which preembryos will not be placed in a uterus.

Such requests will be helpful to researchers who need discarded preembryos to conduct studies that will benefit infertile couples and others in the future. Donation of preembryos for research may also provide meaning for couples when the preembryo cannot be placed in the woman or donated to an infertile couple. It will also lessen the need to create preembryos solely for research, although it will not eliminate this controversial issue altogether.

Collaborative reproduction: donors and surrogates

An important component of noncoital or assisted reproduction is the use of donor gametes and surrogacy. With donor sperm, there is ordinarily no creation or manipulation of preembryos, though sometimes IVF is used for various forms of male factor infertility. However, egg donation, preembryo donation, and the use of a surrogate gestator necessarily involve IVF-created preembryos. Surrogacy arrangements in which the surrogate also provides the egg will also usually not involve the creation of preembryos.

The main issues that arise with these forms of noncoital reproduction, as with those forms discussed above, are whether they may legally be done at all, what the resulting rearing rights and duties are with regard to offspring, and whether anonymity and confidentiality are required or may be assured. Although donor sperm has been explicitly legally recognized in 28 states, and a few states have legislated on some aspects of surrogacy,

many legal issues in the use of donor gametes and surrogacy have not yet been addressed by the courts or legislatures. As noted above, a strong case for a constitutional right to treat infertility through the use of donor gametes and surrogacy can by made and is likely to be recognized, with the possible exception of cases of surrogacy. A brief discussion of each form of collaborative reproduction follows.

Donor sperm

In the United States some 28 states have legislation that gives legal recognition to the use of donor sperm (17). These statutes typically require the husband's consent in writing, require that a physician do the insemination, and make the offspring the legitimate child of the consenting husband, with the donor having no rearing rights or duties with regard to the offspring. States without explicit legislation are likely to follow this model. These laws also attempt to be very protective of anonymity and confidentiality.

Some legal issues that are likely to arise with the use of donor sperm are most salient with regard to single persons, to parties who do not use a physician, and to parties, whether married or unmarried, who have agreed that the sperm donor will have some rearing rights and duties in offspring. Questions about the legal liability of physicians and sperm banks that obtain donor sperm but fail to inspect the sperm for infectious diseases and genetic defects are also likely to arise.

Donor eggs

Donor eggs may soon be a medically viable option for the thousands of women who are unable to provide genetically suitable oocytes for fertilization. Although donor eggs are not likely to be as widely used as donor sperm, many IVF programs will offer the technique.

The ethical, legal, and policy issues presented by egg donation arise from the separation of the female genetic and gestational bond, and from the relative scarcity and inaccessibility of ova as compared with sperm. Neither of these differences, however, makes egg donation for overcoming infertility or for use in research ethically or legally unacceptable.

Indeed, egg donation may be the least problematic of noncoital collaborative reproductive techniques because each rearing parent has a biologic connection with the offspring (18). Although the gestating and rearing mother will not be the genetic mother, and the genetic mother neither gestates nor rears, the resulting family situation should not pose major problems for offspring, families, or donors. The law is likely to recognize agreements to exclude the egg donor from rearing rights and duties, and may enforce some agreements for the donor to participate in rearing.

Egg donation does involve the possibility of greater risk for donors than occurs with sperm donation, at least when donors are not also undergoing IVF. Yet the risks are not so much greater than those of other accepted activities that egg donation should be discouraged. Nor would payments to donors be illegal or unethical, though some persons would disagree and ban paying egg donors as morally offensive.

Surrogate gestators

IVF programs cryopreserving preembryos may occasionally be asked to thaw the preembryo and place it in the uterus of a woman who has agreed to be a surrogate carrier for the woman providing the egg.

The main indication for surrogacy arises when the woman providing the egg lacks uterine function or is unable to complete pregnancy because of hysterectomy, endometriosis, incompetent cervix, or other medical factors. (Surrogacy for career or lifestyle "convenience" is theoretically possible, but there is no real demand for it at present, and it is widely frowned upon.) Surrogacy is thus an alternative to preembryo discard or donation

when the woman providing the egg is unable to maintain a pregnancy herself. Cryopreservation greatly facilitates gestational surrogacy because it avoids the need for synchronizing the surrogate's cycle with retrieval of the egg from its source.

Surrogacy is the most controversial of all the new collaborative reproductive techniques because of the intensity and length of the surrogate's contribution and the importance of the gestational bond to mothers, offspring, and society. Such a placement is not illegal and is not necessarily unethical or undesirable if the surrogate has knowingly chosen this role. Although most surrogates to date have also provided the egg (in essence a preconception agreement to be inseminated and relinquish rearing rights and duties at birth to the father and his partner), the use of surrogates to gestate the preembryo of another couple has occurred and will increase with cryopreservation.

The legal issues in surrogate gestation are still being clarified, and controversy remains (19). Although the birthing woman has always been considered the legal rearing mother, the separation of female genetic and gestational parentage will cause this presumption to be reevaluated. In several instances American courts have permitted the genetic mother to be listed as the mother on the birth certificate and recognized as the rearing mother. In the one case in which the surrogate gestating mother objected, a trial court in California ruled that the agreement should be honored and the genetic mother be recognized as the rearing mother. Although the discussion above of the constitutional status of noncoital reproduction would recognize this outcome as the correct result, further experience is necessary to establish whether this result will be accepted on appeal and in other jurisdictions. When the "surrogate mother" has also provided the egg, it may be that courts will be less likely to honor the preconception agreement for rearing, as occurred in the *Baby M* case in New Jersey.

Surrogate gestation itself is not illegal in most countries, although some American states may penalize payments of money to surrogates under state baby-selling laws or refuse to enforce custody or behavior provisions of surrogate contracts. However, such laws may be subject to constitutional challenge, because payment and contract enforcement are usually necessary to enable an infertile couple to reproduce in this way. Other countries may not permit surrogacy at all. The Warnock Committee in Great Britain, for example, condemned surrogacy and recommended criminal penalties for persons arranging surrogate transactions.

A major issue with surrogate gestation is whether the surrogate who changes her mind can abort or refuse to relinquish the child at birth. A surrogate who has not provided the egg is less likely to be free legally to breach her agreement. If she aborts contrary to contract, she would probably be liable for damages for destruction of the couple's preembryo. Her claim to retain custody at birth is also less compelling, because she never would have received the couple's preembryo of gestation unless she had agreed to relinquish the child at birth. When the surrogate has provided the egg, however, courts may follow the precedent set by the New Jersey Supreme Court in the *Baby M* case and refuse to honor the preconception contract concerning rearing rights and duties in the resulting child.

Gestational surrogacy is best viewed, as the Ethics Committee of the American Fertility Society recommended, as a clinical experiment until more data on its effects are available. It is not unethical for a program to offer surrogacy as an option for placement of stored preembryos when a valid need arises and the surrogate is adequately informed. In such cases the couple and their brokering agents, rather than the IVF program storing preembryos, will probably recruit the surrogate. The IVF program should ensure that the surrogate is freely consenting and is medically fit to carry a child. A copy of the agreement between the parties should be examined and placed in the medical records of each. The program should also cooperate with research studying the effects of surrogacy on the parties involved. Physicians who object to such arrangements or who have doubts about the validity of the surrogate's consent may choose not to participate in surrogate gestation.

Conclusion

This survey of major ethical and legal issues in noncoital and assisted reproduction shows that the law presents few barriers to physicians and couples using these techniques to resolve problems of infertility. Although a number of legal issues remain, and more disputes are likely, careful planning and attention to the informed, voluntary consent of the parties should enable assisted reproductive techniques to be used to form biologically related families in a socially accepted and legitimate way.

References

1. Robertson J. Procreative liberty and the control of conception, pregnancy and childbirth. Virginia Law Review 1983;69:405–414.

2. Robertson J. Embryos, families and procreative liberty: the legal structure of the new reproduction. Southern California Law Review 1986;59:939, 957–962.

3. Ibid, 964–967.

4. Ethics Committee of the American Fertility Society. Ethical considerations of the new reproductive technologies. Fertil Steril 1986; 46(3, Suppl 1):1S, 29S–30S.

5. Walters L. Ethics and new reproductive technologies: an international review of committee statements. Hastings Center Report 1987;17:53–59.

6. Robertson J. In the beginning: the legal status of early embryos. Virginia Law Review 1990;76:437, 450–454.

7. Ibid, 455–458.

8. Ibid, 459.

9. Ibid, 461–463.

10. Robertson J. Prior agreements for disposition of frozen embryos. Ohio State Law Journal 1990;51:407, 414–420.

11. Robertson J. Virginia Law Review 1990;76:473–476.

12. Robertson J. Divorce and disposition of cryo-preserved preembryos. Fertil Steril 1991;55:681–683.

13. Robertson J. Virginia Law Review 1990;76:498, n 159.

14. Ibid, 499–501.

15. Ibid, 501–503.

16. Robertson J. Embryo research. Western Ontario Law Review 1986;24:15–37.

17. Robertson J. Southern California Law Review 1986; 59:1004–1008.

18. Robertson J. Ethical and legal issues in human egg donation. Fertil Steril 1989;52:353–364.

19. Robertson J. Southern California Law Review 1986; 59:1011–1115.

11

The Future of Assisted Reproductive Technologies

James P. Toner
Gary D. Hodgen

Introduction

The birth of Louise Brown on July 25th, 1978, is widely hailed as the advent of assisted reproductive technologies (ART) in human medicine. In 12 short years, there has been a burgeoning of the technology's application as well as of the technological progress itself. What began as a technique to bypass damaged or absent fallopian tubes has become a series of approaches that can be applied to many types of infertility and to certain clinical problems other than infertility.

In the United States and Canada more than 24,000 cycles of assisted reproduction were initiated in 1989, with at least 3472 births of 4736 babies in that year alone (1). Even more such procedures are performed annually in Britain and France (2), with large numbers also being performed in Australia, Israel, South Africa, Japan, and elsewhere in Europe each year. The growth of this technology in the United States and Canada is indicated in Fig. 11.1. It would not be surprising to find that these results will double by the mid–1990s, with a concurrent enhancement in the efficacy of these new treatments.

Such explosive growth is, however, only one facet of this field. Another, perhaps more important feature is the increasing variety of techniques and their applications to a broader mix of clinical situations. In this chapter we shall review some of these newer leads, many explored partially, others barely conceived.

The crucial scientific observations of the 1920s, '30s, '40s, and '50s by Zondek, Pincus, Chang, Hisaw, Hartman, Gemsell, Lunenfeld, and dozens of other outstanding scientists prepared the way for these great clinical advances. If history foretells the future, so it will be again that basic experimentation will precipitate practical applications in clinical medicine. We should also recognize that the evolution of individual procreative rights progressed rapidly in the decades immediately preceding in vitro fertilization (IVF), gamete intrafallopian transfer (GIFT), and so on, manifest in the oral contraceptive, intrauterine device (IUD), and intra-uterine fetal diagnosis via ultrasound and genetic tests of developmental normalcy. Concurrently, the *Roe vs. Wade* decision recognized procreative choice, now stridently affected by RU486 (4). Thus, social conditioning and criteria for ethical behaviors prepared the way for societies to accept the new reproductive technologies, either to adore each heralded "advance" or to fear it.

Techniques such as preimplantation genetic diagnosis and the ability to extract and store oocytes, only a dream a decade ago, are becoming practical possibilities. Such techniques as the use of somatic cell genetic material (rather than DNA from gametes) to establish fertilization, germ line DNA therapy, and the develop-

ment of an artificial womb are surely decades away, but are nonetheless foreseeable scientific objectives in the early twenty-first century. Of course, social responsibility and ethical considerations must be attended along the way.

This chapter is divided into three major parts, according to our perception of temporal events that set forth where we have been, where we are, and where we will be. Assisted reproductive technologies (ART), as used here, means any techniques designed to produce pregnancy which require the involvement of third parties for success. The technical advances "expected" to become practical and clinically available within the next 5 years are called "expected advances." Others we consider less certain are discussed under "probable advances." These seem farther-off and may be available

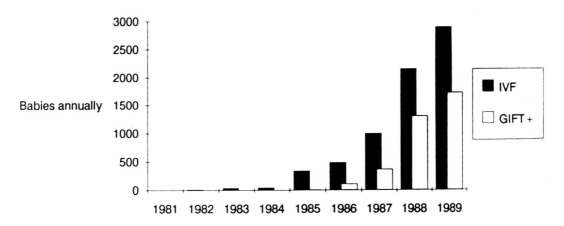

Growth of ART in North America

Fig. 11.1 Number of babies born in North America following the use of in vitro fertilization (IVF) and gamete intrafallopian transfer (GIFT) over the indicated years. Only those pregnancies registered with the Society of Reproductive Technologies' IVF Registry are indicated (1,3). The first North American child was born December 28, 1981, in Norfolk. Continent-wide statistics from 1982 to 1984 are not available; in lieu Norfolk babies are shown for these years. "GIFT+" indicates all nonstandard IVF cases (i.e., GIFT, ZIFT, TET, donor egg, cryopreservation).

clinically in 5 to 10 years. Still others are achievable theoretically but depend on the development of certain techniques and knowledge not yet in evidence. We refer to these as "possible advances," but do not expect clinical applications until more than 10 years from now, and in some instances perhaps much longer. When possible, we have distinguished technologies that are transitional from those that are definitive.

> Prognostics do not always proof prophecies—at least the wisest prophets make sure of the event first.
>
> (Thomas Walpole, February 19, 1785)

Accordingly, we have taken a broad license to speculate here on "The Future of Assisted Reproductive Technologies," and apologize in advance for the inevitable arrival of findings that will surely reveal our myopia at the time of this writing.

Areas of expected advancement: up to 5 years

Favored stimulation protocols

Benefits of stimulation: Though the very first in vitro fertilization attempts used the natural cycle, it became clear early on that having only one oocyte available per cycle hampered progress at both the clinical level (i.e., pregnancy outcome) and experimental level (limited material). Most teams moved rapidly to controlled ovarian stimulation with clomiphene citrate or human menopausal gonadotropin (hMG) or a combination of them. Ultimately, hMG proved most efficacious, especially with the gonadotropin-releasing hormone (GnRH) agonists (see below). The subsequent emergence of GIFT followed similarly (5).

In general, the benefits of controlled ovarian hyperstimulation have been clearly and repeatedly demonstrated. And in conjunction with a successful cryopreservation program, the value of excess pre-embryos in producing pregnancy has also been convincingly demonstrated (Fig. 11.2) (6).

Choosing a stimulation regimen: The ideal stimulation, one that would yield numerous healthy and competent oocytes in all women, has not yet been discovered. Rather, the ability to stimulate folliculogenesis is often limited to some extent. Women differ from one another in this regard; some are innately lower responders and others higher responders to present forms of stimulation. Moreover, sometimes even those women who produce many eggs are faced with a reduction in egg quality that has not yet been overcome. To be sure, the goal of ovarian stimulation depends on whether the oocytes will be collected before fertilization. When ovulation induction (without IVF) is contemplated, a limited ovarian response is intended to minimize the risk of multiple pregnancy. However, when IVF or GIFT procedures are being performed, higher numbers of oocytes are desirable. Various stimulation regimens have been used in an effort to improve the number and quality of oocytes obtained; and these efforts are ongoing.

Pure follicle-stimulating hormone (FSH) has been advocated for use in oligoovulatory women who have tonic elevations of luteinizing hormone (LH), to minimize further increases in LH tone that may have detrimental effects. Though this procedure is logical on theoretical grounds, there has been no apparent clinical benefit; nor has any decrease in androgen production been observed (7). Even when combined with GnRH agonist suppression, no benefit over conventional hMG stimulation has been observed (8). Low-dose FSH (75 IU IM daily) was able to bring about limited follicular development rather than the usual excessive response in women with polycystic ovarian disease (9). It may be that a certain low-dose gonadotropin regimen that achieves limited follicular development could be identified for each high responding patient.

Recombinant human FSH (rechFSH) has been engineered by several groups (10) and may be available for clinical evaluation shortly. Earlier, recombinant human LH (rechLH) was synthesized and shown to act equivalently to native LH in terms of ovulation induction, oocyte maturation, and luteal support (11). One potential advantage of these recombinant forms is that they provide a control over dose not previously available: any ratio between FSH and LH doses can be achieved for individualizing treatment regimens. This fine-tuning may improve oocyte recovery rates in low responders and provide for a more controlled stimulation in high responders. But a second advantage of recombinant gonadotropins is perhaps more important in the long view. Genetic engineering of these glycoprotein hormones can be performed such that molecular variants (isohormones) with differential activities from the par-

ent hormone are achieved (12). "Designer hormones" have been developed for other protein hormones and can have a variety of potencies and valences (agonist, antagonist, or mixed effects) relative to the parent hormone. Naturally occurring in vivo molecular variants of FSH with less than normal activity have been described in women (13) and may be etiologic for their lack of normal follicular development. Recombinant gonadotropins may be more easily monitored for quality control than present extracts from urine, thereby diminishing the interlot variability in biopotency (14), which further complicates current dosage regimens.

GnRH agonists have been successfully applied in two fashions in ART, the so-called long and short regimens (15). As gonadotropin suppressors, they have reduced treatment cancellation rates (fewer LH surges) and increased follicular cohort synchrony (16). Both an increase in the average numbers of oocytes collected and an increase in the percentage of oocytes that are

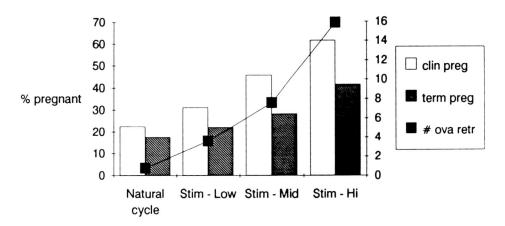

Fig. 11.2 Comparison of results from unstimulated, natural cycle IVF and stimulated IVF in the Norfolk program (6). Patients stimulated with gonadotropins were subdivided into groups by the number of preovulatory oocytes collected.

meiotically mature are reported in all categories of responsiveness (17). In a gonadotropin stimulation mode ("flare-up" protocols), the agonists have maintained good oocyte recovery rates at lower cost per egg in at least this low responding group. Whether the occasional reactivation of the corpus luteum impairs oocyte or endometrial quality is debated. GnRH agonists can have direct effects on ovarian and follicular physiology independent of their influence on the gonadotropin milieu (18); however, the clinical consequences of this possibility are apparently very limited.

In high responding women with polycystic ovarian disease, the role of a *GnRH pump* has been evaluated. This approach was prompted by the observation of increased LH pulse frequency in such patients (19). Its use after suppression with a GnRH agonist has met with some success in that 2 of 6 patients ovulated on this combined therapy (20). This is not surprising since prolonged GnRH agonist therapy produces a "down-regulation" of pituitary GnRH receptors. Another attempt using GnRH pump and exogenous gonadotropins produced fewer large follicles in 6 of 9 cases than without the GnRH agonist (21).

GnRH antagonists are reaching clinical evaluation and offer some potential advantages over GnRH agonists (15). These advantages stem especially from two properties. One is the lack of a "flare effect" of gonadotropin secretion. This means that the "medical hypophysectomy" is virtually immediate, allowing a simultaneous start of the GnRH antagonist and the gonadotropins (22,23). The other is that the antagonists do not "down-regulate" pituitary GnRH receptor functions (24). Consequently, the pituitary remains responsive to exogenous GnRH (24), allowing for the efficient concurrent use of the antagonist and the GnRH pump (25). This combination of the antagonist plus GnRH via a pump may have application in women who manifest chronic hyperandrogenemia, both to control the se-

quellae of the endocrinopathy and, if desired, to induce ovulation (26).

Human chorionic gonadotropin (hCG) has been used to mimic the LH surge since very early in ovulation induction therapy (27). It serves two roles. One is to contribute to the luteal phase support, which is otherwise inadequate in IVF. In one large, randomized, double-blind study, ongoing pregnancy rates were cut in half when no luteal support was provided (28). The other role is to induce final maturation of the oocytes. As a consequence of hCG, about 70% of all eggs are in metaphase at aspiration in the Norfolk program. Oocytes from follicles containing at least 2 ml of fluid (about 13 mm diameter) at the time of hCG administration are most frequently mature when collected 34 hours later (29).

However, at least three issues concerning the role of hCG in oocyte maturation have yet to be resolved. One is whether this maturational signal need be given at all. It is clear from our own work and from that of a Korean group (30) that immature oocytes, once removed from the unstimulated ovary, undergo spontaneous resumption of meiosis through polar body extrusion without exposure to any hCG or LH surge. In the Korean group's work, oocytes came from small antral follicles (1–5 mm) and had a surrounding cumulus. In the presence of mature follicular fluid, half of these oocytes matured meiotically, 92% fertilized, and 86.9% of them cleaved; one triplet pregnancy is reported (30). In our own hands, preantral follicles containing fully grown but meiotically immature oocytes have been matured in vitro, yielding metaphase I oocytes. A cumulus oophorus was not necessary for this development, though no such in vitro maturation has been observed in the absence of a zona pellucida. This may indicate that such in vitro maturation works for all but primary follicles. On the other hand, primary follicles have been successfully transplanted from one mouse to another whose own oocytes were inactivated by irradiation, with subsequent ovulation and even pregnancy resulting from the transplanted oocytes (31). Thus the present limitation for in vitro maturation of primary oocytes may ultimately be overcome as we learn more about the normal process of meiotic arrest and the ongoings of gonadotropin-independent follicle and oocyte growth (see below).

The second issue is whether hCG does any harm. Clearly, hCG does induce morphologic maturity in certain oocytes. However, it can be erroneous to equate morphologic signs of egg maturity with functional maturity. If this distinction is valid, then the hCG-induced maturity of eggs from smaller follicles may be falsely reassuring. Indirect evidence in support of this notion comes from an evaluation of the relative performance of metaphase eggs derived from follicles of different sizes. In one report, miscarriages were observed only in cases in which mature eggs had come from small follicles (2 mm or less; 46% miscarriage rate); no miscarriages were observed in pregnancies established from oocytes of larger follicles (7).

The third issue is whether hCG is an optimal stimulus for oocyte maturation. The normal midcycle gonadotropin surge has both LH and FSH components; hCG acts as surrogate for only the LH component. If the midcycle FSH surge serves any contributory function, that function is missing when hCG is used alone. GnRH agonists can produce a more normal LH-FSH surge (32). Consequently, the role of the midcycle FSH surge is currently open to direct experimental evaluation. If the FSH component is shown to be helpful, then the ovulatory trigger of choice may shift from hCG to a GnRH agonist. However, most existing evidence points away from this possibility.

Treatment of the low responding patient: From the very start of exogenous ovarian stimulation, responsive-ness among women has been recognized as highly individualized; given the same amount of gonadotropins, some are high responders, some mid or low responders. Low responders have remained the most difficult group to treat.

Therapy for low responders has been directed primarily at increasing the amount of stimulation provided to the ovarian follicles in an attempt to stimulate more of them into orderly folliculogenesis. The simplest approach of *increased gonadotropin dose* has met with limited success: the ongoing pregnancy rate of 5% using 4 ampules of gonadotropin daily increased to 12% when 6 ampules were used (33). The use of GnRH agonists in a *"flare-up" protocol* is another variation on this theme and may produce higher levels of gonadotropin (for a few days) than are practical using exogenous gonadotropins alone. This approach has yielded similar pregnancy results to the "6 FSH" protocol described above (33), but in fewer treatment days at less expense (34).

Two other experimental approaches have been proposed. One is to use, in addition to gonadotropins, adjunctive substances to enhance folliculogenesis. Some of these substances are produced within the ovary and may have a paracrine (or autocrine) effect that synergizes with gonadotropin stimulation. Others are not produced locally but nonetheless can play an upward modulatory role (see Table 11.1).

Inhibitory intraovarian regulators have been inferred from observations such as the differential growth of nondominant follicles in the dominant ovary only (42). Once better characterized, these active inhibitors of follicular growth (43) might present new opportunities to enhance the follicular cohort through intraovarian antagonism of their actions.

One tactic for low responding women who have elevated gonadotropin levels has been to *reduce gonadotropin levels* before proceeding with stimulation (44).

The rationale is that under chronic exposure to high levels of gonadotropins, the gonadotropin receptors on the granulosa and theca cells are "down-regulated" to the point that even high-dose gonadotropin stimulation is destined to have only limited effect. Although this is an attractive theory, there is no direct evidence that receptor concentrations are in fact modified by this approach. Furthermore, the clinical results have not demonstrated efficacy (44).

All the strategies outlined above for low responders are predicated on the assumption that the oocytes obtained from low responders are worth obtaining. This may be unrealistic. It is clear that *impaired egg quality* is a factor in low responding patients (45,46). Substitution of donated eggs from younger women for eggs from low responding women reliably increases the implantation and ongoing pregnancy rates: for instance, implantation rates rose from 7% to 36% in one report (45) and from 6% to 25% in another following this substitution (46). In the Norfolk donor egg program, of the 16 transfers in women age 40 and over (range 40–44), 6 pregnancies have been established and 4 term

pregnancies (6 babies, 2 sets of twins). Successful pregnancy following use of donated eggs in a 49-year-old is reported (47). Thus there seems to be little reason to attribute the poor outcome of the low responder to anything but the eggs themselves.

For this reason, serious attention needs to be given to increasing the quality of a woman's own eggs. Certainly, the substitution of *donated oocytes* from a younger woman of proven fertility is an effective remedy, but it misses the mark for women interested in passing on their own genetic material. In low responder patients who decline donated eggs, ooplasmic transfusion may be a useful strategy. This technique involves removing some ooplasm from the compromised oocyte and replacing it with some ooplasm from a healthier oocyte. This technique has proved effective for transforming a morphologically immature oocyte into a functionally mature oocyte with enhanced capability to cleave and even produce pregnancy (48). It is possible that ooplasm from younger mature eggs may increase the ability of eggs from these low responding women to produce viable pregnancy. At present it is not clear whether the age-related factor is contained within the ooplasm, the nucleus, the zona pellucida, or all of them. Such study would help resolve this issue and may provide a practical means to increase the pregnancy potential of aged oocytes for women who find the use of donated eggs unacceptable. If further work determined that certain proteins were deficient in oocytes of perimenopausal women, then this factor might be incorporated by iontophoresis (49). This refinement of technology represents moving beyond transitional technologies (here ooplasmic transfusion), whose efficacy is demonstrated but whose mechanism is unclear, to ultimate technologies (here iontophoretic enzyme injection) in which understanding the mechanism allows a more direct and simpler technique to be applied.

Natural cycle IVF has not been popular in programs

Table 11.1 Paracrine and autocrine factors influencing folliculogenesis

Agent	Effect
Insulin-like growth factor-1	Enhances FSH-stimulated aromatase activity (35)
Insulin-like growth factor-2	Taken up by ovary (36)
Insulin	Stimulates steroidogenesis (37)
Growth hormone	Stimulates steroidogenesis (38)
Activin-A	Increases gonadotropin release (39)
α-Inhibin	Decreases gonadotropin release (40)
Metoclopromide	Increases prolactin secretion (41)

of ART, but may become more common as its indications become better defined and its technique more refined. Often low responding women can do at least as well without expensive stimulation. Couples whose finances are quite limited may be able to use this approach when the standard approach is beyond their reach financially. The chance for ongoing pregnancy per collection in published series ranges from 10% (50) to 18% (51), which is hardly worse than the results of stimulated cycles. The putative superior egg quality (or endometrial normalcy) in cycles without exogenous stimulation has been difficult to demonstrate clearly but is nonetheless suspected to play a role. In conjunction with efforts to obtain additional immature oocytes for maturation in vitro (see below), this procedure may become more attractive to a wider patient population. Among good responders, the natural cycle's attraction is avoidance of multiple pregnancies, especially with more than three concepti. However, stimulation with gonadotropin therapy is likely to remain the more common approach for the foreseeable future.

In vitro culturing of preembryos

Coculture of oocytes with other cell types has been advantageous in many different systems. Perhaps surprisingly, there does not appear to be strong hormone dependency or tissue specificity to these effects. In various coculture systems, all of the following have been effective: cells from tubal (52,53), endometrial (54), granulosa (55), trophoblast (56), and kidney cell lines (52). Species used have included mice (52), humans (53,57), cows (52), and monkeys (52). For each type of preembryo, certain cell supports have been found to be better than others; the best support in one preembryo system is not necessarily the best in another. In humans, one effective and convenient preembryotrophic support is monkey kidney cells (58). Efforts are also directed at developing compound cocultures with both secretory

and stromal cell components. Still others have examined simply placing all oocytes together in the same dish. Another possible refinement would involve sequential coculture systems in which oocytes would be exposed in turn to cells from peritoneum, oviduct, and endometrium in a pattern similar to that experienced in vivo. The source of this benefit in all of these systems is not well understood. Cells may be providing important factors that stimulate oocyte and preembryo health, may remove toxins from the local environment, or both. It is clear that the presence of cells is not critical to the benefit seen in short-term culture. Until the cause for the benefit is clearly identified, work will continue to identify practical and efficacious coculture systems.

Coculture systems, however, will probably be a transitional technology. Once the particular *cytokines or hormones* critical to the coculture advantage are identified, supplying these products may prove simpler and equally effective. As of this writing, several cytokines and hormones have shown some benefit (Table 11.2).

Table 11.2 Cytokines influencing preembryo growth in vitro

Cytokine	Effect on preembryo growth
FSH	Increased rate of blastocyst formation (59)
LH	Increased rate of blastocyst formation (59)
Sequential FSH-LH	Additive increase in blastocyst formation (59)
Platelet-activating factor (PAF)	Enhances growth and implantation (60,61)
Epidermal growth factor (EGF)	Stimulates granulosa cell activity and oocyte development (62)
	Increases blastocyst and implantation rate (S.K. Dey, personal communication)

Several of these also augment the fertilization potential of sperm (e.g., FSH) and are secreted by reproductive tract tissues or by the preembryos themselves (e.g., PAF, EGF).

Many other cytokines are secreted by preembryos, often at specified developmental stages. These include human placental lactogen (hPL), hCG, estradiol (E_2), progesterone (P_4), and histamine (63), prostaglandin E_2 (PGE_2) (64), early pregnancy factor (EPF) (65), plasminogen activator (PA) (66), PA inhibitor (PAI) (66), interleukin-1 (IL-1) (67), IL-6 (67), tumor necrosis factor (TNF) (67), colony-stimulating factor (CSF) (67), and transforming growth factor–β (TGF-β). At later stages, trophoblasts secrete, in addition to the factors just listed, secretory protein 1 (SP1), fibronectin, and laminin. Minimum roles for these factors are that PA and PAI appear to facilitate implantation; histamine and PGE_2 augment decidualization; hCG supports the corpus luteum; and E_2 and P_4 support the endometrium. The roles of EPF, hPL, IL-1, IL-6, CSF, TGF-β, and TNF in preembryo growth and implantation are largely undefined.

Extra pronuclei are not uncommonly observed in IVF. They are more common in aged oocytes and with high sperm concentrations (68). Most cases are thought to represent polyspermy (humans have only a slow block to polyspermy). At present, most programs do not transfer these preembryos. If one of the extra pronuclei could be removed reliably and safely (69), these preembryos could again become useful to the infertile couple. It is generally believed that the male pronucleus is larger than the female pronucleus and is located farther from the second polar body, and that these differences might permit accurate identification of a male pronucleus. At present, this characterization has not been adequately tested (70), though this step is clearly a prerequisite to widespread application of such techniques. A more accurate alternative would involve

DNA hybridization. Direct probes of Y-specific sequences contained in the biopsied pronucleus (via polymerase chain reaction [PCR] amplification and DNA hybridization) would permit correct identification of only half of the male pronuclei. However, it is not clear how X-bearing male pronuclei could be easily distinguished from their X-bearing female counterparts. At present, those restriction fragment length polymorphisms (RFLPs) or other diagnostic systems that are instructive (i.e., allow maternal and paternal X-chromosomal DNA to be distinguished from one another) would need to be determined for each couple individually and applied to each pronucleus (via PCR amplification and RFLP analysis).

Implantation and transfer technology

Implantation remains one of the most significant puzzles in the IVF process. Most patients undergoing IVF can be successfully stimulated, their oocytes can be collected and fertilized, and preembryos can be transferred. However, only a fraction of patients who have preembryos transferred become pregnant. The chance that a particular preembryo leads to a gestational sac is approximately 8% to 13% at most IVF centers. Though some of the IVF failures that are not recognized until the time of implantation are surely due to unrecognized oocyte or preembryo problems, it is not clear whether this preembryo problem is a large or small part of the overall poor performance typically observed.

The source of the inefficiency in implantation has been heuristically divided by Paulson and colleagues into three areas: egg quality, transfer efficiency, and endometrial receptivity (71). Though none of these areas is probably optimized in the standard IVF situation, it has been very difficult to estimate the contribution that each area makes to the overall inefficiency of the process.

Gamete/preembryo quality: Clearly a fraction of the sperm, oocytes, and resulting preembryos are chromosomally abnormal; estimates for preembryos range from 17.3% to 32.7% (72–74). Undoubtedly there are some preembryos with lethal genetic traits that are not amenable to diagnosis by karyotyping. And there may be other growth-limiting deficiencies not related to genetic material (i.e., acquired) that are not apparent during fertilization or early cleavage stages but are nonetheless ultimately lethal. All these reduce the potential implantation rate.

Transfer efficiency: Transfer efficiency is the relative ability of preembryos to implant when artificially introduced into the genital tract relative to their chances under normal circumstances. Potential sources of inefficient transfer include disruptions in cervical mucus architecture, minor trauma to the endometrium, and any adverse effect of the fluid used to transfer the preembryos (volume or content). The inefficiency related to their transfer is difficult to estimate. Whether using a smaller volume would alter this outcome is not clear at present. A preliminary report using a fibrin sealant to plug both tubal and cervical channels produced a 26% pregnancy rate in the treated group ($n = 38$) versus a 19% rate in the control group (75).

The optimal time and site for preembryo transfer depend on several factors. In patients with normal fallopian tubes, tubal replacement of gametes (GIFT), zygotes (zygote intrafallopian transfer [ZIFT] or pronuclear stage transfer [PROST]), or later cleavage stages (tubal embryo transfer [TET]) is more physiologic, and in many studies, but not all (76), appears to have increased efficacy. However, this effect is not overwhelming, and it is difficult to be certain of the inferiority of standard intrauterine preembryo transfer in patients with normal tubes. Conversely, the CO_2 exposure that occurs during laparoscopy (i.e., during GIFT, ZIFT, TET, and PROST) may be detrimental to preembryo health (77). If the transcervical placement of gametes and preembryos becomes reliable (78), it may rapidly replace laparoscopic GIFT, ZIFT, and related procedures. Falloposcopy may permit evaluation of the suitability of tubal placement of gametes or preembryos (79).

Endometrial receptivity: The endometrium has intervals of greater receptivity and lesser receptivity to preembryo implantation. During the receptive interval, Paulson and colleagues (71) have estimated that the maximum value for preembryo implantation in IVF is 36%, since the maximum transfer efficiency and preembryo quality in a stimulated IVF attempt are each about 60% ($.60 \times .60 = .36$). This figure is much below the implantation rate observed in contemporary animal husbandry, where rates in the 50% to 75% range are anticipated (80). This difference is not clearly understood, but may relate to the intense selective breeding in animal husbandry for individuals that reliably establish pregnancy with few coital exposures.

Biology of implantation. In humans, blastocyst implantation follows an interval of apposition and attachment approximately 7 or 8 days beyond fertilization (81). Once attached, the preembryo invades the endometrium to form a hemochorial placenta: endometrial glands are destroyed, and maternal vascular integrity is ultimately interrupted and brought into direct contact with placental villi (Fig. 11.3).

The molecular events that mediate the various phases of implantation and early placentation are being aggressively investigated. One useful working model of implantation has been proposed by Kliman and associates (82). The stages of this model are outlined in Table 11.3 and correspond to Fig. 11.3. Note that the specific factors mediating each stage are being identified.

Other features of the interval of endometrial

receptivity have been described (Table 11.4). Their role in mediating implantation are being defined presently.

Clinical aspects. The "window" of optimal implantation is not unlimited. In one review (100) this span was judged to last at least 3½ days: from preembryos 36 hours ahead of cycle time to 48 hours behind it. On the other hand, efforts to define the window by using endometrial explants showed that cytotrophoblasts attached to the surface endometrium only when the explant was derived from a day 19 endometrium (82). An interesting report indicates that the time of implantation is largely determined by the preembryo rather than the endometrium (101): the stage of preembryo maturity at the time of transfer was a better predictor of the first rise in β-hCG than the day on which transfer occurred. This suggests that the timing of transfer may play a limiting role, but that within the window of receptivity, the particular time of implanta-

tion depends largely on the preembryo's developmental stage.

Noninvasive tests of endometrial receptivity with the use of vaginal ultrasound are being developed (102,103); perhaps some distinct patterns will be recognized as favorable and others unfavorable. If so, therapies might be developed that would produce the favorable ultrasonographic patterns.

From the first use of ovarian stimulation regimens, there was an appropriate concern that the supraphysiologic levels of sex steroids might adversely influence endometrial receptivity. Similar levels of estrogen, for instance, have been used postcoitally to prevent pregnancy (the classic "morning-after pill"). However, it has been difficult to find evidence of a similar adverse effect in IVF programs. In fact, the implantation rate (i.e., per preembryo sac rate) may even be higher in this circumstance: In Norfolk, the implantation rate for

Table 11.3 Proposed stages of implantation

Step	Proposed features	Observed features
1. Trophoblast–endometrial epithelial interaction	Specific cell adhesion molecules	Cell surface glycoconjugates interact with concanavalin A (83)
2. Trophoblast–extracellular matrix (ECM) protein interaction	Contact with fibronectin, laminin, collagen types I and IV, proteoglycans via substrate adhesion molecules	Fibronectin and laminin promote attachment and outgrowth of mouse blastocysts (84); human trophoblasts have fibronectin receptors and attach to laminin and several collagens (85)
3. Controlled degradation of the ECM by proteases	Protease release prompted by contact and controlled by inhibitors	Chorionic villi secrete plasminogen activator (86) and can degrade ECM (87); trophoblasts secrete tissue plasminogen activator (t-PA) and PA inhibitor types 1 and 2 (66)
4. Resynthesis of the ECM	New ECM proteins by trophoblasts	Cultured trophoblasts synthesize fibronectin (88) and laminin (82)

Reproduced by permission from Kliman HJ, Coutifaris C, Reinberg RF, Strauss JF III, Haimowitz JE. Implantation: in vitro models utilizing human tissues. In: Yoshinaga K, ed. Blastocyst implantation. Boston: Adams Publishing Group, 1989.

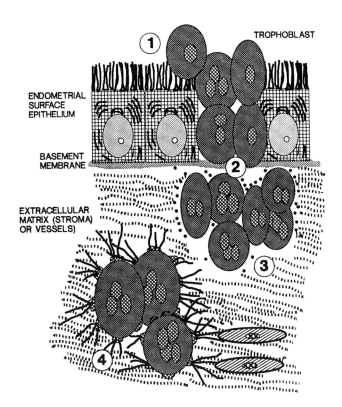

Fig. 11.3 Model of human implantation. Trophoblasts attach to the endometrial surface epithelium through cell adhesion molecules (CAMs) (*1*). The trophoblasts interdigitate between epithelial cells. Eventually, the trophoblasts make contact with the basement membrane (*2*), initiating the secretion of proteases (*3*). The extent of proteolysis is regulated by membrane-associated and secreted protease inhibitors. Once the trophoblasts have reached their final destination (e.g., a maternal spiral artery), they synthesize extracellular matrix (ECM) proteins which firmly attach them to their surroundings (*4*).

Reproduced by permission from Serono Symposia, USA. Blastocyst implantation. Boston: Adams Publishing Group, 1989.

cycles in which the peak E_2 exceeds 1000 pg/ml is higher than the rate in average responders (500–1000 pg/ml): 14.2% versus 10.3% in cycles with GnRH agonist

pretreatment ($p < 0.01$), 11.9% versus 7.8% in cycles with flare-up GnRH agonist use ($p < 0.01$), and 12.2% versus 6.4% without GnRH agonist use ($p < 0.05$) (104). In other work, when controlling for the number of pre-embryos transferred ($n = 5$), the highest pregnancy rates were in the highest response group (Fig. 11.4) (105).

Further evidence that these high steroid levels are not harmful comes from histologic evaluation of the endometrium at the time of biopsy. We have observed in some 28 biopsy specimens a strong relationship between the steroid response and the dating of endometrial maturity (104). The higher the steroid response, the more advanced was the endometrium. Given the fact that the preembryo transfer occurs earlier than is natural in a cycle, on theoretical grounds there may be some advantage to this advanced endometrial status.

As a consequence of findings such as those described above, *pharmacologic manipulation* of endometrial receptivity is currently being attempted and may prove

Table 11.4   Features of periimplantation endometrium

Physical properties
Reduced luminal surface negativity (89)
Increased glycocalyx thickness (90)
Increased lectin binding (91)
Pinopod expression (92)

Antigen expression
Glycoproteins (42 and 145 kilodaltons) differentially
  glycosylated in midluteal phase (93)
Absent HLA-DR expression (94)

Secretory products
α_2-PEG (95)
24 kilodalton protein (95)
IGF-binding protein (96)
prostaglandins E_2 and $F_{2\alpha}$ (97)
S1, S3 (EP11), S4 (98)
Prolactin (99)

beneficial. This result suggests that exogenous delivery of extra E_2 or progesterone (P_4) or both may foster implantation in low responding women. (Experimentally, P_4 alone sufficed to support the endometrium once secretory patterns were established [106].) Clinically, provision of supplemental P_4 from the day after hCG administration in a low responder led to the only case of in-phase endometrial histology in our series of biopsy specimens described above (104). Others have experimented with this approach; some have reported increased implantation and pregnancy rates (107). If the goal instead is a certain ratio of estrogen and progestin (108), then antagonists of these hormones (e.g.,

tamoxifen, mifepristone [RU486]) may be used to achieve such ends. In practice, adequate preparation of the endometrium has proved rather flexible (109).

Since placentation in humans is invasive, some method of direct placement of preembryos under the surface of the endometrium might be effective: it might eliminate failures due to unsuccessful apposition and attachment.

At present the positive identification of pregnancy is delayed in most IVF programs because of the use of high-dose hCG as an ovulatory trigger and a luteal support. The hCG can be detected 8 to 10 days after injection of 10,000 IU, and therefore interferes with the

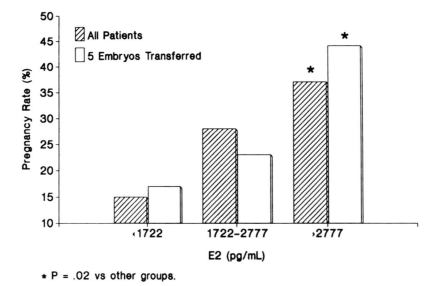

* P = .02 vs other groups.

Fig. 11.4   Clinical pregnancy rates for three levels of estradiol responsiveness in IVF. In all open bars five preembryos were transferred. Accordingly, preembryo implantation does not show any impairment in cases of very high estradiol response.

Adapted from Chenette PE, Sauer MV, Paulson RJ. Very high serum estradiol levels are not detrimental to clinical outcome of in vitro fertilization. Fertil Steril 1990;54:860.

goal of early pregnancy detection. Perhaps other early markers of pregnancy such as early pregnancy factor (EPF) (65,110) may prove convenient in this effort. Alternatively, the use of rechLH for the "ovulatory trigger" would permit the assay of β-hCG without interference (11).

In addition to histologic and secretory features of uterine receptivity, there may be muscular features that could be exploited clinically. In humans preliminary work reveals changes in peristaltic activity over the menstrual cycle and in response to ovarian hyperstimulation (111). In other species analogous activity is essential for sperm transport and pregnancy itself (112).

Male factor

IVF and related procedures have allowed some couples with male factor infertility to conceive when natural reproduction failed. However, the gains have been limited: couples with severe male factor infertility do the poorest of all groups in IVF (113). With current technologies, most of the benefit from IVF may come from the ability to increase the concentration of available sperm about the egg. And although this simple technique appears to increase the zona binding and fertilization rates in cases of severe male factor infertility (114), the increased ongoing pregnancy rate is still well below the rate for most other types of infertility.

The importance of sperm morphology is becoming apparent as more sophisticated means of evaluating sperm are proposed. In collaboration with the Tygerberg group in South Africa, we in Norfolk have reported that a stricter definition of normal morphology is a much more sensitive indicator of failed and successful fertilization in IVF than the conventional World Health Organization criteria (115,116).

Enhanced diagnostic ability to define the particular deficiencies in cases of male infertility will be helpful in designing therapy (117,118). For instance, the hemizona assay (HZA) has proved to be a useful indicator of the adequacy of the sperm-zona binding. In this test, two matched human zona hemispheres are created by microdissection; one half is exposed to the patient's sperm, the other half to sperm from a known fertile male. The ratio between the numbers of sperm bound for each male provides an index of zona binding capacity. This unique homologous bioassay, the HZA, has been used to identify cases in which the only identifiable explanation of fertilization failure is zona binding: semen analysis and hamster egg penetration are normal (119). The HZA has a sensitivity of 95%, specificity of 83%, and positive and negative predictive values of 95% and 83%, respectively, for in vitro fertilization of human oocytes (118). An adaptation from the HZA is an office test kit, using either a human hemizona preparation or recombinant ZP3, the zona protein responsible for sperm binding (120), is being developed to make this test more widely available (121).

Further gains in treating male factor infertility will follow from new understanding of the process of spermatogenesis, the function of the epididymis in enhancing sperm function, of the physiology of capacitation (including hyperactivated motility and the acrosome reaction), and the interaction with the egg.

Biology of spermatogenesis: The hormones FSH, LH, inhibin, activin, and testosterone may all interact to orchestrate spermatogenesis. Within the testis itself, many factors may regulate spermatogenesis by inhibitory or stimulatory influences. For instance, various products of proopiomelanocortin production have contradictory effects on Sertoli cell function: adrenocorticotropic hormone (ACTH) (122), α-melanotropin-stimulating hormone (α-MSH) (123), β-MSH (123), and des–acetyl–α-MSH (124) all stimulate Sertoli cell division, increase cyclic adenosine monophosphate (cAMP), and increase aromatase activity. But β-endorphin appears to play an inhibitory role on Sertoli cell proliferation (125) and cAMP and protein (126) production. At the same time, β-endorphin stimulates Leydig cell testosterone production (127). Sertoli cell secretory proteins include androgen binding protein, IGF-1, testibumin, and many others. The secretion of some of these proteins is tied to the stages of the seminiferous epithelial cycle (128) and may ultimately reveal the mechanism of controlled growth.

Biology of epididymal effects: It is clear from both animal and human studies that the epididymis plays a crucial role in the process of sperm maturation; see review by Cooper (129). Newly formed, immotile sperm are moved through the seminiferous tubules into the epididymis by secretory flow, peristalsis, and ciliary action. During their transit through the epididymis, sperm acquire motility, zona-oolemma-binding capacity, and fertilization capacity. These functional attributes are associated with (and perhaps causally related to) alterations in the lipid and glycoprotein composition (130) of the sperm plasma membrane. Stabilizing, maturational, and aging changes are described. Glycoprotein particles exhibit regular and changing spatial distributions over the surface of the sperm plasma membranes as they move through the epididymis (131). The lipid content of the plasma membrane (especially cholesterol) increases with epididymal transit and alters the plasma membrane stability (132). Sperm also acquire their motility (both amplitude and frequency) as they traverse the epididymis (133). The surface redistribution of a fibronectin component appears to be essential for oolemmal binding (134), while another surface protein (PH-20) is essential for zona binding (135).

Biology of "capacitation": Capacitation of ejaculated sperm in the female genital tract (or in appropriate culture media) will permit sperm to fertilize oocytes. Capacitation is associated with changes in the acrosome and sperm plasma membrane (loss of cholesterol). Although they are commonly associated, capacitation and hyperactivation can be mechanistically distinguished in vitro. Both involve activation of a G protein mechanisms (136) that activate both the cAMP/protein kinase A and Ca^{2+}/ protein kinase C (137) second messenger systems, leading to alterations in sperm protein phosphorylation (138) and hyperactivated motility.

Huge gaps remain in our understanding of all the processes outlined above. For instance, the control of epididymal effects is unclear. Sympathetic nervous innervation of the epididymis seems important for normal sperm motility (139), but why? Whether different areas of the epididymis provide different functions (140) or whether there is just one process common to the entire length is not clear. The relative importance of time spent in the epididymis is unresolved. Whether the sperm participate in or influence epididymal function is unresolved. The normal in vivo triggers of capacitation, acrosome exocytosis, and hyperactivation are not clearly defined (though genital tract fluids, the cumulus oophorous, and the zona pellucida are all in vitro enhancers of these processes).

Sperm-egg interaction: Appropriate sperm-egg interaction is required for successful fertilization. Some of the components of this interaction are listed in Table 11.5. Under normal conditions sperm contact with the cumulus oophorus and/or zona pellucida initiates the acrosome reaction. Sperm binding to the oolemma has been described to depend on a fibronectin component on the sperm surface that has characteristics of a common system of receptor-substrate recognition (RGD tripeptide) (134). Deficiencies at each step are possible; therapy will depend first on being able to define the pathophysiology, then on having a remedy. Such diagnostics are beyond present capabilities in most cases.

Table 11.5 Sequence of events in fertilization process

Event	Time after fertilization	Mediator
1. Plasma membrane depolarization	<5 s	Increased permeability to Na^+ (and Ca^{2+})
2. Hydrolysis of phosphotidylinositol biphosphate	<10 s	Activation of phospholipase C
3. Increased free cytosolic Ca^{2+}	10–40 s	Inositol triphosphate-induced Ca^{2+} release from intracellular compartment
4. Cortical granule exocytosis	10–50 s	Increased intracellular Ca^{2+}
5. Increased intracellular pH	60 s	Activation of Na^+-H^+ exchange by protein kinase C
6. Increased protein synthesis	8 min	Increased intracellular pH
7. Initiation of DNA replication	30–45 min	Increased intracellular pH

Enhancing sperm performance: In vivo attempts to increase sperm output in cases of hypothalamic hypogonadism by administering clomiphene, tamoxifen, and gonadotropins (141) have been helpful only in small series. In vitro techniques to improve the performance of available sperm have been attempted (see Table 11.6), with limited improvements. In the case of follicular fluid, the steroid component appears critical to the observed benefit (142,143). Importantly, no controlled study has been able to show improved pregnancy rates (118).

Sperm maturation changes that occur in the epididymis are passively transferred, since there is no cellular connection between the sperm and epididymal structures. This makes the in vitro substitution of epididymal effects likely, once these effects are understood.

Micromanipulation: Other relatively new techniques involve mechanically assisting the entry of sperm into oocytes. Variations from zonal disruptions ("drilling" or "dissection"), to placement of sperm under the zona (subzonal insertion), to direct injection of sperm into the ooplasm (microinjection) are under evaluation. In general, these relatively primitive techniques have not proved to be very efficacious; see review by Ng et al. (151). One obstacle has been the need to have acrosome-reacted sperm to allow for oolemmal binding. Partial zona dissection (152), especially in conjunction with immunosuppression, has shown promise in one small series of male factor patients (153). As of this writing, no babies have resulted from microinjection, though early cleavage stages have been observed (154). Subzonal insertion has proved successful in some cases of severe oligospermia or oligoasthenospermia: a fertilization rate of 15% per egg (36% per patient) and an ongoing pregnancy rate of 7.8% per preembryo

Table 11.6 Agents that influence sperm performance in vitro

Agent	Effect
Follicular fluid	Increases AR, HA motility, and fertilization rate (142,144,145)
Apoprotein-1/Ig complex	Activates sperm motility (130)
Estradiol	Increases AR, HA motility, and fertilization rate (142,143)
Progesterone	Increases AR, HA motility, and fertilization rate (142,143)
Pentoxifylline (via cAMP)	Increases fertilization rate (146,147)
Potassium	Increases motility (148)
Platelet-activating factor	Increases AR, HPA, and fertilization rate (149,150)

AR, acrosome reaction; HA, hyperactivated; HPA, hamster penetration assay transferred (and 9.7% per patient) (155). In general, oocyte damage and the low rates of fertilization, cleavage, and pregnancy prohibit wide application of the technology (72). Assisted hatching of blastocysts from their zonae (156) may have a role if present stimulations or culture conditions do indeed cause abnormally hard zonae.

On the other hand, these techniques have been applied only in cases of severe male factor infertility for which more conservative measures had failed. If applied to fertile men and found successful, then this technology could allow precise control of which sperm fertilizes the egg. If techniques developed to allow individual sperm to be evaluated for a certain trait (sex, for instance), then these micromanipulative techniques could become an essential element in the control of fertilization.

In cases of obstructive azoospermia, epididymal sperm aspiration has produced some pregnancies (157). Whether particular etiologies or durations of obstruction affect the expectation of pregnancy remains to be explored.

Sperm separation for selection of gender and other traits: Sperm selection has been an ongoing effort and has met some success in the area of sex selection. However, to date it has not been possible to separate X- and Y-bearing sperm completely from one another: significant overlap in the populations exists after various separation techniques (158). The underlying principle of separation in most cases has been on the basis of differential motility or DNA content. A superior technology might involve specific DNA probes to genes of interest. Binding of the probe, visualization with a fluorescent or chemoluminescent agent, and separation by flow cytometry would allow cleaner separation of two populations. More importantly, it would allow a wide range of traits to be examined, thereby expanding the utility of such a technique beyond that of sex

selection. Preembryo selection may be more suitable in many situations of trait selection (see below).

Cryopreservation

Preembryo cryopreservation has proved a useful adjunct in the overall program of IVF, as excess preembryos can be stored for later use without the need for repeat ovarian stimulation. Overall take-home baby rates as high as 58% can be achieved from a single stimulation in women treated with GnRH agonist suppression who produce 10 or more preovulatory oocytes (6).

However, cryopreservation of preembryos has produced some difficult ethical and legal situations that might be avoidable if the technology to freeze oocytes were available. One apparent difficulty in freezing mature eggs has to do with the mitotic spindle, which is disrupted during conventional cryopreservation techniques (159). Only 5 pregnancies have resulted from oocyte freezing (160). Two strategies to circumvent this problem have been identified. One is to freeze eggs at an earlier stage of development. The problem with this approach is that the performance of immature eggs is poor even without freezing; perhaps with improved culture techniques these eggs would no longer be of marginal value. The second approach involves vitrification of the mature oocytes. In contrast to standard cryopreservation, vitrification (161) is a form of ice-free preservation. High concentrations of aqueous cryoprotectants are used, which become so viscous at low temperatures that they solidify into a glass-like state (*vitri* is Latin for glass) in which damaging ice crystals cannot form. Preliminary work has shown higher survival and unaltered implantation rates compared with those for other methods of cryopreservation in one mouse model (162).

Other roles for cryopreservation are anticipated. In women undergoing oophorectomy or radiation or chemotherapy for cancer, treatments might be able to store their eggs for future use, in much the same way that men store their sperm in similar circumstances (163). This opportunity has been limited by the inability to successfully freeze eggs and by the inability to remove the large majority of the oocytes from the ovaries being treated. Both these limitations may soon be overcome.

Is there a limit to the time gametes or preembryos can be cryopreserved? In principle, there may be a limit (164), but it is not practically relevant. In animal husbandry, sperm have been successfully cryopreserved for as many as 30 years; preembryos for 20 years. In the Norfolk program, preembryos stored for 2 to 4 years have a 78% survival and a 45% pregnancy rate following transfer. As of this writing, the preembryo frozen longest which led to a term pregnancy in the Norfolk program was cryopreserved for 913 days.

What is the penalty in preembryo cryopreservation? In our center approximately 30% of preembryos do not survive the thaw, but those that do survive go on to produce an implantation rate equal to that of eggs in the same cohort when transferred fresh (6). Too, there are ethical issues to be confronted with so many preembryos stored and the likelihood that many will never be transferred.

Preembryo biopsy for preimplantation genetic diagnosis

Preimplantation genetic diagnosis is becoming a reality in the clinical arena. A recent study reported successful pregnancy following sexing of preimplantation human preembryos to avoid the X-linked disorders of adreno-leukodystrophy and mental retardation (165). The feasibility of this effort hinged on devising a means of identifying the presence or absence of specific genes in a time frame short enough to allow biopsied pre-embryos to be evaluated before the time of transfer to the uterus. This tool has been the polymerase chain reaction (PCR), which allows amplification of even a single copy of the gene nearly a millionfold within 6 to 10 hours (Fig. 11.5).

Mutation detection is to be preferred over simple sexing of preembryos because it provides positive identification of the gene sequence of interest rather than an index of simple association. Specific point mutation and short insertions were rapidly, reliably, and accurately detected in single human lymphocytes and blastomeres in recent work by Hodgen and associates (manuscripts submitted).

The PCR technology can be applied to any disease or characteristic in which the actual nucleic acid sequence or flanking sequences responsible for the trait are known. At least 71 genes responsible for genetic diseases have been sequenced (166); some of the more familiar ones are given in Table 11.7. Thus, many conditions that are "invisible" to karyotypic analysis are identifiable after PCR amplification. At present, conditions that have a multifactorial inheritance pattern are not amenable to this approach.

Currently, this technology will likely be used only

Table 11.7 Examples of conditions amenable to preembryo biopsy and amplification by polymerase chain reaction

Direct detection of mutation	Sex-linked disorders
Tay-Sachs disease	Duchenne muscular dystrophy
Sickle cell anemia	Becker muscular dystrophy
α_1-Antitrypsin	Lesch-Nyhan syndrome
Cystic fibrosis (some mutations)	Hemophilia A
Duchenne muscular dystrophy (some mutations) (167)	Chromosomal sex
Huntington's chorea	
β-Thalassemia	

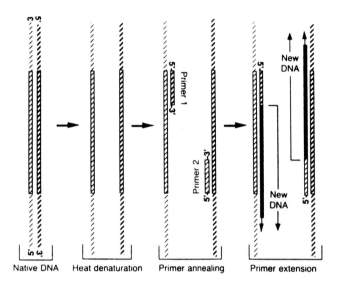

Native DNA Heat denaturation Primer annealing Primer extension

Fig. 11.5   First round of polymerase chain reaction. The basic polymerase-chain-reaction cycle consists of three steps performed in the same closed container but at different temperatures. The elevated temperature in the first step melts the double-stranded DNA into single strands. As the temperature is lowered for the second step, the two oppositely directed oligonucleotide primers anneal to complementary sequences on the target DNA, which acts as a template. During the third step, also performed at a lower temperature, the *Taq* polymerase enzymatically extends the primers covalently in the presence of excess deoxyribonucleoside triphosphates, the building blocks of new DNA synthesis. The native DNA target sequences, which will be massively amplified as "short products" in ensuing cycles, are boxed. The vector of action of the DNA polymerase is denoted by the arrows projecting from the newly synthesized DNA, indicated by the dark bars.

Reprinted by permission of the New England Journal of Medicine, from Eisenstein BI. The polymerase chain reaction. A new method of using molecular genetics for medical diagnosis. N Engl J Med 1990;322:179.

when combined with ovarian hyperstimulation as for conventional IVF. This is because some fraction of the analyzed preembryos will be afflicted with or carriers of the disease, and because no remedy for these affected preembryos is currently available. Once a means of effectively maturing immature eggs in vitro is discovered or a cure is available, this requirement for ovarian stimulation may disappear.

Noninvasive methods of preimplantation diagnosis may be possible for disorders that secrete characteristic compounds into the culture media (168). Coculturing to the four- or eight-cell stage would be necessary to allow expression of nonmaternal messenger RNAs.

Should we cryopreserve those preembryos that carry the genotype for disease expression? The ethical problem of what to do with affected preembryos with and without the availability of gene therapy to repair DNA mutations will require discussion (see below).

At present genes *can* be introduced into other cells. Several techniques are available. To produce transgenic animals by using oocytes, direct microinjection of foreign DNA into a pronucleus is most effective (as many as 25% of offspring will have stably incorporated the new gene, usually in a transcriptionally active form) (169). Transfection via retroviral vectors is another common technique in work with populations of target cells (Fig. 11.6). Electroporation and Sendai virus–mediated cell (or organelle) fusion are other techniques. These approaches have been used to great advantage in the investigation of the function of various hormones and growth factors. The problems of current technologies relative to "fixing" a particular preembryo are that 1) only a fraction of the target cells incorporate the transfected gene, 2) only a limited number of transfected cells receive the entire gene, 3) some of the transfected cells do not stably incorporate the gene, 4) the site of DNA insertion cannot be controlled reliably, so that even in transfectant in which the entire gene is stably incorporated, there is no

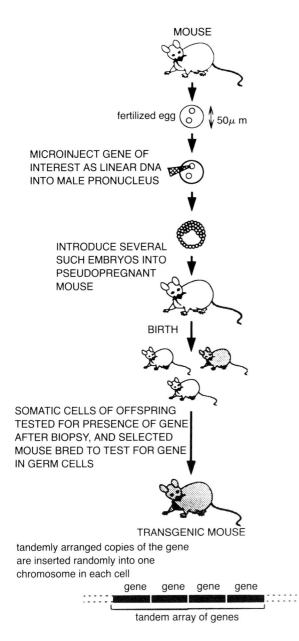

MOUSE

fertilized egg 50μ m

MICROINJECT GENE OF
INTEREST AS LINEAR DNA
INTO MALE PRONUCLEUS

INTRODUCE SEVERAL
SUCH EMBRYOS INTO
PSEUDOPREGNANT
MOUSE

BIRTH

SOMATIC CELLS OF OFFSPRING
TESTED FOR PRESENCE OF GENE
AFTER BIOPSY, AND SELECTED
MOUSE BRED TO TEST FOR GENE
IN GERM CELLS

TRANSGENIC MOUSE

tandemly arranged copies of the gene
are inserted randomly into one
chromosome in each cell

gene   gene   gene   gene

tandem array of genes

Fig. 11.6   Procedure for the production of transgenic mice.
Following microinjection of gene into male pronucleus, some

reliable means to control gene expression, and 5) the gene insertion event (which is a random event) may disrupt an essential gene (insertional mutagenesis). First steps toward site-specific gene insertion have been taken by exploiting homologous DNA recombination, in which the inserted gene actually replaces one of the DNA strands in the region of the original gene, but this occurs no more frequently than in one of 30,000 cells at present (170). Thus, with present technologies, the chance that a particular preembryo is successfully transfected with a gene restoring normal function is vanishingly small. Only with improved transfection rates and site-directed insertions will gene therapy for the germ cell line become possible. The consequences of this technology, once mastered, are discussed below.

Prediction of response

Couples with infertility typically have a variety of therapeutic options, from simple to complex. Given the investment of money, emotions, and time involved in ART, selection of the most appropriate therapy beforehand based on well-founded predictions is desirable.

Refinements in this predictive ability in ART have been achieved. On the male side, critical analysis of morphology has helped identify men with poor chances of success in IVF ($<$ 4% normal forms = low fertilization rate) (115). The number of sperm available after swim-up is also highly predictive of success ($<$ 1.5 million = poor outcome) (171). The hemizona assay can identify men whose sperm demonstrate impaired binding to the zona pellucida despite normal results on all

of the offspring will have incorporated the gene stably and in an active configuration. Some but not all of these animals will also have incorporated the gene into the germ line.

Adapted from Alberts B, Bray D, Lewis J, et al., eds. Molecular biology of the cell. New York: Garland Publishing, 1989:268.

other tests of sperm function; in such cases sperm performance in IVF is poor (172). All these tests can be performed before any attempt at IVF is undertaken and can influence whether the therapy is advisable.

Prediction of female response in IVF has also improved. The standard guide of female age (173) is helpful, but an evaluation of basal FSH level on cycle day 3 is better (174,175). Together, age and basal FSH level can predict pregnancy rates as low as 0% to as high as 40% (175). Women with one ovary do worse than expected based on age and basal FSH (176). Two defects are apparent in the one-ovary case: first, these women have higher levels of basal FSH, which itself predicts poor performance; but second, even when considering the same basal FSH levels, those with one ovary do less well than those with two.

Other predictors of response that rely on a provocation or stimulation test are probably more sensitive indicators but are not as simple as those described above. Low E_2 level after 5 days of gonadotropin stimulation is related to poor performance (177). A clomiphene challenge had predictive value (178). An early follicular phase GnRH agonist stimulation test (179) distinguished certain patterns of E_2 change over cycle days 2–5 which predicted different pregnancy rates. We find that the initial increase in E_2 after GnRH agonist administration (from day 2 to 3) is strongly related to the number of oocytes ultimately collected and available for transfer: $r = 0.51$, $r = 0.49$, respectively (34). This one-day test may prove to be a more sensitive assay of ovarian reserve than basal FSH or the pattern of E_2 change over a few days.

Areas of probable advancements: 5 to 10 years

Protecting gamete supply

Oocyte atresia appears to be a constant feature of normal ovarian physiology in the life of females beyond 20 weeks' gestation. Any mechanism that could arrest this process until the oocytes are needed would provide a dramatic benefit for many women. To date no such technologies have been identified: neither exogenous hormone manipulations (e.g., oral contraceptives) endogenous hormone derangements (e.g., polycystic ovary syndrome/congenital adrenal hyperplasia) are known to influence the rate of oocyte atresia. There are both environmental and genetic factors that do accelerate oocyte atresia: Tobacco use (180) and deletions of X-chromosomal material (the limit defined by Turner's syndrome, 45,X, but intermediate states also exist, e.g., 46,XXp$^-$ [181]) have this effect.

Of more immediate clinical usefulness in women undergoing cancer therapy with radiation or chemotherapy are oral contraceptives. Premature ovarian failure has been shown to depend on ovarian activity at the time of chemotherapy (182). Suppression of normal ovarian activity by this means during the period of active treatment appears to reduce the incidence of ovarian failure after treatment (183). Without treatment ovarian failure is related to radiation dose and chemotherapeutic agent (Table 11.8). Some cases of late

Table 11.8 Effect of ionizing radiation and chemotherapy on ovarian function

Radiation dose (rad)	Age of ovarian failure
250–400	>40 years
450–750	<25 years
2000–3000	childhood

Chemotherapeutic agent	Risk of ovarian failure
Methotrexate	0%
Cyclophosphamide	50%
Chlorambucil	20%
Alkylating agents and radiotherapy	70%

recovery of ovarian function even in untreated cases may occur despite short-term ovarian failure (184).

This approach probably does not protect all oocytes during treatment; the normal process of atresia goes on. Nonetheless, the modest protection that this technique affords will continue to play an important role in gamete protection until such time as alternative methods are available.

In the case of male gametes, cryopreservation is of proven utility when cancer treatment is required. It is important to be aware that treatment does not always lead to sterility (185), so posttreatment semen analyses are important.

Ooplasmic transfusion for aged and immature oocytes

Ooplasmic transfusion from mature oocytes has been shown to provide functional capacity to immature oocytes in humans (48). Whether the same technique could restore functional capacity to aged and atretic oocytes is not yet tested, but is a possibility. This exercise would also help establish the relative roles of ooplasmic and nuclear factors in the process of oocyte aging.

Maturing immature oocytes

But ooplasmic transfusion may not work. Furthermore, for those in need of pelvic irradiation or chemotherapy, techniques to remove and cryopreserve the entire pool of oocytes from these ovaries before treatment would be welcome. Obviously significant advances on several fronts would be needed to make this reality: reliable separation of all oocytes from their stroma (perhaps by collagenase treatment after mincing [31]), the ability to cryopreserve oocytes, and the ability to mature immature (even primary [30]) oocytes in vitro in a way that preserves their full pregnancy potential.

Primordial oocytes are not meiotically competent. If removed from their surrounding cell supports, they do not resume meiosis as do larger oocytes. During their transition to meiotic competence, many changes occur. In humans, the oocytes enlarge from approximately 50 mm to between 80 and 100 mm. Intense transcriptional activity is initiated. Some of the mRNA is immediately translated to support the rapid growth of the oocyte itself and the production of zona proteins. Another portion of the mRNA produced during the growth phase is stored for translation later, shortly after fertilization. The larger oocyte remains metabolically quiescent until the surrounding granulosa cells become well developed. The control of primordial oocyte activation is not well understood. Though gonadotropins may hasten activation, they are not required.

The molecular biology that underpins the resumption of meiosis in competent oocytes is becoming clearer. Much of the work has been done on the *Xenopus* (frog) oocyte, but many of the factors identified are highly conserved and thus may operate in human oocytes as well. What is apparent is that a multiplicity of pathways can regulate the resumption of meiosis (Fig. 11.7). Both phosphorylating and dephosphorylating processes are activated. The cAMP path is down-regulated (186), which normally leads to reduced phosphorylation (via protein kinase A inactivation). The phosphotidylinositol system, however, is up-regulated (187), which activates the C kinase system. Other important factors in this process include the proto-oncogenes *ras* (187) and *mos* (188) and the M-phase promoter (MFP), all of which become activated. The MFP is now described to be a heterodimer composed of a protein kinase (similar to cdc2) and a cyclin (189). Cyclins normally appear at the G_2-M interface, and are degraded at the end of the M phase. Microinjection of cyclins, *ras, mos,* or cAMP action blockade are each sufficient to trigger meiosis.

Important loose ends remain in our understanding

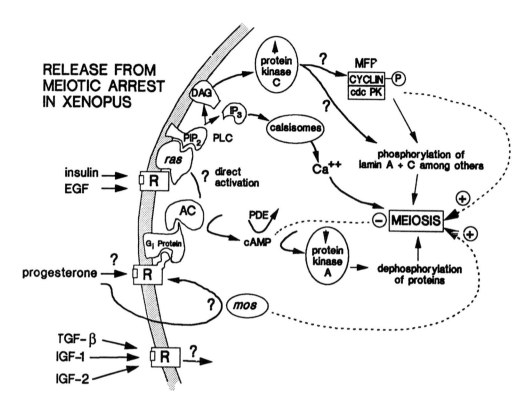

Fig. 11.7 Controls of meiotic arrest in *Xenopus* oocytes. Multiple types of control appear to operate to hold oocytes in meiotic arrest. Certain factors are inhibitory to meiosis (e.g., cAMP) while others are stimulatory. The stimulatory factors normally do not appear until meiosis is about to resume (e.g., M-phase promoter [MFP], *mos, ras*). Experimentally, *mos, ras,* and the MFP are sufficient when injected into arrest oocytes to induce the resumption of meiosis, though it is not clear that the induced meiosis is normal in all respects. Similarly, removal of cAMP activity in and of itself will permit the resumption of meiosis. Exactly how the various physiologic stimulators of meiosis influence the intracellular machinery depicted here is not clear. Nor has the intracellular interaction of these pathways been elucidated. The hypothetical connections depicted here represent our best guess based on the present literature. As indicated, both insulin and EGF activate *ras* through a membrane receptor. *Ras,* in turn, permits phospholipase C (PLC) to cleave phophotidylinositol diphosphate (PIP_2) into diacylglycerol (DAG) and inositol triphosphate (IP_3). DAG activates the protein kinase C system, which may play a crucial role in the phosphorylation of MFP and nuclear lamins either directly or indirectly. IP_3 stimulates the release of calcium from specialized calcium-storing vesicles called calcisomes; such calcium release does influence meiosis, but the mechanisms are not clear. Other receptor systems interact with G proteins (probably the inhibitory form); progesterone may have its effect here. The subsequent activation of adenylate cyclase (AC) leads to increased cAMP concentrations, which

of meiotic control. How does P_4 activate a cAMP pathway? How is c-*mos* tied into either pathway? Does insulin, another known stimulus to meiosis in *Xenopus,* have a role in the normal physiology? How is *ras* action blocked by inhibitors of cAMP degradation (e.g., cholera toxin)? How do the cAMP and phosphotidy-linositol pathways interact? Which pathway alters MFP activity (or do both)? What controls cyclin production and activity? Do the growth factors EGF, TGF-β, IGF-1, and IGF-2, which influence meiosis in vitro, play physiologic roles in vivo? One hopes that more work in these areas will elucidate the mechanisms more precisely. This would then provide clues to allow the system to be exploited to clinical advantage.

Even with a full understanding of meiosis resumption, however, it will still be important to understand the factors that suppress and then initiate the growth of primordial oocytes into meiotically competent ones. Examining differences in the intracellular mRNAs for these two cell types via subtractive hybridization may be an important first step. Gaining control of this transition would lend clinical utility to these primordial oocytes.

Managing impaired sperm

As discussed above, male factor infertility remains a very difficult obstacle in IVF. At present, sperm with impaired motility or zona binding have been subjected to micromanipulative procedures with little success. It is possible (if not probable) that many sperm with these defects have entirely normal chromosomal complements. Since only the chromosomes are needed to establish a diploid cell, procedures that provide the egg with this material would be welcome. To date micro-

fertilization has not been successful in humans, in part because the process of decondensation is not reliable with this procedure.

Sperm are not capable of fertilization as soon as they leave the Sertoli cells. As detailed above, modifications of the sperm membrane protein coat occur in the epididymis, and appear to be critical for normal fertilizing capacity. Once the specific functions of the epididymis are better understood, it may be possible to remedy certain deficiencies of epididymal processing. It may be that simple incubations with proteins or other components rectify poor sperm performance in some cases. In other cases, it may be necessary to remove sperm before they come into contact with abnormal substances in the epididymis to achieve the desired result.

Alloplastic spermatoceles can be crafted in cases of obstructive azoospermia (190). Whether they provide any advantage over direct epididymal aspiration is uncertain.

Cells can be fused with the aid of viruses or electricity. Consequently, it may be possible to effect fertilization of oocytes by sperm even when the sperm are incapable of normal penetration. It is even possible that immature sperm (spermatids or spermatozoa never exposed to epididymal secretions) could be fused in this way (151).

Multiplying preembryos

In mammal studies to date, blastomeres retain their totipotency to at least the four-cell stage (cases as high as 32-cell stage are reported). This means that blastomeres from early cleavage stages can be separated, each can be

---

normally prevent the resumption of meiosis through the protein kinase A system. Cyclic AMP activity is also modulated by phophodiesterase (PDE) activity. The position of *mos* in the mechanism of meiosis resumption is not clear though its importance is certain. The mechanisms by which TGF-β, IGF-1, and IGF-2 have their effects are also unclear.

placed within a new zona, and a completely normal individual can result from each. In principle, this procedure can be repeated when the separated blastomeres have undergone several rounds of cleavage. Depending on the species, the production of new mRNAs and new proteins might be a limiting factor in the number of times this blastocyst amplification can be repeated. To circumvent this limit, the blastomere's nuclei might be transferred into enucleated oocytes temporarily. In either case, at least four clonal blastocysts could be obtained in this way. Such a technology would be appealing to couples who have few embryos to work with. And depending on the number of times this division can be performed, it might make repeated ovarian stimulations unnecessary.

Present technical obstacles include reliable and atraumatic means of extracting blastomeres. It is not known for humans how long preembryos' blastomeres retain their totipotency; this would need to be established. Furthermore, whether this division could be performed more than once is not known.

Ethical constraints could be overcome. Though the idea of multiple copies of the same genetic person (perhaps even of different ages!) is startling, it is formally not very different from identical twinning. Furthermore, the number of clones could easily be controlled by cryopreserving all but one copy of each clone; only if pregnancy is unsuccessful would additional copies of the clone be transferred.

"Gene therapy" substitutes

As discussed above, specific, directed gene therapy currently faces several significant obstacles. In brief, genes cannot be introduced reliably or accurately into cells presently. An interim strategy is deliberate chimera formation. In this procedure, some of the blastomeres from an affected blasotcyst are removed and replaced by blastomeres from an unaffected blastocyst. (Apparent spontaneous chimera formation in vitro has been reported [191].) Such a technology has worked in a mouse system (192). What begins as two homozygous preembryos, one with a disease and one without it, ends up as two heterozygous (technically chimeric) preembryos, each having some cells expressing the disease state and others not. Usually the cells still expressing the disease are compensated by the healthy cells. This solution works only for recessive disorders. Whether the germ cells of this individual contain the gene for the disease or not is unpredictable and random.

Areas of possible advancement: beyond 10 years

Use of genetic material from somatic cells

All cells in the body contain a full complement of chromosomes. Somatic cells have a maternal and paternal copy of each chromosome; gametes have only one of each, and that one is a hybrid of maternal and paternal DNA following crossing-over. Gametes, having a haploid number of chromosomes, can easily combine to form the diploid number typical of somatic cells. For the present, assisted reproduction will most likely be restricted to the use of these haploid cells. However, since each somatic cell does contain each of the chromosomes required for reproduction, if a means to extract a haploid set of chromosomes from somatic cells were discovered, then the current restriction to the genetic material from gametes will be removed. This ability to use somatic cell genetic material will come from one of two techniques: some way to turn on meiosis in somatic cells, or some means to directly separate the paired chromosomes (or destroy one set). The resulting haploid set of chromosomes could then be transferred into an egg for subsequent fertilization. In theory, this technique would allow the "mating" of any two individuals. In the case of two men, one would have his genetic material placed into an enucleated egg, which would then be fertilized by sperm from the partner. In the case of two women, one would have her genetic material microinjected into an egg from her partner. In either case the egg receiving the chromosomes would probably need to be human to avoid the problem of nonhuman mitochondrial DNA.

Such a technology would remove the current problem of aging gametes. Women and men of any age could reproduce. Perhaps cryopreservation of some somatic tissue could even lead to the banking and subsequent use of genetic material from people long since dead.

Missing from the essential technology are the ability to separate a haploid set of chromosomes from a diploid complement, the ability to induce meiosis, and the ability to confirm that the correct sorting has occurred.

There are huge moral issues to consider in applying such technologies to human reproduction; some are raised below.

Increasing gamete numbers

Oocytes have undergone terminal differentiation before birth. This means that under normal circumstances, these cells cannot be induced to divide or change their morphology. Consequently, there has been no means of increasing the supply of female gametes. Furthermore, oocytes have already begun meiosis, a process that is not repeated. However, this restriction may be temporary as we learn the normal controls of the cell cycle, and those that produce a meiotic rather than mitotic division.

At birth oocytes have a double diploid chromosomal complement (duplicated sister chromatids; 4n), and are arrested in the diplotene phase of the first meiotic prophase: duplicated chromosomes have lined up in homologous pairs along the spindle (rather than lining up independently as they do in mitosis) and have undergone crossing-over, and the synaptonemal complexes have dissolved (Fig. 11.8). Thus oocytes are committed to undergoing a meiotic, rather than mitotic, division.

It is difficult to imagine how this process of meiosis could be reversed. However, the process might be interrupted to advantage: at the conclusion of the first meiotic division, oocytes have a diploid set of chromosomes (2n). If the sister chromatids could be separated at their centromere or later freed from the spindle apparatus, it might be possible to induce additional mitotic divisions before a haploid chromosomal complement (1n) is produced. Since crossing-over has already occurred, none of the daughter cells will have pure paternal or maternal chromosomes that would have resulted from mitosis alone. Nonetheless, the appropriate number of chromosomes would be available for subsequent mitotic divisions. For this strategy to be effective, the signals that initiate a meiotic division would need to be understood and controllable (as discussed in the section above). Control of the M-phase-promoting factor (MFP) would be one factor to evaluate, since it is required both in normal mitosis to permit exit from the G_2 phase into the M phase and in meiosis for the exit from meiotic arrest (Fig. 11.9) (193). The report of parthenogenic activation of human (194) and mouse (195) oocytes lends plausibility to this idea, as does the observation of isodisomy for two different chromosomes in humans (196,197).

As more information is gained about the molecular biology of terminal differentiation, which is the condition in which resting oocytes are maintained in the ovarian stroma, it is becoming apparent that terminally differentiated cells acquire factors which block replication. Terminally differentiated cells have not "accidentally" lost their replicative ability through accumulation of gene defects or abnormal proteins, but deliberately stop making proteins essential for replication and begin

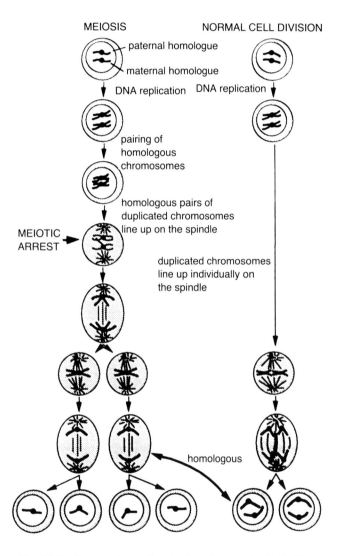

MEIOSIS   NORMAL CELL DIVISION

paternal homologue

maternal homologue

DNA replication   DNA replication

pairing of
homologous
chromosomes

homologous pairs of
duplicated chromosomes
line up on the spindle

MEIOTIC
ARREST

duplicated chromosomes
line up individually on
the spindle

homologous

Fig. 11.8   Comparison of meiosis and normal cell division. For clarity, only one set of homologous chromosomes is shown. The pairing of homologous chromosomes (homologues) is unique to meiosis. Each chromosome has been duplicated and exists as attached sister chromatids before the pairing occurs, so that two nuclear divisions are required to produce the haploid gametes. Each diploid cell that enters meiosis therefore produces four haploid cells.

making proteins that enhance this block to replication. Study of this condition may provide insight into the types of controls that are operating and the interventions that may override them.

For instance, in human fibroblasts, replicative senescence (the in vitro analogue of terminal differentiation) is associated with the dephosphorylation of retinoblastoma gene product (RB1), a tumor repressor gene product (198). Underphosphorylated RB1 prevents transcription of the c-*fos* gene (199), a growth stimulation gene, which in turn is essential for the production of other proteins required to synthesize DNA such as c-*ras*, actin, c-*myc*, and histones (200). In addition, these cells begin to produce a type of histone that is polyadenylated (normal histones are not) and may independently inhibit DNA synthesis (200). Thus this block to further replication is an active process and not necessarily an irreversible one (201).

Once the specific gene products responsible for the replication block are identified, their effects can probably be reversed in vitro. Missing proteins may be provided by diffusion (if small) or via transfection (see Fig. 11.6). Active suppressors can be negated by preventing their transcription (oligonucleotide primers that cover the transcription initiation site; Fig. 11.10) or translation (antisense messenger RNA that hybridizes the native RNA, making it unavailable for translation; Fig. 11.11). Once this is accomplished, oocytes might be induced to undergo several rounds of mitosis before again inducing meiosis.

The chromosome pairing in meiosis involves crossing-over between homologous chromosomes and occurs before meiotic arrest. Between their first and second cell divisions, cells undergoing meosis are diploid, a fact that might be exploited in an effort to induce further cell divisions.

Adapted from Alberts B, Bray D, Lewis J, et al, eds. Molecular biology of the cell. New York: Garland Publishing, 1989:846.

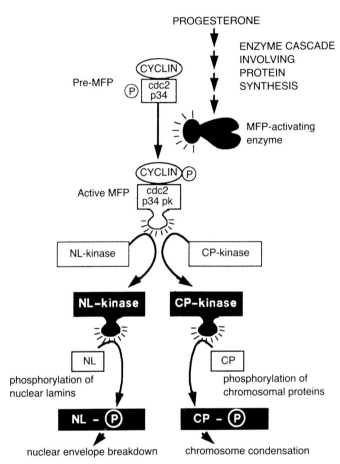

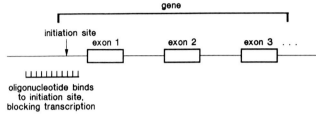

Fig. 11.10 Oligonucleotides can be used to block gene transcription. To transcribe any gene, RNA polymerase must be able to bind to the initiation site, which is close to the site where RNA synthesis will begin. If this site is covered by an exogenously administered oligonucleotide complementary to the DNA sequence in this region, then the RNA polymerase cannot bind and transcription cannot occur.

If control over meiosis can be gained, perhaps the ultimate contraceptive, one that would reversibly inhibit the progression of meiosis, could be devised.

The multiplication of sperm may be simpler. Seminiferous tubules contain active primordial germ cells capable of producing spermatazoa. To date, in vitro cultures of seminiferous tubule explants have not been successful in supporting in vitro spermatogenesis. Nonetheless, this approach has much promise and should be practical once the appropriate tissue culture technique is discovered.

Gene therapy

Germ line gene therapy is surely a decade or more in the future in terms of practical clinical application. Primary tasks are ways to increase the transfection rate and to provide for site-specific gene insertion. Once these are accomplished, the adverse potential of defective genes

Fig. 11.9 A model showing how the M-phase promoter (MFP) may act to trigger a frog oocyte (*Xenopus*) to progress out of prophase I into metaphase following stimulation by progesterone. It is hypothesized that progesterone indirectly activates MFP by mechanisms which result in the phosphorylation of cyclin and the dephosphorylation of cdc2–protein kinase, producing the active form of MFP. This activation of MFP leads to the activation both of more MFP (greatly amplifying the response) and of protein kinases which phosphorylate nuclear lamins and chromosomal proteins. This causes the nuclear envelope to break down and chromosomes to condense, thereby driving the cell into metaphase. A subsequent inactivation of MFP al-

lows the nuclear envelope to re-form and chromosomes to decondense so that the cell can proceed into meiosis II.

Adapted from Alberts B, Bray D, Lewis J, et al, eds. Molecular biology of the cell. New York: Garland Publishing, 1989:861.

whose expression is normally recessive could be overcome by providing a copy of the normal gene.

The problem of defective genes that are dominantly
expressed is more difficult. Techniques to excise the
mutant gene, prevent its expression, or negate the
activity of the mutant mRNA or protein would be
required to prevent the manifestations of disease.
Antisense mRNA to cover the transcription initiation
site on the DNA or to complex with the sense mRNA is
a likely vehicle (Figs. 11.9 and 11.10).

Lastly, the ethical ramifications of such an approach
become enormous when it is considered that this

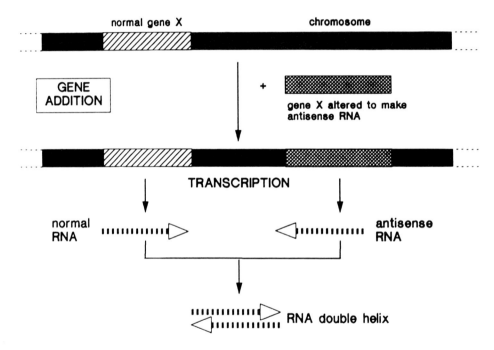

formation of RNA/RNA helix prevents the synthesis
of a protein product from normal gene X

Fig. 11.11 The antisense RNA strategy for generating dominant mutations. As illustrated, mutant genes that have been engineered to produce RNA that is complementary in
sequence to the RNA made by the normal gene can cause double-stranded RNA to form
inside cells. If a large excess of the antisense RNA is produced, it can hybridize with—and
thereby inactivate—most of the normal RNA produced by gene X. In the future it may be
possible to inactivate any gene in this way. At present the technique seems to work for
some genes but not others.

Reproduced by permission from Alberts B, Bray D, Lewis J, et al, eds. Molecular biology
of the cell. New York: Garland Publishing, 1989:195.

technique can be used to select any genetically defined trait. Introduction of this new trait into the germ line (vs. somatic line insertion) leads to propagation of this gene in all offspring. Once the genes responsible for so-called trivial characteristics (e.g., height, eye color, intelligence) are sequenced, this approach can be immediately applied to select for the "desirable" forms of these traits. This will allow for a much more efficient form of directed evolution ("positive eugenics") than that practiced in contemporary animal breeding. The process of human evolution would no longer depend on "random" matings and environmental challenges but on the selections made by humans themselves. Is this the "medicine" of the twenty-first century? Do we have the capacity to manage these technologies for net benefits to humanity? Are there unforeseen side effects that may not become apparent for several generations? All these issues need resolution over the decades ahead.

Artificial tube and/or womb

The largest group of women in IVF programs is still those with impaired tubal function. While IVF is an effective strategy in these cases, it is expensive and does not allow increased chances for pregnancy once treatment has been given. Hunter and collaborators in Utah have been working on an artificial fallopian tube that, once placed, would allow increased chances for pregnancy thereafter. Short-term success in a mouse model is reported (202).

The uterus is the only location where pregnancy is successful from the stages beginning at preembryo hatching until about 25 weeks of pregnancy. As the physiology of pregnancy and placentation is better understood, it may be possible to devise a system that could support pregnancy within a uterus. Since abdominal pregnancies are sometimes successful (i.e., they go to term and a healthy infant is surgically delivered without any maternal complications), it may be possible

for males to carry pregnancy in this way. Since there is normally significant risk of bleeding (the site of implantation is currently not controlled), it is not a type of pregnancy that one would elect to produce without first gaining control of the process in light of its risks and their management. Nonetheless, once these complications can be controlled, it may offer a way for men to carry pregnancies successfully.

Parthenogenesis

Parthenogenic humans are not yet a reality. There are cases where humans have obtained both copies of a particular chromosome from the same parent (uniparental isodisomy), but probably not the entire genome. Two individuals with cystic fibrosis have isodisomic chromosome 7s (196). Uniparental isodisomy has also been observed in two families with Prader-Willi syndrome (197). It is not clear whether any other chromosomes in these individuals were isodisomic, since this issue was not examined. It is clear, however, that parthenogenesis per se is not incompatible with life for some species: some lizards and turtles use this form of reproduction exclusively. And some species use parthenogenesis intermittently: in one type of salamander, sexual reproduction occurs at high ambient temperatures while gynogenesis (sperm activate the egg but the paternal genome is not incorporated) occurs at lower temperatures (203). In human IVF, spontaneous activation of an oocyte by acid Tyrode's solution is reported (194). But in studies of mammalian parthenogenesis, such embryos have limited capacity for growth; no offspring have been produced. Both maternal and paternal genomes are apparently required for orderly embryogenesis (204).

Ethical issues

Many of the topics reviewed above will create ever greater opportunities for controversy. Some of these are points raised in chapter 10 of this book. We possess only a limited perspective on the variables that will be considered in resolving these dilemmas. The findings of the Ethics Committee of the American Fertility Society (205) are highly influential upon our present thinking. However, ultimately, an independent national board composed of various experts in ethics, religion, law, science, and medicine may provide a consistency of review on ethical issues, thereby amounting to a national policy. We see the following as some of the fundamental and inevitable ethical issues to be faced:

1. Who decides?
2. How do they decide?
3. What spheres of responsibility and authority can be defined?
4. How do we incorporate new knowledge or process change based on newly recognized patient needs or scientific advancements?
5. Should guidelines, policies, rules, laws, and punitive measures be differentially applied?

So often today debate about procreative rights hinges on when human life is judged to begin. From an evolutionary perspective, such debates miss an important feature of life on this planet: life does not "begin" or "end" with the individual organism; rather, in the genes of gametic and germ cell lines of the preembryo, life is extended on a continuum, renewing replication and expression in the next generation.

Acknowledgments: We thank Drs. Howard W. Jones, Jr., Robert G. Brzyski, and Sergio Oehninger for critical review of portions of this manuscript.

References

1. Medical Research International, Society for Assisted Reproductive Technologies, American Fertility Society. In vitro fertilization–embryo transfer (IVF-ET) in the United States: 1989 results from the IVF-ET registry. Fertil Steril 1991;55:14–23.

2. Edwards RG, Plachot M, Renard JP, Questiaux N, Testart J. Discussion on ethical and judicial aspects of embryo research. Hum Reprod 1990;4:206–217.

3. Medical Research International, American Fertility Society Special Interest Group for Assisted Reproductive Technologies. In vitro fertilization–embryo transfer in the United States: 1988 results from the IVF-ET registry. Fertil Steril 1990;53:13–20.

4. Baulieu E-E. RU-486 as an antiprogesterone steroid: from receptor to contragestion and beyond. JAMA 1989; 262:1808–1814.

5. Guzick DS, Balmaceda JP, Ord T, Asch RH. The importance of egg and sperm factors in predicting the likelihood of pregnancy from gamete intrafallopian transfer. Fertil Steril 1989;52:795–800.

6. Toner JP, Muasher SJ, Brzyski RG, et al. Combined impact of the number of preovulatory oocytes and cryopreservation on IVF outcome. Hum Reprod Human Reprod 1991;6:284–289.

7. Larsen T, Larsen JF, Schiler V, Bostofte E, Felding C. Comparison of urinary human follicle-stimulating hormone and human menopausal gonadotropin for ovarian stimulation in polycystic ovarian syndrome. Fertil Steril 1990;53:426–431.

8. Edelstein MC, Brzyski RG, Jones GS, Simonetti S, Muasher SJ. Equivalency of human menopausal gonadotropin and follicle-stimulating hormone stimulation after gonadotropin-releasing hormone agonist suppression. Fertil Steril 1990;53:103–106.

9. Buvat J, Buvat-Herbaut M, Marcolin G, Dehaene JL, Verbecq P, Renouard O. Purified follicle-stimulating hormone in polycystic ovary syndrome: slow administration is safer and more effective. Fertil Steril 1989;52:553–559.

10. Galway AB, Hsueh JW, Keene JL, Yamoto M, Fauser BCL, Boime I. In vitro and in vivo bioactivity of recombinant human follicle-stimulating hormone and partially deglycosylated variants secreted by transfected eukaryotic cell lines. Endocrinology 1990;127:93–100.

11. Simon JA, Danforth DR, Hutchison JS, Hodgen

GD. Characterization of recombinant DNA derived-human luteinizing hormone in vitro and in vivo. JAMA 1988;259: 3290–3295.

12. Chappel S. Biological to immunological ratios: reevaluation of a concept. J Clin Endocrinol Metab 1990;70: 1494–1495.

13. Layman LC, Roach DJ, Plouffe L Jr, McDonough PG, Wilson JT. The detection of *Hind-III* restriction-fragment length polymorphisms using a deoxyribonucleic acid probe for the beta subunit of follicle-stimulating hormone. Fertil Steril 1990;53:261–265.

14. Stone BA, Quinn K, Quinn P, Vargas JM, Marrs RP. Responses of patients to different lots of human menopausal gonadotropins during controlled ovarian hyperstimulation. Fertil Steril 1989;52:745–752.

15. Hodgen GD. Uses of GnRH analogs in IVF/ET. Contemp Ob Gyn 1990;35:10.

16. Thanki KH, Schmidt CL. Follicular development and oocyte maturation after stimulation with gonadotropins versus leuprolide acetate/gonadotropins during in vitro fertilization. Fertil Steril 1990;54:656–660.

17. Droesch K, Muasher SJ, Brzyski RG, et al. Value of suppression with a gonadotropin releasing-hormone agonist prior to gonadotropin stimulation for in vitro fertilization. Fertil Steril 1989;51:292–297.

18. Pellicer A, Miró F. Steroidogenesis in vitro of human granulosa-luteal cells pretreated in vivo with gonadotropin-releasing hormone analogs. Fertil Steril 1990;54:590–596.

19. Yen SSC. The polycystic ovary syndrome. Clin Endocrinol (Oxf) 1980;12:177–208.

20. Surrey ES, deZeigler D, Lu JKH, Chang RJ, Judd HL. Effects of gonadotropin-releasing hormone (GnRH) agonist on pituitary and ovarian responses to pulsatile GnRH therapy in polycystic ovarian disease. Fertil Steril 1989;52:547–552.

21. Homburg R, Kilborn J, West C, Jacobs HS. Treatment with pulsatile luteinizing hormone-releasing hormone modulates folliculogenesis in response to ovarian stimulation with exogenous gonadotropins in patients with polycystic ovaries. Fertil Steril 1990;54:737–739.

22. Gordon K, Williams RF, Danforth DR, Hodgen GD. The use of a GnRH antagonist (Antide) as adjunctive therapy with gonadotropins for ovulation induction in cynomolgus monkeys [abstract 42]. Presented at the Annual Meeting of the Canadian Fertility and Andrology Society, Ville D'Estrerel, Quebec, Canada, October 3–6, 1990.

23. Kenigsburg D, Littman BA, Hodgen GD. Medical hypophysectomy. I. Dose-response using a gonadotropin-releasing hormone antagonist. Fertil Steril 1984;42:112–115.

24. Leal JA, Gordon K, Williams RF, Danforth DR, Roh SI, Hodgen GD. Probing studies on multiple dose effects of Antide (Nal-Lys) GnRH antagonist in ovariectomized monkeys. Contraception 1989;40:623–633.

25. Gordon K, Williams RF, Danforth DR, Hodgen GD. A novel regimen of gonadotropin-releasing hormone (GnRH) antagonist plus pulsatile GnRH: controlled restoration of gonadotropin secretion and ovulation induction. Fertil Steril 1990;54:1140–1145.

26. Filicori M, Campaniello E, Michelacci L, et al. Gonadotropin-releasing hormone (GnRH) analog suppression renders polycystic ovarian disease patients more susceptible to ovulation induction with pulsatile GnRH. J Clin Endocrinol Metab 1988;66:327–333.

27. Jones GS. Induction of ovulation. Annu Rev Med 1968;19:351–372.

28. Belaisch-Allart J, De Mouzon J, Lapousterle C, Mayer M. The effect of hCG supplementation after combined GnRH agonist/hMG treatment in an IVF program. Hum Reprod 1990;5:163–166.

29. Simonetti S, Veeck LL, Jones HW Jr. Correlation of follicular fluid volume with oocyte morphology from follicles stimulated by human menopausal gonadotropin. Fertil Steril 1985;44:177–180.

30. Cha KY, Koo JJ, Ko JJ, Choi DH, Han SY, Yoon TK. Pregnancy after in vitro fertilization of human follicular oocytes collected from nonstimulated cycles, their culture in vitro and their transfer in a donor oocyte program. Fertil Steril 1991;55:109–113.

31. Godsen RG. Restitution of fertility in sterilized mice by transferring primordial ovarian follicles. Hum Reprod 1990;5:117–122.

32. Gonen Y, Balakier H, Powell W, Casper RF. Use of gonadotropin-releasing hormone agonist to trigger follicular

maturation for in vitro fertilization. J Clin Endocrinol Metab 1990;71:918–922.

33. Hofmann GE, Toner JP, Muasher SJ. Supraphysiologic FSH doses in low responder IVF patients. J In Vitro Fert Embryo Transf 1990;6:285–289.

34. Winslow K, Toner JP, Brzyski RG. Prediction of response to stimulation from initial estradiol response to leuprolide acetate in a "flare-up" stimulation regimen for in vitro fertilization [abstract P-138]. Presented at the 46th Annual Meeting of the American Fertility Society, Washington, D.C., October 15–18, 1990.

35. Adashi EY, Resnick CE, Hernandez ER, et al. Insulin-like growth factor-I as an amplifier of follicle stimulating hormone action: studies on mechanism(s) and site(s) of action in cultured rat granulosa cells. Endocrinology 1988;122:1583–1591.

36. Jesionowska H, Hemmings R, Guyda HJ, Posner BI. Determination of insulin and insulin-like growth factors in the ovarian circulation. Fertil Steril 1990;53:88–91.

37. Magoffin DA, Erickson GF. An improved method for primary culture of ovarian androgen-producing cells in serum-free medium: effect of lipoproteins, insulin, and insulinlike growth factor-I. In Vitro Cell Dev Biol 1988;24:862–810.

38. Homburg R, West C, Torresani T, Jacobs HS. Cotreatment with human growth hormone and gonadotropins for induction of ovulation: a controlled clinical trial. Fertil Steril 1990;53:254–260.

39. McLachlan RI, Dahl KD, Bremner WJ, et al. Recombinant human activin-A stimulates basal FSH and GnRH-stimulated FSH and LH release in the adult male macaque, *Macaca fascicularis*. Endocrinology 1989;125:2787–2789.

40. Mizumachi M, Voglmayr JK, Washington DW, Chen C-L, Bardin CW. Superovulation of ewes immunized against the human recombinant inhibin α-subunit associated with increased pre- and post-ovulatory follicle-stimulating hormone levels. Endocrinology 1990;126:1058–1063.

41. Lissak A, Dirnfeld M, Sorokin Y, Kahana L, Abramovici H, Koch Y. The effect of metoclopromide on ovarian response to gonadotropin administration in patients with severe polycystic ovarian syndrome. Fertil Steril 1990;54:585–589.

42. Pache TD, Wladimiroff JW, de Jong FH, Hop WC, Fauser BCJM. Growth patterns of nondominant ovarian follicles during the normal menstrual cycle. Fertil Steril 1990;54:638–642.

43. Lee DW, Shelden RM, Reichert LE. Identification of low and high molecular weight follicle-stimulating hormone receptor-binding inhibitors in human follicular fluid. Fertil Steril 1990;53:830–835.

44. Check JH, Nowroozi K, Chase JS, Nazari A, Shapse D, Vaze M. Ovulation induction and pregnancies in 100 consecutive women with hypergonadotropic amenorrhea. Fertil Steril 1990;53:811–816.

45. Sauer MV, Paulson RJ, Lobo RA. A preliminary report on oocyte donation: extending reproductive potential to women over 40. N Engl J Med 1990;323:1157–1160.

46. De Ziegler D, Frydman R. Different implantation rates after transfers of cryopreserved embryos originating from donated oocytes or from regular in vitro fertilization. Fertil Steril 1990;54:682–688.

47. Jacobson A, Galen DI. Letter: a successful term pregnancy in a 49-year-old woman using donated oocytes. Fertil Steril 1990;54:546.

48. Flood JT, Chillik CF, van Uem JFHM, Iritani A, Hodgen GD. Ooplasmic transfusion: prophase germinal vesicle oocytes made developmentally competent by microinjection of metaphase II egg cytoplasm. Fertil Steril 1990;53:1049–1054.

49. Douglas JW, Kim MH, Batten BE. Electric field mediated transfer of enzymes into human oocytes. Fertil Steril 1990;53:1044–1048.

50. Lim JH, Kim SH, Kim KC, Moon SY, Chang YS. In vitro fertilization–embryo transfer program in natural ovulation cycles [abstract O-023]. Presented at the 46th Annual Meeting of the American Fertility Society, Washington, D.C., October 15–18, 1990.

51. Foulot H, Ranoux C, Dubuisson J-B, Rambaud D, Aubriot F-X, Poirot C. In vitro fertilization without ovarian stimulation: a simplified protocol applied in 80 cycles. Fertil Steril 1989;52:617–621.

52. Ouhibi N, Hamidi J, Guillaud J, Mènèzo Y. Coculture of 1-cell mouse embryos on different cell supports. Hum Reprod 1990;5:737–743.

53. Takeuchi K, Yamamoto S, Oki T, Nagata Y, Sandow BA. Primary culture of human fallopian tube epithelial cells and co-culture of early mouse pre-embryos [abstract P-214]. Presented at the 46th Annual Meeting of the American Fertility Society, Washington, D.C., October 15–18, 1990.

54. Goodeaux LL, Voelkel SA, Anzalone CA, Mènèzo Y, Graves KH. The effect of rhesus uterine epithelial cell monolayers on in-vitro growth of rhesus embryos. Theriogenology 1989;31:197.

55. Baird WC, Johnson CA, Williams SR, Godke RA, Jenkins CL, Schmidt G. Increased blastocyst formation in the mouse following culture on hamster cumulus cell monolayers [abstract O-020]. Presented at the 46th Annual Meeting of the American Fertility Society, Washington, D.C., October 15–18, 1990.

56. Camous D, Heyman Y, Meziou W, Mènèzo Y. Cleavage beyond the block stage and survival after transfer of early bovine embryos cultured with trophoblastic vesicles. J Reprod Fertil 1984;72:479–485.

57. Sathananthan H, Bongso A, Ng S-C, Ho J, Mok H, Ratnam S. Ultrastructure of preimplantation human embryos co-cultured with human ampullary cells. Hum Reprod 1990;5:309–318.

58. Mènèzo Y, Guerin JF, Czyba JC. Improvement of human early development in vitro by co-culture on monolayers of Vero cells. Biol Reprod 1990;42:301–306.

59. Jinno M, Sandow BA, Iizuka R, Hodgen GD. Full physiologic maturation in vitro of immature mouse oocytes induced by sequential treatment with follicle-stimulating hormone and luteinizing hormone. J In Vitro Embryo Transf 1990;7:285–291.

60. Collier M, O'Neill C, Ammit AJ, Saunders DM. Measurement of human embryo-derived platelet-activating factor (PAF) using a quantitative bioassay of platelet aggregation. Hum Reprod 1990;323–328.

61. O'Neill C, Collier M, Saunders DM. Embryo-derived platelet-activating factor. Its diagnostic and therapeutic future. Ann N Y Acad Sci 1988;541:398–406.

62. Downs SM, Daniel SAJ, Eppig JJ. Induction of maturation in cumulus cell-enclosed mouse oocytes by follicle-stimulating hormone and epidermal growth factor: evidence for a positive stimulus of somatic cell origin. J Exp Zool 1988;245:86–96.

63. Dey SK, Johnson DC. Histamine formation by mouse preimplantation embryos. J Reprod Fertil 1980;60:457–460.

64. Holmes PV, Gordashko BJ. Evidence of prostaglandin involvement in blastocyst implantation. J Embryol Exp Morphol 1980;55:109–122.

65. Mesrogli M, Schneider J, Mas DHA. Early pregnancy factor as a marker for the earliest stages of pregnancy in infertile women. Hum Reprod 1988;3:113–115.

66. Feinberg RF, Strauss JF III, Wun T-C, Kliman HJ. Plasminogen activators (PAs) and plasminogen activator inhibitors (PAIs) in human trophoblasts: markers of trophoblast invasion [abstract]. Presented at the 36th Annual Meeting of the Society for Gynecologic Investigation, 1989.

67. Ben-Rafael Z, Zolti M, Meirom R, et al. Can the early human embryo communicate? [abstract O-127]. Presented at the 46th Annual Meeting of the American Fertility Society, Washington, D.C., October 15–18, 1990.

68. Dandekar PV, Martin MC, Glass RH. Polypronuclear embryos after in vitro fertilization. Fertil Steril 1990;53:510–514.

69. Malter H, Hunt P, Cohen J. A non-traumatic enucleation method for correction of polyspermic human zygotes [abstract O-013]. Presented at the 45th Annual Meeting of the American Fertility Society, San Francisco, Calif., November 13–16, 1989.

70. Wiker S, Malter H, Wright G, Cohen J. Recognition of paternal pronuclei in human zygotes. J In Vitro Fertil Embryo Transf 1990;7:33–37.

71. Paulson RJ, Sauer MV, Lobo RA. Factors affecting implantation following human in vitro fertilization: a hypothesis. Am J Obstet Gynecol 1990;163:2020–2023.

72. Tarin JJ, Pellicer A. Consequences of high ovarian response to gonadotropins: a cytogenetic analysis of unfertilized human oocytes. Fertil Steril 1990;54:665–670.

73. Maca E, Floersheim Y, Hotz E, Imthurn B, Deller PJ, Walt H. Abnormal chromosomal arrangements in human oocytes. Hum Reprod 1990;5:703–707.

74. De Sutter P, Vanluchene E, Dhont M, Vande-

kerckhove D. Correlations between follicular fluid steroid analysis, maturity and cytogenetic analysis of human oocytes which remained unfertilized after in vitro fertilization. J In Vitro Ferti Embryo Transf 1990;7:9–15.

75. Feichtinger W, Barad D, Feinman M, Barg P. The use of two-component fibrin sealant for embryo transfer. Fertil Steril 1990;54:733–734.

76. Tanbo T, Dale PO, Abyholm T. Assisted fertilization in infertile women with patent fallopian tubes. A comparison of in-vitro fertilization, gamete intrafallopian transfer and tubal embryo stage transfer. Hum Reprod 1990;5:266–270.

77. Mastroyannis C, Hosoi Y, Yoshimura Y, Atlas SJ, Wallach EE. The effect of a carbon dioxide pneunoperitoneum on rabbit follicular oocytes and early embryonic development. Fertil Steril 1987;47:1025–1030.

78. Scholtes MCW, Roozenburg BJ, Alberda AT, Zeilmaker GH. Transcervical intrafallopian transfer of zygotes. Fertil Steril 1990;54:283–286.

79. Kerin J, Daykhovsky L, Segaowitz J, et al. Falloposcopy: a microendoscopic technique for visual exploration of the human fallopian tube from the uterotubal ostium to the fimbria using a transvaginal approach. Fertil Steril 1990;54:390–400.

80. Anderson GB. Embryo transfer in domestic animals. Adv Vet Sci Comp Med 1983;27:129–162.

81. Hertig AT, Rock J, Adams EC, Menkin MC. Thirty-four fertilized human ova, good, bad and indifferent, recovered from 210 women of known fertility. Pediatrics 1959;23:202–212.

82. Kliman HJ, Coutifaris C, Reinberg RF, Strauss JF III, Haimowitz JE. Implantation: in vitro models utilizing human tissues. In: Yoshinaga K, ed. Blastocyst implantation. Boston: Adams Publishing Group, 1989.

83. Guillomot M, Flechon JE, Wintenberger-Torres S. Cytochemical studies of uterine and trophoblastic surface coats during blastocyst attachment in the ewe. J Reprod Fertil 1982;65:1–8.

84. Armant DR, Kaplan HA, Lennarz WJ. Fibronectin and laminin promote in vitro attachment and outgrowth of mouse blastocysts. Dev Biol 1986;116:519–523.

85. Kao L-C, Caltabiano S, Wu S, Strauss JF III, Kliman HJ. The human villous cytotrophoblast: interaction with extracellular matrix proteins, endocrine function, and cytoplasmic differentiation in the absence of syncytium formation. Dev Biol 1988;130:693–702.

86. Queenan JT Jr, Kao L-C, Arboleda CE, et al. Regulation of urokinase-type plasminogen activator production by cultured human cytotrophoblasts. J Biol Chem 1987;262:10903–10906.

87. Fisher SJ, Cui TY, Zhang L, et al. Adhesive and degradative properties of human pacental cytotrophoblast cells in vitro. J Cell Biol 1989;109:891–902.

88. Ulloa-Aguirre A, August AM, Golos TG, et al. 8-Bromo-3′5′-adenosine monophosphate regulates expression of chorionic gonadotropin and fibronectin in human cytotrophoblasts. J Clin Endocrinol Metab 1987;64:1002–1009.

89. Nilsson BO, Lindkvist I, Ronqvist G. Decreased surface charge of mouse blastocysts at implantation. Exp Cell Res 1973;83:421–423.

90. Chavez DJ. Anderson TL. The glycocalyx of the mouse luminal epithelium during estrus, early pregnancy, the peri-implantation period, and delayed implantation. I. Acquisition of *Ricinus communis-I* binding sites during pregnancy. Biol Reprod 1985;32:1135–1142.

91. Chavez DJ, Enders AC. Lectin-binding of mouse blastocysts: appearance of *Dolichos befloris* binding sites on the trophoblast during delayed implantation and their subsequent disappearance during implantation. Biol Reprod 1982;21:545.

92. Martel D, Frydman R, Sarantis L, Roche D, Psychoyos A. Scanning electron microscopy of the uterine luminal epithelium as a marker of the implantation window. In: Yoshinaga K, ed. Blastocyst implantation. Boston: Adams Publishing Group, 1989.

93. Anderson TL, Sieg SM, Hodgen GD. Membrane composition of the endometrial epithelium: molecular markers of uterine receptivity to implantation. In: Iizuka R, Simm K, eds. Human reproduction: current status/future prospect. Amsterdam: Elsevier, 1988.

94. Tabizadeh SS, Sivarajah A, Carpenter D, Ohlsson-Wilhelm BM, Satyaswaroop PG. Modulation of HLA-DR expression in epithelial cells by interleukin 1 and estradiol-17β. J Clin Endocrinol Metab 1990;71:740–747.

95. Manners CV. Endometrial assessment in a group of

infertile women on stimulated cycles for IVF: immunohisto-chemical findings. Hum Reprod 1990;5:128–132.

96. Bell SC. Decidualization and insulin-like growth factor (IGF) binding protein: implications for its role in stromal cell differentiation and the decidual cell in hae-mochorial placentation. Hum Reprod 1990;4:125–130.

97. Kasamo M, Harper MJK. Prostaglandin release in vitro from rabbit endometrial epithelial and stromal cells during peri-implantation period [abstract 443]. Presented at the 37th Annual Meeting of the Society for Gynecologic Investigation, St. Louis, Mo., March 21–24, 1990.

98. Bell SC, Fazleabas AT, Verhage HG. Comparative aspects of secretory proteins of the endometrium and decidua in the human and non-human primates. In: Yoshinaga K, ed. Blastocyst implantation. Boston: Adams Publishing Group, 1989.

99. Zhu HH, Huang JR, Mazella J, Rosenberg M, Tseng L. Differential effect of progestin and relaxin on the synthesis and secretion of immunoreactive prolactin in long term cultures of human endometrial cells. J Clin Endocrinol Metab 1990;71:889–899.

100. Rogers RAW, Murphy CR. Uterine receptivity for implantation: human studies. In: Yoshinaga K, ed. Blastocyst implantation. Boston: Adams Publishing Group, 1989.

101. Bergh PA, Kaplan P, Hofmann GE, et al. Timing of the earliest embryonic signal (hCG) is determined by embry-onic development rather than endometrial receptivity [abstract P-229]. Presented at the 46th Annual Meeting of the American Fertility Society, Washington, D.C., October 15–18, 1990.

102. Gonen Y, Casper RF. Prediction of implantation by the sonographic appearance of the endometrium during controlled ovarian stimulation for in vitro fertilization. J In Vitro Fert Embryo Transf 1990;7:146–152.

103. Grunfeld L, Walker B, Williams MA, Hofmann GE, Navot D. High resolution endovaginal ultrasound of the endometrium, a non-invasive test for endometrial receptivity [abstract 441]. Presented at the 37th Annual Meeting of the Society Gynecologic Investigation, St. Louis, Mo., March 21–24, 1990.

104. Toner JP, Hassiakos D, Muasher SJ, Jones HW Jr. Endometrial receptivities after leuprolide suppression and gonadotropin stimulation: endometrial histology, steroid re-ceptor concentrations and implantation rates. Ann N Y Acad Sci 1991;622:220–229.

105. Chenette PE, Sauer MV, Paulson RJ. Very high serum estradiol levels are not detrimental to clinical outcome of in vitro fertilization. Fertil Steril 1990;54:858–863.

106. Hodgen GD. Surrogate embryo transfer combined with estrogen-progesterone therapy in monkeys: implanta-tion, gestation, and delivery without ovaries. JAMA 1983;250:2167–2171.

107. Ben-Nun I, Ghetler Y, Jaffe R, Siegal A, Kaneti H, Fejgin M. Effect of preovulatory progesterone administration on the endometrial maturation and implantation rate after in vitro fertilization and embryo transfer. Fertil Steril 1990;53:276–281.

108. Maclin VM, Radwanska E, Binor Z, Dmowski WP. Progesterone:estradiol ratios at implantation in ongoing preg-nancies, abortions, and nonconception cycles resulting from ovulation induction. Fertil Steril 1990;54:238–244.

109. Navot D, Anderson TL, Droesch K, Scott RT, Kreiner D, Rosenwaks Z. Hormonal manipulation of en-dometrial maturation. J Clin Endocrinol Metab 1989;68:801–807.

110. Maas DHA, Mesrolgi M. Early pregnancy factor in patients after in vitro fertilization [abstract P-213]. Presented at the 46th Annual Meeting of the American Fertility Society, Washington, D.C., October 15–18, 1990.

111. Abramowicz JS, Archer DF. Uterine endometrial peristalsis—a transvaginal ultrasound study. Fertil Steril 1990;54:451–454.

112. Van Demark NL, Hays RL. Rapid sperm transport in the cow. Fertil Steril 1954;5:131–137.

113. Jones HW Jr, Jones GS, Hodgen GD, Rosenwaks Z, eds. In vitro fertilization: Norfolk. Baltimore: Williams & Wilkins, 1986.

114. Franken DR, Kruger TF, Menkveld R, Oehninger S, Coddington CC, Hodgen GD. Hemizona assay and teratozoospermia: increasing sperm insemination concentra-tions to enhance zona pellucida binding. Fertil Steril 1990;54:497–503.

115. Kruger TF, Acosta AA, Simmons KF, Swanson

RJ, Matta JF, Oehninger S. Predictive value of abnormal sperm morphology in in vitro fertilization. Fertil Steril 1988;49:112–117.

116. Menkved R, Oettle EE, Kruger TF, Swanson RJ, Acosta AA, Oehninger S, eds. Atlas of human sperm morphology. Baltimore: Williams & Wilkins, 1991.

117. Menkveld R, Franken T, Oehninger S, Hodgen GD. Sperm selective capacity of the zona pellucida under hemizona assay conditions. Mol Reprod Dev 1991;30(4): 346–352.

118. Oehninger S, Hodgen GD, DeCherney, AH.

119. Oehninger S, Franken D, Kruger T, Toner JP, Acosta AA, Hodgen GD. Hemizona assay: sperm defect analysis, a diagnostic method for assessment of human sperm-oocyte interactions, and predictive value for fertilization outcomes. Ann NY Acad Sci 1991;626:111–124.

120. Dean J, Chamberlin ME, Millar S, Baur AW, Lunsford RD. Developmental expression of the sperm receptor of the mouse zona pellucida. Ann N Y Acad Sci 1989;564:281–288.

121. Hodgen GD, Burkmann LJ, Coddington CC, et al. The hemizona assay (HZA): finding sperm that have the "right stuff." J In Vitro Fert Embryo Transf 1988;5:311–313.

122. Brinkmann AO, Leemborg FG, Roodnat EM, deJong FH, Van der Molen HJ. A specific action of estradiol on enzyme involvement in testicular steroidogenesis. Biol Reprod 1980;23:801–809.

123. Morris PL, Mather JP. Modulation of steroidogenic responsiveness in Leydig cells in vitro. Recent progress in cellular endocrinology of the testis. INSERM 1984;123:187.

124. Boitani C, Mather JP, Bardin CW. Stimulation of adenosine 3',5'-monophosphate production in rat Sertoli cells by α-melanotropin-stimulating hormone (αMSH) and des-acetyl αMSH. Endocrinology 1986;118:1513–1518.

125. Orth JM. FSH-induced Sertoli cell proliferation in the developing rat is modified by β-endorphin production in the testis. Endocrinology 1986;119:1876–1878.

126. Gerendai I, Shaha C, Gunsalus GL, Bardin CW. The effect of opioid receptor antagonists suggests that testicular opiates regulate Sertoli and Leydig cell function in the neonatal rat. Endocrinology 1986;118:2039–2044.

127. Morris PL, Bardin CW. Intratesticular opiates as regulators of Leydig cell function. Ann N Y Acad Sci 1987;513:380–382.

128. Wright WW, Parvinen M, Musto NA, et al. Identification of stage-specific proteins synthesized by rat seminiferous tubules. Biol Reprod 1983;29:257–270.

129. Cooper TG. In defense of a function for the human epididymis. Fertil Steril 1990;54:965–975.

130. Ricker DD, Tillman SL, Billups K, Chang TSK. Protein changes in rat caudal epididymal fluid following partial denervation of the epididymis [abstract O-035]. Presented at the 46th Annual Meeting of the American Fertility Society, Washington, D.C., October 15–18, 1990.

131. Suzuki F. Morphological aspects of sperm maturation: modification of the sperm plasma membrane during epididymal transport. In: Bavister BD, Cummins J, Roldan ERS, eds. Fertilization in mammals. Norwell, Mass.: Serono Symposia, 1990.

132. Parks JE, Ehrenwald E. Cholesterol efflux from mammalian sperm and its potential role in capacitation. In: Bavister BD, Cummins J, Roldan ERS, eds. Fertilization in mammals. Norwell, Mass.: Serono Symposia, 1990.

133. Ishijima S. Changes in the beating pattern of spermatozoa during maturation and capacitation. In: Bavister BD, Cummins J, Roldan ERS, eds. Fertilization in mammals. Norwell, Mass.: Serono Symposia, 1990.

134. Bronson RA, Fusi F. The GRDV-mediated inhibition of oolemmal binding and oocyte penetration of zona-free hamster eggs by human spermatozoa is reversed by fibronectin derived peptide GRGES [abstract O-147]. Presented at the 46th Annual Meeting of the American Fertility Society, Washington, D.C., October 15–18, 1990.

135. Myles DG, Koppel ED, Primakoff P. Sperm surface domains and fertilization. In: Bavister BD, Cummins J, Roldan ERS, eds. Fertilization in mammals. Norwell, Mass.: Serono Symposia, 1990.

136. Lee MA, Check JH, Kopf GS. A guanine nucleotide-binding regulatory protein in human sperm mediates acrosomal exocytosis induced by the human zona pellucida [abstract O-102]. Presented at the 46th Annual Meeting of the American Fertility Society, Washington, D.C., October 15–18, 1990.

137. Fahmy NW, Bissonnette F, Benoit J, Girard Y, Sullivan R. Activation of protein kinase C induces acrosomal reaction of the human sperms [abstract P-170]. Presented at the 46th Annual Meeting of the American Fertility Society, Washington, D.C., October 15–18, 1990.

138. Suzuki S, Komatsu S, Furuya S, Endo Y. Changes in protein phosphorylation during capacitation and acrosome reaction of mouse sperm [abstract P-168]. Presented at the 46th Annual Meeting of the American Fertility Society, Washington, D.C., October 15–18, 1990.

139. Billups KL, Tillman SL, Chang TSK. Reduction of epididymal sperm motility after ablation of the inferior mesenteric plexus in the rat. Fertil Steril 1990;53:1076–1082.

140. Vreeburg JTM, Holland MK, Cornwall GA, Orgebin-Crist M-C. Secretion and transport of mouse epididymal proteins after injection of ^{35}S-methionine. Biol Reprod 1990;43:113–120.

141. Acosta AA, Oehninger S, Ertunc H, Philput C. Possible role of pure human follicle-stimulating hormone (FSH) in the treatment of severe male-factor infertility: a preliminary report. Fertil Steril 1991;55(6):1150–1156.

142. Mbizvo MT, Burkman LJ, Alexander NJ. Human follicular fluid stimulates hyperactivated motility in human sperm. Fertil Steril 1990;54:708–712.

143. Mbizvo MT, Thomas S, Fulgham DL, Alexander NJ. Serum hormone levels affect sperm function. Fertil Steril 1990;54:113–120.

144. Fakih H, Vijayakumar R. Improved pregnancy rates and outcome with gamete intrafallopian transfer when follicular fluid is used as a sperm capacitation and gamete transfer medium. Fertil Steril 1990;53:515–520.

145. Suarez SS, Wolf DP, Meizel S. Induction of the acrosome reaction in human spermatozoa by a fraction of human follicular fluid. Gamete Res 1986;14:107–121.

146. Yovich JM, Edirisinghe WR, Cummins JM, Yovich JL. Influence of pentoxifylline in severe male factor infertility. Fertil Steril 1990;53:715–722.

147. Tash JS, Means AR. Cyclic adenosine 3′,5′ monophosphate, calcium and protein phosphorylation in flagellar motility. Biol Reprod 1983;28:75–104.

148. Roblero LS, Guadarrama A, Ortiz ME, Fernandez E, Zegers-Hochschild F. High potassium concentration and the cumulus corona oocyte complex stimulate the fertilizing capacity of human spermatozoa. Fertil Steril 1990;54:328–332.

149. Minhas BS, Palmer TV, Roudebush WE, Fortunato SJ, Dodson MG. Platelet activating factor treatment of human spermatozoa enhances fertilization potential [abstract 236]. Presented at the 37th Annual Meeting of the Society Gynecologic Investigation, St. Louis, Mo., March 21–24, 1990.

150. Angle MJ, Tom R, Jarvi K, McClure RD. PAF enhancement of the acrosome reaction and hamster egg penetration by human sperm: modulation by calcium [abstract O-078]. Presented at the 46th Annual Meeting of the American Fertility Society, Washington, D.C., October 15–18, 1990.

151. Ng S-C, Bongso A, Sathananthan H, Ratnam SS. Micromanipulation: its relevance to human in vitro fertilization. Fertil Steril 1990;53:203–219.

152. Cohen J, Malter H, Wright G, Kort H, Massey J, Mitchell D. Partial zona dissection of human oocytes when failure of zona pellucida penetration is anticipated. Hum Reprod 1989;4:435–442.

153. Cohen J, Malter H, Elsner C, Kort H, Massey J, Mayer MP. Immunosuppression supports implantation of zona pellucida dissected human embryos. Fertil Steril 1990;53:662–665.

154. Bongso TA, Sathananthan AH, Wong PC, et al. Human fertilization by micro-injection of immobile spermatozoa. Hum Reprod 1990;4:175–179.

155. Fishel S, Jackson P, Antinori S, Johnson J, Grossi S, Verasci C. Subzonal insemination for the alleviation of infertility. Fertil Steril 1990;54:828–835.

156. Cohen J, Elsner C, Kort H, et al. Impairment of the hatching process following IVF in the human and improvement of implantation by assisting hatching using micromanipulation. Hum Reprod 1990;5:7–13.

157. Jequier AM, Cummins JM, Gearon C, Apted SL, Yovich JM, Yovich JL. A pregnancy achieved using sperm from the epididymal caput in idiopathic obstructive azoospermia. Fertil Steril 1990;53:1104–1105.

158. Beckett TA, Martin RH, Hoar DI. Assessment of

the sephadex technique for selection of X-bearing human sperm by analysis of sperm chromosomes, deoxyribonucleic acid and Y-bodies. Fertil Steril 1989;52:829–835.

159. Mazur P. Limits to life at low temperatures and at reduced water contents and water activities. Orig Life 1980;10:137–159.

160. Surrey ES, Quinn PJ. Successful ultrarapid freezing of unfertilized oocytes. J In Vitro Fert Embryo Transf 1990;7:262–266.

161. Rall WF, Fahy GM. Ice free cryopreservation of mouse embryos at −196°C by vitrification. Nature 1985;313: 573–575.

162. Nakagata N. High survival rate of unfertilized mouse oocytes after vitrification. J Reprod Fert 1989;87:479–483.

163. Davis OK, Bedford JM, Berkeley AS, Graf MJ, Rosenwaks Z. Pregnancy achieved through in vitro fertilization with cryopreserved semen from a man with Hodgkin's disease. Fertil Steril 1990;53:377–378.

164. Schneider U. Cryobiological principles of embryo freezing. J In Vitro Fert Embryo Transf 1986;3:3–9.

165. Handyside AH, Kontogianni EH, Hardy K, Winston RML. Pregnancies from biopsied preimplantation embryos sexed by Y-specific DNA amplification. Nature 1990; 344:768–770.

166. Antonarakis SE. Diagnosis of genetic disorder at the DNA level. N Engl J Med 1989;320:153–163.

167. Sanyal M, Fenton W, Bale A, Grifo J, Lavy G, Mahoney MJ. Amplification of deletion prone Duchenne muscular dystrophy gene segments by multiplex polymerase chain reaction in human oocytes [abstract 390]. Presented at the 37th Annual Meeting of the Soc Gynecol Invest, St. Louis, Mo., March 21–24, 1990.

168. Hardy K, Hooper MAK, Handyside AG, et al. Non-invasive measurement of glucose and pyruvate uptake by individual human oocytes and preimplantation embryos. Hum Reprod 1989;4.188–191.

169. Palmiter RD, Brinster RL. Germ-line transfection of mice. Annu Rev Genet 1986;20:465–499.

170. Capecchi MR. Altering the genome by homologous recombination. Science 1989;244:1288–1292.

171. Acosta AA, Oehninger S, Morshedi M, Swanson RJ, Scott R, Irianni F. Assisted reproduction in the diagnosis and treatment of the male factor. Obstet Gynecol Surv 1988;44:1–18.

172. Oehninger S, Franken D, Kruger T, Toner JP, Acosta AA, Hodgen GD. Hemizona assay: sperm defect analysis, a diagnostic method for assessment of human sperm-oocyte interactions, and predictive value for fertilization outcome. Ann N Y Acad Sci (in press).

173. Piette C, De Mouzon J, Bachelot A, Spira A. In-vitro fertilization: influence of woman's age on pregnancy rates. Hum Reprod 1990;5:56–59.

174. Scott RT, Toner JP, Muasher SJ, Oehninger S, Robinson S, Rosenwaks Z. Follicle-stimulating hormone levels on cycle day 3 are predictive of in vitro fertilization outcome. Fertil Steril 1989;51:651–654.

175. Toner JP, Philput C, Jones GS, Muasher SJ. Basal follicle stimulating hormone (FSH) level is a better predictor of in vitro fertilization (IVF) performance than age. Fertil Steril (in press).

176. Toner JP, Khalifa E, Acosta AA. Interpretation of basal FSH levels in women with one ovary [abstract]. Presented at the 7th World Congress of IVF and Assisted Medical Reproduction, Paris, France, June 28–30, 1991.

177. Hershlag A, Asis RC, Diamond MP, DeCherney AH, Lavy G. The predictive value and the management of cycles with low initial estradiol levels. Fertil Steril 1990;53: 1064–1067.

178. Loumaye E, Billion J-M, Mine J-M, Psalti I, Pensis M, Thomas K. Prediction of individual response to controlled ovarian hyperstimulation by means of a clomiphene citrate challenge test. Fertil Steril 1990;53:295–301.

179. Padilla SL, Bayati J, Garcia JE. Prognostic value of the early serum estradiol response to leuprolide acetate in in vitro fertilization. Fertil Steril 1990;53:288–294.

180. Jick H, Porter J, Morrison AJ. Relation between smoking and age of natural menopause. Lancet 1977;1: 1354–1355.

181. Krauss CM, Turksoy RN, Atkins L, McLaughlin C, Brown LG, Page DC. Familial premature ovarian failure due to the interstitial deletion of the long arm of the X chromosome. N Engl J Med 1987;317:125–131.

182. Rivkees SA, Crawford JD. The relationship of gonadal activity and chemotherapy-induced gonadal damage. JAMA 1988;259:2123–2125.

183. Chapman RM, Sutcliffe SB. Protection of ovarian function by oral contraceptives in women receiving chemotherapy for Hodgkin's disease. Blood 1981;58:849–851.

184. Pydyn EF, Ataya KM. Recovery of mouse oocyte in vitro fertilizability and cleavage after cyclophosphamide injection [abstract P-050]. Presented at the 46th Annual Meeting of the American Fertility Society, Washington, D.C., October 15–18, 1990.

185. Fossa SD, Theodorsen L, Norman N, Aabyholm T. Recovery of impaired pretreatment spermatogenesis in testicular cancer. Fertil Steril 1990;54:493–496.

186. Downs SM, Daniel SAJ, Bornslaeger EA, Hoppe PC, Eppig JJ. Maintenance of meiotic arrest in mouse oocytes by purines: modulation of cAMP levels and cAMP phosphodiesterase activity. Gamete Res 1989;23:323–334.

187. Pan B-T, Cooper GM. Role of phosphotidyl-inositide metabolism in ras-induced Xenopus oocyte maturation. Mol Cell Biol 1990;10:923–929.

188. Sagata N, Oskarsson M, Copeland T, Brumbaugh J, Vande Woude GF. Function of c-mos proto-oncogene product in meiotic maturation of Xenopus oocytes. Nature 1988;335:519–525.

189. Draetta G, Luca F, Westendorf J, Brizuela L, Ruderman J, Beach D. cdc2 protein kinase is complexed with both cyclin A and B: evidence for proteolytic inactivation of MPF. Cell 1989;56:829–838.

190. Müller-Tyl E, Deutinger J, Reinthaller A, Fischl F, Riss P, Lunglmayr G. In vitro fertilization with spermatozoa from alloplastic spermatocele. Fertil Steril 1990;53:744–746.

191. Van de Leur SJCM, Zeilmaker GH. Double fertilization in vitro and the origin of human chimerism. Fertil Steril 1990;54:539–540.

192. Palmiter RD, Brinster RL, Hammer RE, et al. Dramatic growth of mice that develop from eggs microinjected with metallothionein–growth hormone fusion genes. Nature 1982;300:611–615.

193. Cyert MS, Kirschner MW. Regulation of MPF activity in vitro. Cell 1988;53:185–195.

194. Johnson MH, Pickering SJ, Bruade PR, Vincent C, Cant A, Currie J. Acid Tyrode's solution can stimulate parthenogenetic activation of human and mouse oocytes. Fertil Steril 1990;53:266–270.

195. Cuthbertson KSR. Parthenogenetic activation of mouse oocytes in vitro with ethanol and benzyl alcohol. J Exp Zool 1983;226:311–314.

196. Voss R, Ben-Simon E, Avital A, et al. Isodisomy of chromosome 7 in a patient with cystic fibrosis: could uniparental disomy be common in humans? Am J Hum Genet 1989;45:373–380.

197. Nichols RD, Knoll JHM, Butler MG, Karman S, Lalande M. Genetic imprinting by maternal heterodisomy in nondeletion Prader-Willi syndrome. Nature 1989;342:281–285.

198. Stein GH, Beeson M, Gordon L. Failure to phosphorylate the retinoblastoma gene product in senescent human fibroblasts. Science 1990;249:666–669.

199. Robbins PD, Horowitz JM, Mulligan RC. Negative regulation of human c-fos expression by the retinoblastoma gene product. Nature 1990;346:668–671.

200. Seshadri T, Campisi J. Repression of c-fos transcription and an altered genetic program in senescent human fibroblasts. Science 1990;247:205–209.

201. Maier JAM, Voulalas P, Roeder D, Maciag T. Extension of the life-span of human endothelial cells by an interleukin-1α antisense oligomer. Science 1990;249:1570–1574.

202. Hunter SK, Neeld JB, Scott JR, Olsen DB, Urry RL, Cichocki T. Developing an artificial fallopian tube: successful in vitro trials in mice. Fertil Steril 1990;53:1083–1086.

203. Bogart JP, Elinson RP, Licht LE. Temperature and sperm incorporation in polyploid salamanders. Science 1989;246:1032–1034.

204. McGrath J, Solter D. Completion of mouse embryogenesis requires both the maternal and paternal genomes. Cell 1984;37:179–183.

205. Ethics Committee of the American Fertility Society. Ethical considerations of the new reproductive technologies. Fertil Steril 1986;46(3, Suppl 1):1S–88S.

Index